The Borderland between Caries
and Periodontal Disease II

Proceedings of the 2nd European Symposium on the Borderland between Caries
and Periodontal Disease held at Geneva, Switzerland, 28–29 February 1980

The Borderland between Caries and Periodontal Disease II

Edited by

T. Lehner
*Department of Oral Immunology and Microbiology,
Guy's Hospital Medical and Dental Schools, London, U.K.*

and

G. Cimasoni
*Section de Médicine Dentaire,
Université de Genève, Geneva, Switzerland*

1980

Academic Press   London · Toronto · Sydney

Grune & Stratton   New York · San Francisco

ACADEMIC PRESS INC. (LONDON) LTD.
24/28 Oval Road
London NW1 7DX

United States Edition published by
GRUNE & STRATTON INC.
111 Fifth Avenue
New York, New York 10003

Copyright © 1980 by
ACADEMIC PRESS INC. (LONDON) LTD.

All right Reserved

No part of this book may be reproduced in any form by photostat, microfilm, or any other means, without written permission from the publishers

British Library Cataloguing in Publication Data
 Borderland between Caries and Periodontal
 Disease Conference, *2nd, Geneva, 1980*
  The borderland between caries and periodontal
  disease, II.
  1. Dental caries—Congresses
  I. Title II. Lehner, T
  III. Cimasoni, G
  617.6′7   RK331   77–77147

 ISBN 0–12–792506–6

Filmset by Willmer Brothers Limited,
Birkenhead, Merseyside
Printed in Great Britain by
Fletcher and Son Ltd, Norwich

Contributors

J. AINAMO   Department of Periodontology, Institute of Dentistry, University of Helsinki, 172 Mannerheimintie, SF-00280 Helsinki 28, Finland

O. P. DE ALMEIDA   Department of Oral Biology, Dental School, Sao Paulo, Brazil

O. ANKKURINIEMI   First Central Military Hospital, 164 Mannerheimintie, SF-00280 Helsinki 28, Finland

R. ATTSTRÖM   Department of Periodontology, Royal Dental College, Vennelyst Boulevard, 8000 Aarhus C, Denmark

D. E. BARMES   Oral Health Unit, World Health Organisation, 1211 Geneva 27, Switzerland.

J. BJÖRKANDER   Department of Allerogology, First Medical Service, Sahlgren's Hospital, Göteborg, Sweden

E. BOLANOS   Apartado 1668, San Jose, Costa Rica, Central America

D. BRATTHALL   Department of Cariology, University of Lund, Malmö, Sweden

S. J. CHALLACOMBE   Department of Oral Immunology and Microbiology, Guy's Hospital Medical and Dental Schools, London SE1 9RT, England

H. CHURCH   Department of Periodontology, Dental School, Welsh National School of Medicine, Heath Park, Cardiff, Wales

G. CIMASONI   School of Dentistry, Faculty of Medicine, University of Geneva, 19 rue Barthelemy, Menn, 1211 Geneva, Switzerland

A. E. DOLBY   Department of Periodontology, Dental School, Welsh National School of Medicine, Heath Park, Cardiff, Wales

D. GNANASEKHAR   Department of Periodontology, Dental School, Welsh National School of Medicine, Heath Park, Cardiff, Wales

B. GUGGENHEIM   Department of Oral Microbiology and General Immunology, Dental Institute, University of Zürich, Plattenstrasse 11, CH-8028 Zürich, Switzerland

J. S. VAN DER HOEVEN   Institute of Preventive and Community Dentistry, University of Nijmegen, Nijmegen, The Netherlands

L. IVANYI   Department of Oral Medicine, Institute of Dental Surgery, London WC1, England

G. N. JENKINS   Department of Oral Physiology, The Dental School, Framlington Place, Newcastle-upon-Tyne NE2 4BW, England

Y. KOWASHI   School of Dentistry, Toyko Medical and Dental University, Yushima-Bunkyo-Ku, Tokyo, Japan

T. LEHNER   Department of Oral Immunology and Microbiology, Guy's Hospital Medical and Dental Schools, London SE1 9RT, England

H. LÖE   School of Dental Medicine, University of Connecticut, Farmington, Connecticut, U.S.A.

C. E. NORD   Department of Oral Microbiology, Karolinska Institute and National Bacteriological Laboratory, Stockholm, Sweden

K. PARVIAINEN   Department of Periodontology, Institute of Dentistry, University of Helsinki, 172 Mannerheimintie, SF-00280 Helsinki 28, Finland

G. RÖLLA   Department of Periodontic and Preventive Dentistry, Faculty of Dentistry, University of Oslo, Geitmyrsvn. 71, Oslo 4, Norway

H. E. SCHROEDER   Deparatment of Oral and Structural Biology, Dental Institute, University of Zürich, Plattenstrasse 11, 8028 Zürich, Switzerland

C. M. SCULLY   Department of Oral Medicine and Pathology, Glasgow Dental Hospital, Glasgow GT 3JZ, Scotland

G. SINGH   Department of Periodontology, Dental School, Welsh National School of Medicine, Heath Park, Cardiff, Wales

J. M. A. WILTON   Department of Oral Immunology and Microbiology, Guy's Hospital Medical and Dental Schools, London SE1 9RT, England

Preface

The first symposium on the "Borderland between Caries and Periodontal Disease", held at the Royal Society of Medicine in 1977 in London, left little doubt about the desirability to pursue this multidisciplinary approach. The second symposium on this subject was held in Geneva in February 1980 and the 17 contributions are published in this volume.

The multidisciplinary approach to the two most common diseases of mankind has been maintained by bringing together immunologists, microbiologists, biochemists, epidemiologists and clinicians. The rationale for considering caries together with periodontal disease is that the initiating factors in both diseases are the components of dental bacterial plaque and that the host immune responses modulate the effects of plaque antigens. Recent advances in our understanding of the complexities of the microbiology of dental plaque, and the identification of a plethora of new microorganisms in periodontal disease makes this a most challenging subject. The enormous strides in basic immunology which have taken place over the past two decades have also greatly influenced applied immunology. Indeed, oral immunology is a relatively new subject which has caught the imagination of a considerable number of scientists working in the field of oral biology. The interplay between immunological factors, microbial antigens and enzyme functions is seen at its best in the gingival crevicular domain which is the initial site of development of caries and periodontal disease.

The aims of this volume are to present recent concepts of immunology, microbiology and biochemistry of dental plaque components, with direct reference to the epidemiology of caries and periodontal disease, and to the current and prospective preventive measures. The future in prevention of these two chronic diseases lies in a painstaking, systematic investigation of the factors and mechanisms responsible for these diseases. An informed interchange of ideas and of new concepts between the different disciplines is essential in achieving the ultimate aim of preventing dental disease.

May 1980

The Editors

Acknowledgements

The organisers of the Symposium wish to acknowledge financial support from the Swiss National Fund for Scientific Research; GABA AG, Basle; Hawe-Neos, Gentilino; Trisa AG, Triengen; Uhlmann-Eyraud SA (Laroche-Navaron), Geneva; Informationskreis Mundhygiene und Ernährungsverhalten (IME), Frankfurt.

Contents

List of Contributors

Preface

1. Caries and Periodontal Disease as a World Health Problem, by D. E. Barmes 1

2. The Prevalence of Caries and Periodontal Disease in the Same Subjects, by J. Ainamo, O. Ankkuriniemi and K. Parviainen . 9

3. Proteinases of the Gingival Crevice and their Inhibitors, by G. Cimasoni and Y. Kowashi 31

4. Passage of Serum Immunoglobulins into the Oral Cavity, by S. J. Challacombe 51

5. Transport and Function of Polymorphonuclear Leukocytes in Crevicular Fluid, by C. M. Scully 69

6. The Comparative Inflammatory Effect of Dental Plaque, Lipopolysaccharide, Lipoteichoic Acid, Dextran and Levan on Leukocytes in the Mouse Peritoneal Cavity, by J. M. A. Wilton and O. P. de Almeida 83

7. Pocket Formation: An Hypothesis, by H. E. Schroeder and R. Attström 99

8. Stimulation of Gingival Lymphocytes by Antigens from Oral Bacteria, by L. Ivanyi 125

9. Cellular Autoimmunity in Periodontal Disease, by E. Bolanos, D. Gnanasekhar, G. Singh, H. Church and A. E. Dolby . . 135

10. Bacteria and Oral Fluid Components; Report of the Oral Condition in Hypogammaglobulinaemic Patients, by D. Bratthall and J. Björkander. 159

11. Effects of Immunization on Periodontal Disease and Caries in Gnotobiotic Rats Associated with *Actinomyces viscosus*, by B. Guggenheim 175

12. The Role of Serum and Salivary Antibodies in Protection against Dental Caries, *by T. Lehner* 193

13. Microbial Interactions in the Mouth, *by J. S. van der Hoeven*. 215

14. Role of Adherence in the Development of Dental Plaque, *by G. Rölla* 227

15. Anaerobic Microorganisms in Gingival Plaque, *by C. E. Nord* 241

16. Principles and Progress in the Prevention of Periodontal Disease, *by H. löe*. 255

17. Mechanism of Action of Fluoride in the Control of Plaque in Dental Caries, *by G. N. Jenkins* 269

Index 281

1. Caries and Periodontal Disease as a World Health Problem

D. E. BARMES

Despite the vast amount of data in the WHO Oral Disease Data Bank, I still have fundamental difficulties in placing periodontal disease on a priority scale as a world health problem. These difficulties arise because we continue to have doubts about the comparability of our measurement tools, the amount of prevention and treatment needed, the efficacy of our methods of prevention and treatment and the impact on either oral health or general health on existing levels of these diseases. If we keep to the broad canvas, which may be unjust to the large amount of detailed information we have, but is necessary for this paper, one single telling example suffices. Although we continue to say that after 30 years of age the major cause of loss of teeth is periodontal disease, it is impossible yet on a global basis to substantiate that claim with sound data. There is even some inferential data from the International Collaborative Study of Dental Manpower Systems (WHO, 1979) which would question the validity of that statement. Unless sound data on tooth mortality as a result of periodontal disease becomes more plentiful, it is unlikely that we will convince any but the "converted" that it poses a world health problem of some substance, although we can talk endlessly about prevalence of the disease at 90% or more from the age of 15 onwards.

Having commenced in such a gloomy way, and trusting that it will have some beneficial effect on data collection in the future, I can pass to a brighter note, at least in terms of what we *can* claim. Out data shows us clearly that there is a sharp contrast between highly industrialized and developing countries in terms of caries prevalence and trends. In the main, highly industrialized countries have high to very high prevalence of the disease, but some are now experiencing a decrease associated with comprehensive preventive programmes. Developing countries have been experiencing increases in the disease at varying rates and for varying periods, but still, there is a majority of countries at the very low, low or moderate prevalance levels. Thus, of 80 developing countries for which we have data, 51 have a mean DMF index of 3 or less at 12 years of age, but only four out of 25 highly industrialized countries have a DMF index within that range. There is little doubt that data from the 58 countries, most of them developing, for which we do not yet have sufficient information to use as national estimates, would make this contrast even more striking. A further contrast relates to the fact that the D component of DMF means tends to be much higher in most developing countries than in the highly industrialized nations, even to the extent of closely approximating 100%. These data give a very clear picture of the huge caries problem which is growing fast in developing countries.

Notwithstanding the vast differences in the available data for the two major oral diseases, an integrated approach to their prevention, control and residual care, as suggested by the title of this symposium, is an excellent strategy for a number of reasons.

If we look first at manpower implications, we have abundant information for highly developed countries, that even ratios approaching one dental operator (dentist or operating auxiliary) to 1000 in countries where caries prevalence is high have not managed to keep whole populations in a state of optimal oral health, although in some situations successful restoration and rehabilitation have been achieved. International Collaborative Study data for New Zealand, Norway and Denmark illustrate this point in that the DMF mean at 13–14 years is predominantly F.

That tremendously costly manpower supply can be compared with ratios calculated in a recently completed planning manual (WHO, 1980) prepared in the Oral Health unit of WHO. The manual indicates that one dental operator to 30 000 is sufficient for a goal-oriented, preventive first approach, where the DMF index at 12 years of age is no more than 1.5 and periodontal disease prevalence is moderate to high. Where the DMF index is 3 and periodontal disease prevalence again moderate to high; the recommended ratio is about 1:4000. If all countries reached the caries levels so common in highly industrialized countries, while retaining their existing periodontal disease problems, the present world population would thus need 3 500 000 clinical dental personnel to provide the comprehensive treatment coverage needed. However, if all countries stabilized even at the 3 DMF level at 12 years, which is considerably higher than is now experienced by many, only a little more than 800 000 dental personnel would be required. These two figures should be contemplated against the present world dental manpower estimates of about 600 000, plus the data for developing countries which indicates that only about 100 000 of these are employed in such countries, although they account for 80% of the world's population. There is no need to comment further on the economic and equitable distribution reasons for a concerted approach to management of caries and periodontal disease, or on the enormity of the economic/health problem posed on a global level by these two diseases.

Considering next the preventive aspect, upon which manpower economy depends, there is now a massive amount of data on reduction of dental caries incidence by the use of fluorides. Fluoridation of water supplies has been the most safe and economic method used to date and has achieved effective reductions in DMF means at 12 years, from above 6 to slightly below 3 DMF teeth. However, fluoridated water still reaches only 5% of the world's population. Furthermore, its extension over the past few years has been slow, not only because of sociopolitical or technical obstacles, but because many populations are not served by water supplies which could be safely and effectively fluoridated.

Thus, the use of fluoride toothpaste, fluoride tablets, fluoridated salt, fluoride rinses and high fluoride-bearing pastes has grown, and effective national, provincial or local programmes have resulted. Probably the most rapid further growth amongst these methodologies will be related to fluoride rinses, pastes and toothpastes, where the latter are not already universally used. All of those vehicles are best incorporated in school-supervised, individually applied programmes, for which oral hygiene routines are either indispensable or easily added. They are, therefore, ideal for the strategy of preventing and/or controlling the prevalence of dental caries and periodontal disease simultaneously.

Embodied in the reasons supporting the strategy so far is, of course, the improved health of populations. That entails not only a direct effect through a reduction in oral disease experience, but also indirect effects on all health sectors through economy of manpower and essential supporting facilities which can be used for other health achievements. However, the health implications of dental caries and periodontal disease, in isolation from these factors, have not been satisfactorily quantified. The most telling facts are (1) that the public begins to value oral health services when the DMF index rises to moderate or higher levels, 3 DMF teeth at 12 years of age being once more significant in approximating the borderline of rapidly increasing demand, and (2) that higher levels of disease have led to dramatic rises in edentulousness in several highly industrialized countries, even where comprehensive services are available. The triggering mechanism in increased demand for services is clearly dental caries, but, as indicated earlier, it is not clear how much tooth loss is due to one or both diseases. However, from our own clinical observations and the growth of professional concern for periodontal care, it is clear that periodontal disease has a significant to major role in decisions about conserving or losing teeth in adult life and about the radical decision to accept the edentulous state. Similarly, the desire for conservative care of the supporting tissues, as well as the teeth, is evident, even if not well quantified, in any population once the demand for any conservative services develops. Thus, the interrelation of these two major oral diseases and the need for an integrated approach in providing care and, at the same time, secondary prevention is evident.

Satellite reasons for an integrated approach relate to the types of manpower besides the dentist or specialist who might manage prevention and care of both conditions and to the necessary monitoring of trends in incidence of the two diseases at the same time. Obviously, from our Basic Oral Health Survey Methods (WHO, 1977), separate monitoring makes no sense, and the same can be said for manpower dealing with health education and non-manipulative prevention. However, even for the latter, particularly prophylaxis, and for other items of care, it is a fundamental consideration whether auxiliaries should be limited, as they often are, to care of the supporting tissues or care of the teeth. Certainly, such an artificial division is rarely possible in national oral health programmes for less affluent populations, and one must query its basis in human health for any population.

So far we have looked at the global situation briefly in regard to caries and periodontal disease and we have considered and endorsed an integrated approach to prevention, control and care of the two conditions. What then could be a global strategy to apply such an approach to alleviate existing, or to reverse growing problems in oral health?

It will be obvious to all by now that 3 DMF teeth in a 12-year-old child, as a national average, is of special interest to our oral health programme. It is the level which not only represents a crude average for 80% of the world's population living in developing countries, but also approximates the level to which we know, from the experience of a number of highly industrialized countries, that we can reduce high and very high levels of the disease. It is also the level consistent with a need for about one dental operator to every 4000 people. Depending on the national philosophy and resources, that ratio can relate to dentists only or to far fewer dentists supported by operating dental auxiliaries. The planning manual referred to earlier recommends a ratio of one dentist to 12 500 people with approximately two operating auxiliaries to one dentist, making up the overall 1:4000.

Thus, this goal is meaningful for developing countries and highly industrialized countries alike. For the former, it means either halting the trend of increasing caries prevalence so as not to exceed that level, or returning to that level for those which have already exceeded it. For a few fortunate countries it may even be possible to stay below the 3 DMF level, but the rate of increase which has already taken one or two developing countries to the very highest caries prevalence levels recorded in our data must not be underestimated. For the highly industrialized countries, the goal means a practical and economically dramatic return to a reasonable level of oral health. For developing countries it gives some hope of attaining adequate dental manpower levels at reasonable costs and for highly industrialized countries the opportunity to control escalating costs in the oral health sector and redistribute health manpower proportions.

Therefore, 3 DMF teeth at 12 years of age is being proposed as a global goal for the year 2000. Already, leaders of the dental profession have been asked to consider the appropriateness of this goal at the World Congress in Paris last September, in a symposium on "Child Dental Health" in Tokyo last November and in various working groups and meetings within the WHO programme. Thus far it has been very well received. As with any goal, some will achieve more than is targeted, others less: some will achieve it well before the year 2000 while others will be "behind the clock". However, the achievement of that goal, on average, by the year 2000 will have a major impact on oral health and health economics in general for the next century.

Nevertheless, for the subject of this meeting there appears to be a very large deficiency. Where is periodontal disease in all this? The overall goal is not intended to be exclusive. Indeed, it should give rise to many sub-goals relating to all aspects of oral disease and oral health sector activities and organization, all of them, hopefully, practical and measurable. For periodontal disease such a sub-goal is a very high priority and one might even call it a twin goal in line with the philosophy of this symposium. However, this need returns us to the first challenging point in this paper. In what terms shall we express and with what measurements shall we evaluate this twin goal? I have tried to set such a goal in terms of no more than one segment with calculus and one segment with gingivitis, or gingival bleeding, on average, at 15 years, as measured by the Oral Health Surveys Basic Methods, or by the proposed method being tested following the report of the Scientific Group on the Aetiology, Epidemiology and Prevention of Periodontal Diseases (WHO, 1978). That is the type of goal we need, but much work needs still to be done before we are sure that it is relevant as an objective in periodontal health, in preventive capabilities and in treatment resources.

Mention of the need for this development work leads me to the concluding question. What type of programme is needed for our global goal for the year 2000? First, national integrated planning is essential. Already we see penalties at both extremes of failure to plan in an integrated way. Where the oral disease problem and/or awareness is increasing, an already short supply of manpower has reached disaster proportions. Where oral disease prevention programmes are very successful, over-supply of manpower is rapidly becoming a reality and will almost surely cause much hardship and waste before a remedy is found. These penalties can only be avoided if prevention, treatment, manpower production, evaluation and overall administration are integrated for a defined population, be it national or provincial. Therefore, promotion of integrated planning based on periodic standard monitoring is a fundamental pillar of any programme to achieve our goal.

Within that framework the overwhelming priority area is prevention. Where prevention is school-based, using fluoride rinses, pastes or even tablets and gels, oral hygiene will be either an integral or an easily linked part of the activity which will then practise the integrated approach to management of caries and periodontal disease. Where prevention of caries is "remote" in terms of water or salt fluoridation, the oral hygiene activity specially directed to prevention and control of periodontal disease will need to be mounted separately. Health education will be fundamental to either situation and even more important if programmes of individual action in the community are to be the main approach.

Apart from these two main factors there are numerous possibilities in terms of manpower types, targeted or non-targeted services, and standard systems of recording, administering and sustaining oral health programmes, which will support the drive towards target achievement. In particular, carefully selected research endeavours will be necessary to improve our ability in all areas, but particularly to prevent dental caries and periodontal disease. Such endeavours, it is hoped, would show us the way by the year 2000 to formulate a much more ambitious goal for the following generation.

In conclusion, then, it is felt that the borderland between dental caries and periodontal disease is not just a catchy title. It is a fundamental concept which leads us to an integrated approach in planning, preventing, providing treatment and manpower, as well as evaluating our progress to much better oral health on a global basis as we enter the twenty-first century.

Summary

The World Health Organization Data Bank on Oral Disease contains a vast amount of information on the prevalence and trends of dental caries and periodontal disease. In developing countries, the prevalence of dental caries has been low and often extremely low, but increasing incidence in such populations is virtually a constant in data gathered over the past 10–20 years. Those increases have been so great that several developing countries have now entered the high and very high prevalence categories, one of them having returned the highest level of dental caries ever recorded for a whole population at 12 years of age. By contrast, prevalence of dental caries in highly industrialized nations has usually been in the high and very high categories, since reliable national studies commenced in the past two or three decades. Nevertheless, there are signs that some of these populations are now achieving large reductions in incidence of the disease, mainly through preventive programmes using fluorides.

Periodontal disease is shown to be even more prevalent than dental caries, although at a more advanced age. The evidence of an equivalent contrast between developing and developed nations is not clear, but there is a trend for lower prevalence of those diseases, although still at an important level, in developed countries.

1. A World Health Problem

The situation demands a concerted preventive approach to affect these two major problems simultaneously and thus a single numerical measurable goal for the year 2000 is being proposed.

References

WHO (1977). *Oral Health Surveys–Basic Methods*, 2nd edn, WHO, Geneva.
WHO (1978). *Epidemiology, Etiology and Prevention of Periodontal Diseases*, Technical Report Series no. 621, WHO, Geneva.
WHO (1979). *Interim Report of International Collaborative Study of Dental Manpower Systems*, WHO, Geneva.
WHO (1980). *Planning and Evaluation of Oral Health Services*, WHO, Geneva, in press.

2. The Prevalence of Caries and Periodontal Disease in the Same Subjects

J. AINAMO, O. ANKKURINIEMI and K. PARVIAINEN

Introduction

There seem to be few reliable epidemiological data available to determine whether dental caries and periodontal disease occur frequently in the same subjects (Slack, 1977). The lack of information is probably due to the strictly departmental research and teaching programmes in most dental schools.

The question, once raised, is a fascinating one. The answer, however, seems rather complicated. On the one hand, it is common knowledge that dental plaque is the aetiological factor in both diseases. On the other hand, on a global basis it is easy to demonstrate that the highest caries experience scores are, on the average, to be found in those countries in which tooth-brushing and oral cleanliness are most prevalent. In developing countries with poor oral hygiene and low sucrose consumption, periodontal disease is a problem in the absence of dental caries. In industrialized countries, sucrose consumption is high and, in spite of measures taken to promote oral hygiene, people seem to be frequently affected by both dental caries and periodontal disease.

It would seem that periodontal problems represent the genuine plaque-induced oral disease. In addition to plaque, an unfavourable sucrose consumption pattern is required in order for dental caries to develop into a major problem (Ainamo, 1976, 1980). Once caries is established, it seems to complicate further the periodontal condition by creating extra plaque-retentive elements, in the form of actual caries lesions and, subsequently, often defective restorations (Ainamo, 1970).

In theory the two main oral diseases, dental caries and periodontal disease, may either act in synergy or in antagonism to each other. The third possibility would be that there is no relation between the two oral conditions.

A synergistic association has been suggested by those authors who claim that both diseases are caused by the same dental plaque which, in man, tends to colonize specifically the gingival region and contact areas of the tooth surfaces (Löe et al., 1965, 1972; Waerhaug, 1966; Axelsson et al., 1976; Axelsson and Lindhe, 1978). However, in spite of lower plaque and gingivitis scores, higher DMF scores may be found in Western populations than in comparable groups from the Far East (Ainamo and Ainamo, 1978). Improved oral hygiene measures have repeatedly been found to improve gingival and periodontal conditions. It is true that proper plaque control has been reported to reduce the caries activity among children, but the required degree of cleanliness has been assumed to be difficult to achieve by the children themselves (Wright *et al.*, 1979). Good results have been obtained only with professional tooth-cleaning.

An antagonistic association between caries and periodontal disease has been suggested by Schroeder (1969) who emphasized the fact that dental caries represents a demineralization process of the tooth surface while calculus formation represents a mineralization process of dental plaque. This argument also appears to be valid, although no reliable epidemiological data seem to be available on an antagonistic prevalence of these two factors. On the other hand, while no serious doubts about the positive correlation between plaque and periodontal disease have been presented during the last 20 years, no association has been found between the presence of debris and of approximal caries and restorations (Sutcliffe, 1968). Low DMF scores have even been found to increase with regular brushing (Miller, 1961; Miller and Hobson, 1961; Ainamo and Parviainen, 1979). Also, according to Lehner (1977), there is a negative correlation between the DMF and the gingival index (GI) under the immuno-potentiating effect of plaque during experimental gingivitis.

A lack of correlation between dental caries and periodontal disease may have been concealed by the accustomed practice in epidemiological studies of reporting findings as mean scores for population groups. If, for example, in one population one-third of subjects is reported to be affected by severe gingivitis and one-third by rampant caries, there is no way of telling from mean scores if or how often the two diseases occur at the same time in one subject. Even if they did occur in the same subject, it is further possible that different teeth or tooth surfaces of the dentition are differently affected. It thus seems that a close analysis of the prevalence of oral disease is needed for further clarification of the question posed.

Intraoral Distribution of Oral Disease

When no effort is made to clean the teeth, dental plaque seems to colonize all tooth surfaces to the same extent (Sznajder *et al.*, 1968).

With careless tooth-brushing, the plaque scores predominantly of the front teeth seem to decrease (Ainamo, 1970). The severity of gingivitis closely conforms to the amount of dental plaque (Fig. 1). However, neither the intraoral distribution of dental caries (Fig. 2) nor that of dental calculus (Fig. 3) follows the distribution of dental plaque. Especially in the lower anterior

2. Caries and Periodontal Disease in Same Subjects

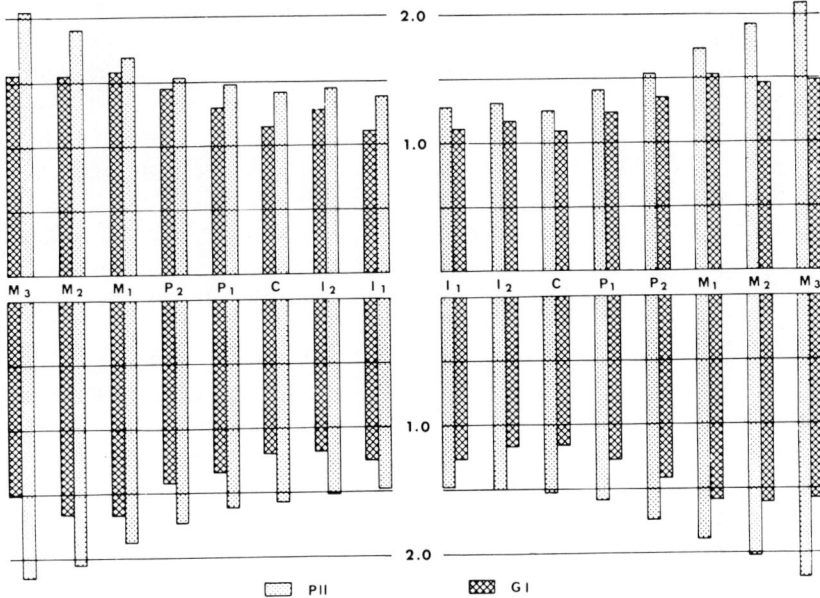

Fig. 1 The mean plaque index (PlI; Silness and Löe, 1964) and gingival index (GI; Löe and Silness, 1963) scores for the different teeth of 154 Finnish male conscripts aged 20 years (Ainamo, 1970).

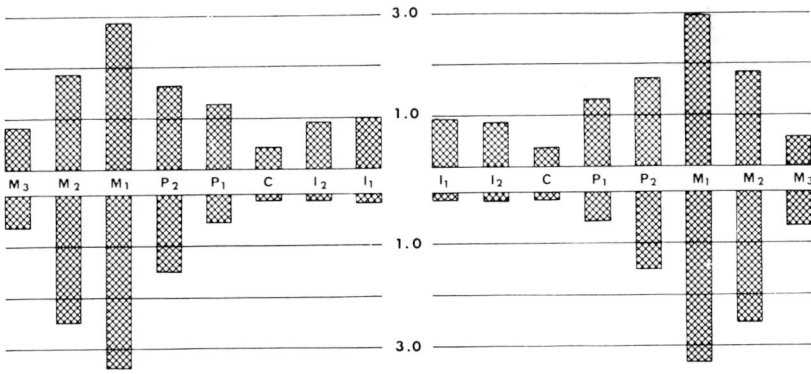

Fig. 2 Mean numbers of DMF (decayed, missing or filled) surfaces in different teeth of 20-year-old Finnish conscripts (Ainamo, 1970).

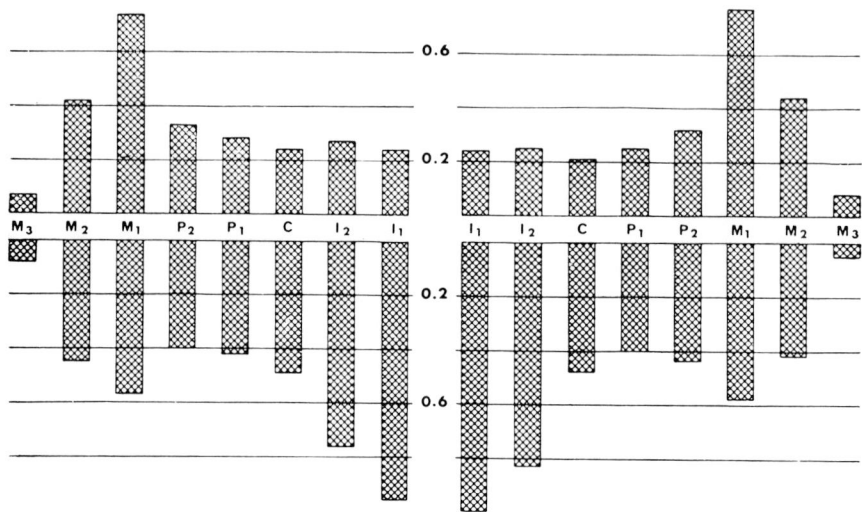

Fig. 3 The mean retention index (Björby and Löe, 1967) scores for dental calculus separately for the different teeth of 154 20-year-old Finnish conscripts (Ainamo, 1970).

region, a marked intraoral antagonism can be observed between the mean scores for caries and calculus. The distribution of loss of tooth attachment seems to fall somewhere in between the distribution curves for the two plaque retentive factors (Fig. 4).

When mean index scores are used either for the entire individual dentition or the individual tooth, as well as when tooth surface scores are utilized, there is always a positive correlation between the occurrence of caries in the gingival region and both gingivitis and loss of tooth attachment (Ainamo, 1970). When the corresponding correlations are calculated for plaque-retentive fillings in the gingival region, a different result is obtained. On the tooth surface the margin of the filling prevents cleaning, which results in a positive correlation between retentive fillings and gingivitis. When the dentition is considered a negative correlation is observed, probably reflecting the better brushing habits of those subjects who also take care of having their cavities filled.

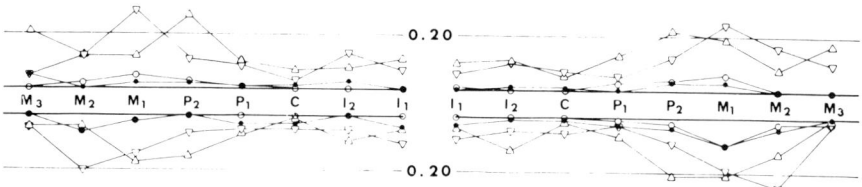

Fig. 4 Mean amount of lost tooth attachment (in millimetres) per surface around the teeth of 154 Finnish Army conscripts. △, distal; ▽, mesial; ○, oral; ●, facial (Ainamo, 1970).

Dental Caries and Periodontal Disease in Young Adult Males

Analyses of intraoral distribution patterns and mutual correlations contribute to the understanding of the relation between periodontal disease and dental caries. However, other approaches are required to clarify further the possible concurrence of the two diseases.

Dental Caries and Periodontal Disease in Young Adult Males

Identification of high-risk subjects for dental caries has become a common practice in community dental health care. A general experience is that 20% of the most caries-active subjects in a given population require as much reparative care as the remaining 80% (Bay and Ainamo, 1974). Identification of the high-risk group thus offers the possibility of directing intensive preventive measures towards those who are in the greatest need of them. According to the synergistic hypothesis, high-risk groups for gingivitis have been assumed to be included in the high-caries groups. In most dental health care systems no separate high-risk groups for gingivitis have therefore been identified.

In 1976 a total of 3344 Finnish conscripts were first interviewed and then subjected to a detailed examination of their oral health (Ankkuriniemi, 1979). The mean age of the young adult males was 20.3 years. The clinical examination was carried out by 34 military dentists. A whole day was used to instruct each dentist in the use of the simple criteria employed. The caries status per tooth was recorded for all teeth according to the DMF criteria, but only the 14 permanent teeth in the right side of the jaws were used to define the presence or absence of visible plaque, supragingival and subgingival calculus, pocket depth of 4 mm or more and gingival bleeding after probing (Ainamo and Bay, 1975; WHO, 1978).

The conscripts examined had left the regular dental care programme for children and adolescents a few years before starting their military service. At the time of the examination one-third of the young men reported not having

TABLE I
Characteristics of the Dental Condition of
3344 Finnish Army Conscripts (Ankkuriniemi, 1979)

Oral health index	Mean	S.D.	Prevalence (%)
No. of teeth	28.17	3.31	99.7
Filled teeth (FT)	10.28	5.73	96.3
Decayed teeth (DT)	4.34	5.03	75.6
Extracted teeth (MT)	1.22	2.77	41.2
DMFT	15.84	6.04	99.4

TABLE II
Characteristics of the Periodontal Condition of
3344 Finnish Army Conscripts (Ankkuriniemi, 1979)

Oral health index	Mean	S.D.	Prevalence (%)
Visible plaque (VPI)	4.84	4.50	75.6
Supragingival calculus (RC_1)	0.78	1.36	32.3
Subgingival calculus (RC_2)	1.18	2.24	34.0
Gingival bleeding (GBI)	4.27	4.31	73.4
Pockets ≥ 4 mm	0.24	0.89	11.0

visited a dentist during the preceding 2 years. Another third had visited a dentist one or two times and the remaining third between three and 10 times during the preceding 2 years. Accordingly, the averages and prevalences of the various oral disease parameters indicated a substantial need for curative and interceptive oral health care (Tables I and II).

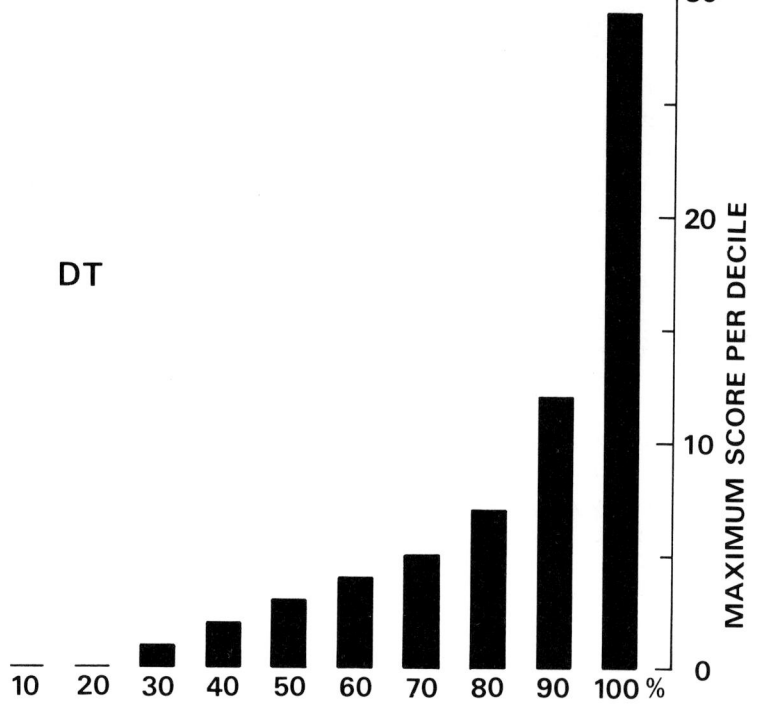

Fig. 5 A group of 3344 Finnish Army conscripts divided into deciles according to increasing need for caries treatment. The peak score in each decile determines the height of the column (Ankkuriniemi, 1979). DT, decayed teeth.

2. Caries and Periodontal Disease in Same Subjects

In Fig. 5 the 3344 conscripts are arranged into sequential deciles according to increasing numbers of teeth in need of reparative dental care. In a separate analysis 16.7% of the subjects were found to have nine or more decayed teeth. The need for reparative care in this high-risk group totalled 52.5% of the caries treatment need in the entire group.

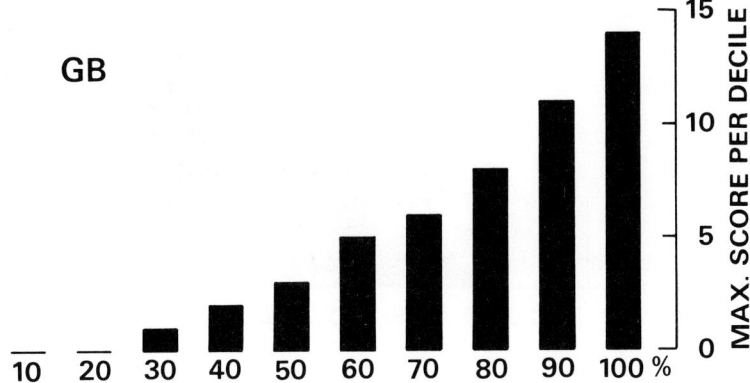

Fig. 6 A group of 3344 Finnish Army conscripts divided into deciles according to increasing numbers of teeth with gingival bleeding after probing. The highest score in each decile determines the height of the column (Ankkuriniemi, 1979).

In Fig. 6 the conscripts have been arranged analogously into sequential deciles according to increasing numbers of teeth with gingival bleeding after probing. It can be calculated that 19.3% of the subjects who had nine or more teeth with gingival bleeding had 51.8% of all the bleeding gingival units of the whole group.

In Fig. 7 the total number of teeth requiring treatment for caries is taken as 100%. The distribution into successive decayed teeth (DT) deciles forms the background of the illustration. The first seven deciles are shown in black and the percentages of DT falling into the last three deciles are indicated by the sums of the solid and the stippled columns. Superimposed on the decile distribution of decayed teeth are the scorings for gingival bleeding in each DT decile (Ankkuriniemi and Ainamo, 1979). The total number of teeth with gingival bleeding is again taken as 100%. The distribution of gingival bleeding units into the successive DT deciles is indicated by the sum of the hatched and solid columns. The black portion of the illustration is indicative of a certain amount of synergism between the prevalence of decay and gingivitis while the separate hatched and stippled parts show that one disease may well be present in the absence of the other.

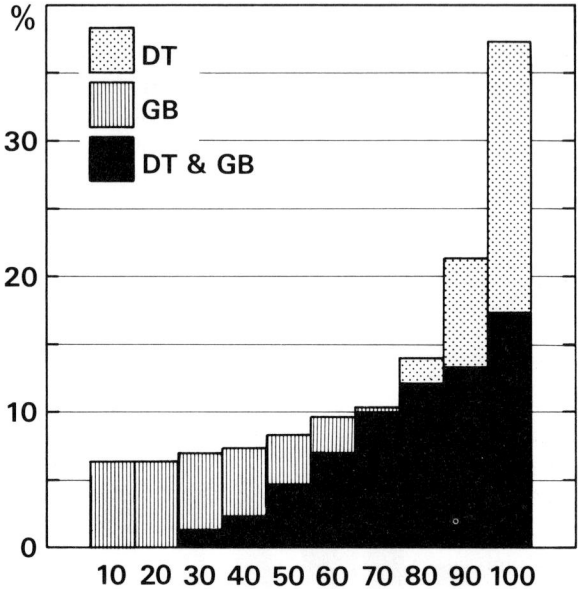

Fig. 7 The mean numbers of decayed teeth (in per cent) falling into each decile are indicated by the sum of the stippled and the solid columns. Superimposed are the mean numbers of teeth (in per cent) with gingival bleeding after probing (sum of striped and black columns) in the respective 334 men of each DT decile.

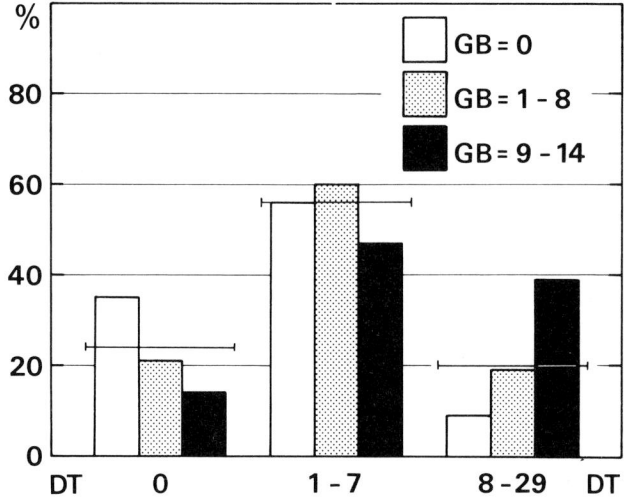

Fig. 8 The cross-bars indicate that the high-risk group for decayed teeth (DT) includes 20%, the medium group 56%, and the low-caries group 24% of the 3344 conscripts. With a total correlation the entire high-risk group for gingivitis (GB = 9–14) should have fallen into the high-risk group for decay. With total lack of correlation the various gingivitis groups should have shown a distribution conforming to the cross-bars.

Figure 8 is drawn on the basis of the same data. The cross-bars indicate that 24% of the conscripts fell into the low-caries group and had no need for reparative care. The high-risk group of 20% had between eight and 29 decayed teeth per subject. The solid columns indicate the distribution of the high-risk group for gingivitis within the three DT groups. Only 39% of those subjects with between nine and 14 teeth with gingival bleeding were found in the high-risk group for decay while 14% were found in the low-risk group needing no caries treatment. Again a certain degree of synergism is seen, but the correlation is far from complete.

Although there is no direct evidence that gingivitis would always lead to progressive breakdown of tooth attachment, there seem to be clinical indications that most of those subjects who, at a young age, suffer from severe gingivitis are at a later stage included in the group with the highest degree of loss of tooth attachment. In the 3344 Finnish conscripts periodontal pockets were found in 11% of the subjects. Of these 11%, one fell into the 30% group with no gingivitis, 7% into the 51% medium group with gingival bleeding of between one and eight teeth and 3% into the 19% high-risk group for gingival bleeding (Table III).

TABLE III

A Cross-tabulation of 3344 Finnish Conscripts, According to the Number of Teeth with Gingival Bleeding and the Number of Teeth with 4 mm or Deeper Pockets

No. of teeth with 4 mm or deeper pockets	No. of teeth with gingival bleeding			
	0	1–8	9–14	Total
0	29	44	**16**	89
1–13	1	7	**3**	**11**
Total	30	51	**19**	100

All numbers are percentages of 3344. Bold print has been used for high-risk groups.

A closer analysis of those conscripts with 4 mm or deeper pockets revealed that 5% had only one out of 14 teeth with a deepened pocket while 6% had pockets in between two and 13 teeth. When pocketing was related to the need for treatment of dental caries (Fig. 9), an essentially similar distribution was found as in the analysis of the high-risk groups for gingival bleeding and dental decay in Fig. 8. Subjects belonging to the high-risk group for caries occurred more frequently than expected in the group with most pockets while the opposite was true for the main group of 89% in which no pockets were recorded (Fig. 9).

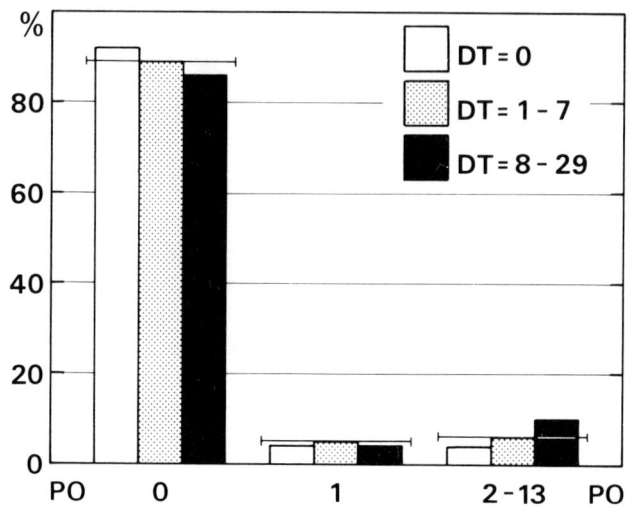

Fig. 9 The cross-bars indicate that the high-risk group for periodontal pockets (PO) contains 6% and the medium group (one pocket per subject) 5% of 3344 subjects. An over-representation of subjects belonging to the high-risk group for dental caries is evident in the high-risk group for pocket formation. The medium DT group conforms exactly to an equal distribution hypothesis.

The degree of overlapping of the high-risk groups for dental caries and gingival bleeding in young adult Finnish males was as follows. If the 19% of subjects with maximal gingival bleeding are pooled with the 20% of subjects with maximal dental caries, a group of $19 + 20 - 8 = 31\%$ of the entire sample of 3344 men is obtained (Table IV). Only 8% (252 subjects) belong to both

TABLE IV
A Cross-tabulation of 3344 Finnish Conscripts According to the Number of Teeth with Gingival Bleeding and the Number of Untreated Decayed Teeth

No. of decayed teeth	No. of teeth with gingival bleeding			
	0	1–8	9–14	Total
0	10	11	3	24
1–7	16	31	9	56
8–29	**3**	**10**	**8**	**20**
Total	30	51	**19**	100

All numbers are given as percentages of 3344 subjects. Bold print has been used for high-risk groups.

high-risk groups at the same time. Of the remaining 23%, 12% belong only to the high-risk group for dental caries and 11% only to the high-risk group for gingival bleeding. These observations are not consistent with either the synergistic or the antagonistic hypothesis. The correct interpretation is to be found somewhere in between these two extreme views (Ankkuriniemi and Ainamo, 1979).

TABLE V

A Cross-tabulation of 3344 Young Adult Finnish Males According to the Number of Teeth with Gingival Bleeding and the Number of Teeth with Fillings

No. of filled teeth	No. of teeth with gingival bleeding			
	0	1–8	9–14	Total
0–5	5	11	**6**	22
6–15	18	31	**10**	59
16–28	**6**	**10**	**3**	**19**
Total	30	52	**19**	100

All numbers are percentages of 3344 subjects. The numbers indicating high-risk groups are printed in bold type.

As a high number of untreated decayed teeth is indicative of low personal interest in oral health care, a further and yet unpublished analysis was performed in which gingival bleeding was related to the number of filled teeth in the mouth. A total of 627 subjects (19%) was found to have from 16 to 28 filled teeth (Table V). Of these 19% only 3% were at the same time found in the equally large 19% high-risk group for gingivitis. That high numbers of fillings are less often associated with gingivitis than are large numbers of decayed teeth confirms the impression obtained from the earlier study on concomitant occurrence of dental caries and periodontal disease (Ainamo, 1970). In the high-risk group for gingivitis the proportion of subjects with only a few fillings was actually greater than the proportion of subjects with the highest number of fillings (Table V), whereas this was reversed when gingival bleeding was related to dental decay (Table IV). Accordingly, a separate cross-tabulation between the number of teeth with gingival bleeding and the number of DMF teeth indicated a 5% overlapping between the 19% high-gingivitis group and the 21% group of subjects with 24–32 DMF teeth.

Caries and Gingivitis in Schoolchildren Receiving Regular Dental Care

The conscripts represented a population with rather a poor level of oral health. It was therfore decided to check the levels of overlap of high-risk groups for dental caries and gingival bleeding at a younger age, in a population still receiving regular school dental care.

This material consists of 366 schoolchildren aged 13–15 years from three different fluoride areas in Finland (Parviainen et al., 1977). For each age group of 13, 14 and 15 years, in each one of the three fluoride areas, 40 children were examined for the number of DMF surfaces. Separate observations were also made for the presence or absence of visible plaque on and gingival bleeding after probing at three surfaces of each permanent tooth in the right side of the jaws (Ainamo and Bay, 1975).

In the group of schoolchildren pocket depth was not recorded. There were also only four permanent teeth missing, which seemed to justify the use of the DFS instead of the DMFS score in tabulations that follow. Because of frequent visits to the school dentist, the DFS of the children included only a few untreated decayed tooth surfaces. The mean scores for the total sample were 43% for the visible plaque index and 40% for the gingival bleeding index. A total mean score of 14.5 was recorded for the DFS index (Parviainen et al., 1977).

Analysis of the highest DFS scores in successive deciles of the goup of schoolchildren are illustrated in Fig. 10. The maximal score of 60 decayed

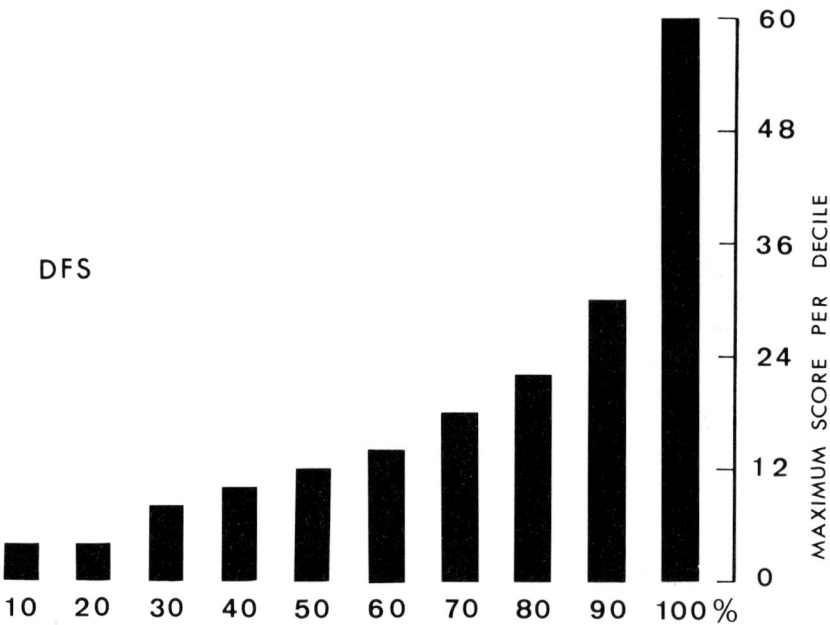

Fig. 10 A group of 366 schoolchildren are arranged into sequential deciles according to the number of decayed or filled tooth surfaces. The maximum score in the worst decile was DFS 60, as compared with the maximum DFS score of 4 in the two first deciles.

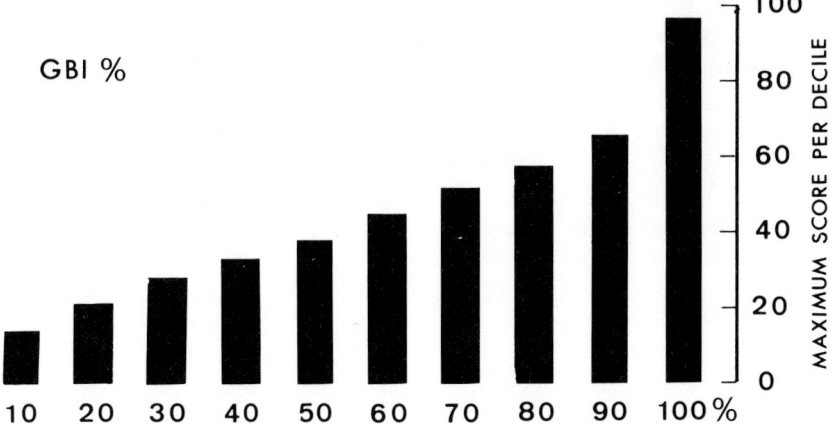

Fig. 11 The gingival bleeding index (GBI: Ainamo and Bay, 1975) scores in successive deciles of 366 schoolchildren are given in per cent of the total of 42 examined surfaces. The maximum score in the worst decile is 97%, as compared with a maximum of 14% in the first decile.

and/or filled surfaces was recorded for one child in the last decile whereas a maximal score of 4 was recorded among the children falling into the first two deciles.

A corresponding illustration of the variance between children with regard to gingival bleeding after probing (GBI) indicates that a maximum of 97% of the gingival units examined were affected in a child belonging to the tenth decile (Fig. 11). The corresponding highest score in the decile with least gingivitis was 14%.

A separate analysis of the data from the 366 children indicated that out of the total of 5338 DF surfaces documented, 2660 (50%) were found in the 85 (23%) worst affected children. Similarly, half of all units with gingival bleeding were found in those 31% of the children who had most gingivitis. If one adheres to the definition that the high-risk group consists of those who are worst affected and who have as high a diseases experience or disease prevalence as the remaining part of the population examined, the trend in those results seems to indicate that with younger age and regular oral health care the high-risk groups are larger than in the group of slightly older conscripts who were in acute need of dental treatment. Whether this situation affects the occurrence of the two diseases in the same subjects was therefore analysed by means of cross-tabulation.

In Table VI the 25% of the subjects having a DFS score of 19–60 are compared with the 34% having bleeding from 49 to 97% of their gingival margins. The cross-tabulation shows that only 9% of the subjects belong to the

TABLE VI
A Cross-tabulation of 366 Finnish Schoolchildren, Aged 13–15 Years, According to the Percentage of Gingival Units with Bleeding after Probing and Past Caries Experience (DFS)

DFS	Percentage of units with gingival bleeding			
	0–27	28–48	49–97	Total
0–8	9	12	**14**	35
9–18	14	14	**12**	40
19–60	**6**	**10**	**9**	**25**
Total	29	37	34	100

All numbers are percentages of 366 children. Bold print has been used for the high-risk groups.

two high-risk groups at the same time. There is, in fact, a larger group of high-gingivitis scores in children in the low-DFS than in the high-DFS group.

A reduction of the high-risk groups to 16% for DFS and to 24% for gingival bleeding does not seem to increase the degree of overlap of the two diseases (Table VII). Now only 4% of the subjects have a DFS score of 25–60 and at the same time a gingival bleeding score of 57–97%. Again there are more 'high-gingivitis' scores in children in the low- than in the high-DFS group. If the reduced high-risk groups of 16% for past caries experience and 24% for prevalence of gingival bleeding are pooled together, a high-risk group of 36% is obtained (16 + 24 − 4 = 36).

If in Table VII this 4% is taken, as a percentage proportion, from the 36%, the final calculation indicates that of those who are most affected by either

TABLE VII
A Cross-tabulation of 366 Finnish Schoolchildren, Aged 13–15 Years, According to the Percentage of Gingival Units which Bleed after Probing and the Past Caries Experience (DFS)

DFS	Percentage of bleeding gingival units			
	0–20	21–56	57–97	Total
0–4	3	11	7	21
5–24	12	38	**14**	63
25–60	**3**	**9**	**4**	**16**
Total	18	58	24	100

All numbers are percentages of the 366 children examined. Bold print has been used for the high-risk groups.

disease only 11% are affected by both diseases at the same time. A similar calculation from Table VI gives a corresponding concurrence of 18%. When these relative numbers are compared with similarly calculated percentages from the conscript material (Tables IV and V), the concurrence of high GBI and DT subjects is found to be 25.8% and that of GBI and FT subjects only 8.6% $((3/(19+19-3)) \times 100)$ (Table V). It thus seems that there is a greater overlap between gingival bleeding and untreated than treated dental caries. In other words, regular reparative care seems to affect the degree of overlap more than the difference in age between the two populations studied.

A final analysis was undertaken in order to clarify further which factors might influence the prevalence of dental caries and periodontal disease in the same subjects, by relating a few background variables to the disease prevalence.

Relation between Oral Disease and Different Background Variables

There are specific background variables which are generally considered to affect oral health in a specific way. Such background variables are, for example, the number of years the subject has spent in education, the frequency of tooth-brushing, the frequency of visits to the dentist, and the fluoride content of the drinking water (Ankkuriniemi, 1980). Another very useful variable would be the sucrose consumption pattern of the individual. However, reliable data on sucrose consumption have proven extremely difficult to obtain, and were therefore not included in this study. On the other hand, a personal history of gingival bleeding while brushing the teeth and of toothache during the preceding 2 years have been used as background variables in the following analyses of the data based on 3344 Finnish conscripts (O. Ankkuriniemi and J. Ainamo, unpublished).

TABLE VIII

Relationship between the Different Oral Health Indices and the Number of Years Spent being Educated in a Population of 3335 Young Adult Males

Years of education	No.	Oral health indices				
		$\bar{x}$ DT	$\bar{x}$ DMFT	$\bar{x}$ VPI	$\bar{x}$ GBI	$\bar{x}$ PP
0–8	489	6.91	16.15	6.46	5.63	0.31
9–11	1247	4.75	15.86	5.27	4.80	0.31
12–14	1336	3.31	15.49	4.12	3.53	0.16
15–	263	2.77	16.96	3.38	3.02	0.26

Nine subjects did not answer the question. DT, number of decayed teeth; DMFT, decayed, missing or filled teeth; VPI, number of teeth with visible plaque; GBI, gingival bleeding index; PP, 4 mm or deeper pockets. Maximum scores for DT and DMFT were 32; maximum scores for periodontal parameters were 14.

The more years spent in education, the significantly smaller is the average number of decayed teeth (Table VIII). As no corresponding decrease of the DMFT scores is observed, the results indicate that those with a long education have the highest number of filled teeth. The highest DMF score for the group with the longest education is explained by the fact that the mean age of this group is higher than that of the others. The decrease of the visible plaque index (VPI) and gingival bleeding index (GBI) scores confirms the superior oral health awareness of those with a long as compared to those with a short education. Nevertheless, there is an increase in the mean prevalence of periodontal pockets ($\bar{x}$ PP) between the two most highly educated groups. This increase may be related either to age or to the high number of fillings in the group with maximum education.

The frequency of tooth-brushing reported by individuals (Table IX) seems to affect the different oral health indices in the same way as did the number of years spent on education. The number of decayed teeth decreases and all the three periodontal parameters improve with increasing frequency of brushing. No corresponding change is noticed with regard to mean DMF scores.

TABLE IX
Relationship between the Different Oral Health Indices and Frequency of Daily Toothbrushing Reported by the Subjects in a Population of 3340 Young Adult Males

Brushing frequency	No.	Oral health indices				
		$\bar{x}$ DT	$\bar{x}$ DMFT	$\bar{x}$ VPI	$\bar{x}$ GBI	$\bar{x}$ PP
Less than once	789	6.87	16.22	7.23	6.16	0.35
Once daily	1476	4.00	15.61	4.49	4.06	0.24
More than once	1075	2.97	15.88	3.55	3.18	0.17

For explanation of abbreviations see Table VIII.

Those who had not visited a dentist during the last 2 years were found to have the highest mean number of decayed teeth (Table X). Interestingly enough, they had at the same time the lowest DMF score. The visits to the dentist thus seem to affect mainly treatment of caries and occasional extractions. The influence of dental visits on the periodontal status is rather modest, being considerably weaker than were the influences of education and self-reported frequency of tooth-brushing.

The fluoride content of domestic drinking water is the first variable which

TABLE X

Relationship between the Different Oral Health Indices and the Number of Visits to the Dentist during the Preceding 2 Years in a Population of 3344 Young Adult Males

No. of visits to dentist	No.	Oral health indices				
		$\bar{x}$ DT	$\bar{x}$ DMFT	$\bar{x}$ VPI	$\bar{x}$ GBI	$\bar{x}$ PP
None	1126	5.68	14.49	5.42	4.86	0.29
1–2	1125	3.96	15.38	4.69	4.08	0.26
3–10	963	2.73	17.39	4.42	3.82	0.17
11–	130	3.12	20.07	4.17	4.15	0.25

For abbreviations see Table VIII.

affects both the DT and DMFT scores in the same direction (Table XI). As the number of both decayed and filled teeth decreases with increasing fluoride content, this variable seems to represent a genuine caries preventive agent which is independent of treatment received. As to the periodontal status, there is no difference between the low and medium fluoride levels. The better periodontal status in the optimal and high fluoride areas may or may not be related to the fluoride itself. A reasonable explanation would be that the low caries experience favourably reduces the plaque retention caused by decay or fillings.

The frequency of self-reported bleeding from the gums correlates to both increasing DT and periodontal scores (Table XII). The association between a history of gingival bleeding and measured gingival bleeding was surprisingly low. This finding may be partly due to the controversy that bleeding from the gums after tooth-brushing is more likely noticed by those who brush their teeth frequently and scrupulously than by those who do not brush at all or

TABLE XI

Relationship between the Oral Health Indices and Fluoride Content of the Domestic Drinking Water of 3266 Young Adult Finnish Males

Fluoride content (mg/l)	No.	Oral health indices				
		$\bar{x}$ DT	$\bar{x}$ DMFT	$\bar{x}$ VPI	$\bar{x}$ GBI	$\bar{x}$ PP
0.0–0.4	2759	4.51	16.11	4.90	4.32	0.25
0.5–0.9	332	3.64	15.10	4.84	4.38	0.26
1.0–3.7	175	3.33	12.83	4.21	3.53	0.18

For explanation of abbreviations see Table VIII. Fluoride content of the drinking water could not be assessed for 78 subjects.

Table XII
Relationship between the Different Oral Health Indices and a History of Bleeding from the Gums while Brushing the Teeth in a Population of 3331 Young Adult Males

Bleeding observed	No.	Oral health indices				
		$\bar{x}$ DT	$\bar{x}$ DMFT	$\bar{x}$ RC$_2$	$\bar{x}$ GBI	$\bar{x}$ PP
Often	184	5.52	16.03	1.98	4.90	0.42
Seldom	1505	4.35	16.08	1.24	4.54	0.25
Not at all	1642	4.16	15.57	1.02	3.95	0.21

RC$_2$, number of teeth with subgingival calculus. For other abbreviations see Table VIII.

who only briefly clean the facial surfaces of their anterior teeth. Much stronger correlations were found between self-reported bleeding and the prevalence of subgingival calculus (RC 2) and 4 mm or deeper pockets. The evident improvement in the latter two indices suggests that a history of gingival bleeding may represent a rather useful criterion for evaluation of periodontal health.

The last variable tabulated is the experience of toothache during the 2 years before the examination (Table XIII). Only 38% of the conscripts had no history of toothache. Interestingly enough, these subjects had mean scores for oral health which were very close to those of frequent tooth-brushers (Table IX), with the one exception that their DMF scores were as low as for those living in an optimal or high fluoride area (Table XI).

If any conclusions are to be drawn from this analysis of oral health as related to background variables, it seems that fluoride in the drinking water has the greatest effect on past caries experience, while its effect on the periodontal conditions is not very pronounced (Table XI). The most effective

Table XIII
Relationship between the Different Oral Health Indices and Historical Frequency of Toothache during the Preceding 2 Years in a Population of 3340 Young Adult Males

History of toothache	No.	Oral health indices				
		$\bar{x}$ DT	$\bar{x}$ DMFT	$\bar{x}$ VPI	$\bar{x}$ GBI	$\bar{x}$ PP
Often	204	9.30	19.13	6.50	5.52	0.34
Seldom	1879	5.09	16.77	5.12	4.52	0.26
Not at all	1257	2.43	13.93	4.16	3.70	0.20

For abbreviations see Table VIII.

variable affecting periodontal health is the reported frequency of toothbrushing which, however, seems to have little or no effect on the average number of DMF teeth per individual (Table IX). The frequency of visits to the dentist during the preceding 2 years was not associated in a convincing way with improved oral health (Table X). A possible explanation for these figures is that those who have most disease to start with are the subjects who most frequently visit the dentist. The modest improvement of the periodontal condition with frequent dental visits allows also the assumption that the visits had been of a more reparative than preventive nature.

Summary

A detailed analysis of the relation between dental caries and periodontal disease is reported. The evidence does not support either a directly synergistic or directly antagonistic correlation in the prevalence of these two diseases in the same subjects. The fact that both diseases are highly prevalent in industrialized countries may have hampered the objective evaluation of their interrelationship. In developing countries poor oral hygiene is known to cause a high prevalence of periodontal disease. With increasing sucrose consumption the prevalence of caries also increases. High caries activity, in turn, causes additional plaque retention and thus contributes to further periodontal involvement.

In industrialized countries the high prevalence of caries related to the diet has successfully been reduced with optimal fluoride programmes, whereas oral hygiene measures prevent caries only when administered at frequent intervals by dental health care personnel. At the same time, mechanical cleaning of the teeth, even when performed by the individual himself, has been shown to reduce the prevalence and severity of periodontal disorders.

According to the data presented, dental caries and periodontal disease, even when occurring in the same subject, may well have different locations in the dentition. When groups of young adults or teenage children were analysed, high-risk groups could be identified separately for both caries prevalence and periodontal disorders. A closer analysis, however, revealed that only in a few cases did the same subjects belong to both high-risk groups. This finding was not influenced by the choice of either past caries experience (DMF) or the number of open carious lesions (DT) as the indicators of caries activity.

Those subjects who had the highest numbers of filled teeth belonged less commonly to the high-risk group for gingivitis than did the subjects with the highest numbers of decayed teeth. This difference appears to be related to individual differences in oral health care patterns and in the amount and type of professional treatment received.

Among those with a high DMF score there seemed to be one group of subjects, usually with a high level of education, who visited their dentist regularly to have their carious lesions treated and who also took better than average care of their oral hygiene. Subjects belonging to this group therefore had, in spite of a high number of fillings, a fairly good gingival status. The other extreme group was formed by individuals who had a high caries experience, yet visited the dentist infrequently and were also less interested in personal oral hygiene measures. Typical of this group was the great number of open carious lesions. Representatives of this group frequently seemed to give a history of toothache. Their periodontal condition was often poor.

Among those subjects with relatively low DMF scores the lack of plaque-retentive decay and fillings contributes to lower scores for periodontal disease. However, a low caries experience seemed by no means to rule out the possibility of high scores for gingivitis and periodontal disease.

In industrialized countries a variety of factors seems to determine the prevalences of dental caries and periodontal disease. Such factors are dietary habits, access to fluorides, efficacy of oral hygiene measures and utilization of professional dental health care services. The fact that many of these variables, in addition, are mutually related, has greatly hampered the intelligent interpretation of epidemiological findings. In the populations described in this review the prevalences of dental caries and periodontal disease appeared to a great extent to be mutually independent. Further analyses of other types of population groups are required in order to confirm the general validity of this statement.

References

Ainamo, J. (1970). *Proc. Finn. dent. Soc.* **66**, 303–366.
Ainamo, J. (1976). *J. Indian dent. Assoc.* **48**, 117–124.
Ainamo, J. (1980). *Int. dent. J.* **30**, 54–66.
Ainamo, J. and Ainamo, A. (1978). *Int. dent. J.* **28**, 427–433.
Ainamo, J. and Bay, I. (1975). *Int. dent. J.* **25**, 229–235.
Ainamo, J. and Parviainen, K. (1979). *Community Dent. oral Epidemiol.* **7**, 142–146.
Ankkuriniemi, O. (1979). *Annls Med. militar. Fenn.* **54**, 37–120.
Ankkuriniemi, O. (1980). *Proc. Finn. dent. Soc.* **76**, in press.
Ankkuriniemi, O. and Ainamo, J. (1979). *J. dent. Res.* **58**, special issue A, 367.
Axelsson, P. and Lindhe, J. (1978). *J. clin. Periodont.* **5**, 133–151.
Axelsson, P., Lindhe, J. and Wäseby, J. (1976).*Community Dent. oral Epidemiol.* **4**, 232–239.
Bay, I. and Ainamo, J. (1974). *Community Dent. oral Epidemiol.* **2**, 75–79.
Björby, Å. and Löe, H. (1967). *J. periodont. Res.* **2**, 76–77.
Lehner, T. (1977). In *Borderland between Caries and Periodontal Disease* (T. Lehner, ed.). pp.129–144, Academic Press, New York and London.
Löe, H., von der Fehr, F. R. and Rindom Schiött, C. (1972). *Scand. J. dent. Res.* **80**, 1–9.
Löe, H. and Silness, J. (1963). *Acta odont. scand.* **21**, 533–551.

Löe, H., Theilade, E. and Jensen, S. B. (1965). *J. Periodont.* **36**, 177–187.
Miller, J. (1961). *Archs oral Biol.* **6**, 70–79.
Miller, J. and Hobson, P. (1961). *Br. dent. J.* **11**, 43–52.
Parviainen, K., Nordling, H. and Ainamo, J. (1977). *Community Dent. oral Epidemiol.* **5**, 287–291.
Schroeder, H. E. (1969). *Formation and Inhibition of Dental Calculus,* Hans Huber Verlag, Berne.
Silness, J. and Löe, H. (1964). *Acta odont. scand.* **22**, 121–135.
Slack, G. L. (1977). In *Borderland between Caries and Periodontal Disease* (T. Lehner, ed.), pp. 1–3, Academic Press, New York and London.
Sutcliffe, P. (1972). *J. periodont. Res.* **7**, 52–58.
Sznajder, N. Carraro, J. J., Otero, E. and Carranza, F. A., Jr (1968). *J. periodont. Res.* **3**, 1–5.
Waerhaug, J. (1966) In *World Workshop in Periodontics* (S.P. Ramfjord, D. A. Kerr and M. M. Ash, eds), pp. 179–211, Ann Arbor, Michigan.
WHO (1978). *Epidemiology, Etiology and Prevention of Periodontal Diseases,* Technical Report Series no. 621, WHO, Geneva.
Wright, G. Z., Banting, D. W. and Feasby, W. H. (1979). *Clin. prevent. Dent.* **1**, 23–26.

3. Proteinases of the Gingival Crevice and their Inhibitors

G. CIMASONI and Y. KOWASHI

Introduction

The rates of renewal of epithelial structures and of passage of leukocytes through the junctional epithelium modulate the concentration of various enzymes in the gingival crevice. This concentration will also depend upon the endogenous production of enzymes, either in the periodontal tissues or transported locally by blood. Furthermore, the presence of bacteria will significantly modify the enzymatic content of the crevice. It is therefore difficult to find out to what extent biochemical measurements of the content of the gingival crevice reflect physiological or pathological functions within the marginal gingiva or the deeper periodontal structures.

With this limitation in mind it seems reasonable to study the presence and characteristics of enzymes in the gingival crevice, taking into account the role that some of them could play in the pathogenesis of periodontal disease (for a review see Cimasoni *et al.*, 1977).

Proteinases have received particular attention in the past few years and their possible role in the destruction of tissue components during inflammation has been extensively reviewed in two recent monographs (Barrett, 1977; Havemann and Janoff, 1978). In periodontology much emphasis has been put on collagenase but as the present review will show, other proteinases, such as the elastase of polymorphonuclear leukocytes, seem to have an important biological function.

Characteristics of Mammalian Proteinases

According to the classification recently reviewed by Barrett (1977) the proteinases of mammalian tissues can be divided into two main categories, the exopeptidases and the endopeptidases. The enzymes of the first category cleave only bonds near the end of short polypeptide substrates; with the exception of aminopeptidase A (Paunio *et al.*, 1971) their presence in the gingival sulcus has received limited attention.

Practically all the proteinases which have been studied in the gingival sulcus belong to the category of endopeptidases. According to the chemical nature of their catalytic groups or cofactors, these enzymes have been divided into four major classes, the "thiol", "carboxyl", "serine" and "metallo" endoproteinases, each class being inhibited by specific inhibitors (Barrett, 1977).

Thiol Endopeptidases

These enzymes are inhibited by alkylating agents, by chloromercuribenzoate and by disulphides. Among others, cathepsins B, H, L and S, as well as insulinase, are found in this class of proteinases, but no data are available concerning their presence in the gingival sulcus.

Carboxylendopeptidases

Of the six proteinases belonging to the group of carboxylendopeptidases, *cathepsin D* (EC 3.4.4.23) has been found in human gingiva and the properties of this enzyme will be discussed in detail below.

Serine Endopeptidases

The group of serine endopeptidases includes a series of 15 enzymes and, among those, three proteinases which have received a great deal of attention by students of inflammation are *neutrophil elastase* (EC 3.4.21.11), *cathepsin G* (EC 3.4.21.20) and *plasminogen activator* (EC 3.4.21.–). The main inhibitor of this group of enzymes is diisopropyl phosphofluoridate (Dip-F), but the less toxic phenylmethane sulphonylfluoride (Pms-F) has almost the same reactivity as Dip-F and is more convenient to use.

Metalloendopeptidases

Vertebrate collagenase (EC 3.4.24.7) and (or) *granulocyte collagenase* (EC 3.4.24.7) belong to the group of metalloendopeptidases. They are inhibited by chelating agents and by various physiological inhibitors. Their presence and activity, together with that of their inhibitors, have been studied in the gingival environment and will be reviewed here.

Studies on Gingival Cathepsin D

Cathepsin D, a carboxyl endopeptidase, is one of the chief acid enzymes in lysosomes, present at high concentrations in inflamed tissues. It is particularly abundant in human mononuclear leukocytes, while polymorphonuclear leukocytes (PMNs) contain relatively less enzyme (Ishikawa and Cimasoni, 1977). Much attention has been devoted to its presence in the gingival environment, as reviewed in detail in the previous symposium (Cimasoni *et al.*, 1977). In summary, the concentration of cathepsin D was 10 times higher in crevicular fluid than in serum and this concentration was positively correlated with periodontal destruction (Ishikawa *et al.*, 1972). In the gingival washings collected from human volunteers, the activities of both free and total cathepsin D were found to increase during a period of experimental gingivitis (Tzamouranis *et al.*, 1977). Finally, homogenates of inflamed gingiva were found to contain more free cathepsin D, when compared to homogenates of biopsies of sound gingiva (Hasegawa *et al.*, 1975).

In spite of its unphysiological pH, the enzyme may be capable of attacking various components of the connective tissue. It is possible that the pH of the extracellular medium at specific sites, for instance along a non-phagocytosable surface, is comparable to that of endocytic vacuoles (Baggiolini, 1972). Sections of gingiva cut in a cryostat and exposed to the granular fraction of human leukocytes at a pH of 3.5, which is optimum for the activity of cathepsin D, showed extensive destruction of both epithelium and connective tissue (Heiniger and Cimasoni, 1980).

Elastase

General Properties

Elastase and cathepsin G are confined to the azurophil granules of PMN which are analogous to lysosomes (Dewald *et al.*, 1975). Neutrophil elastase is a basic glycoprotein, with an isoelectric point of about 10 (Starkey, 1977). It is immunologically identical to spleen elastase, since both human spleen and PMN elastases react with a specific antiserum directed against the neutrophil enzyme (Starkey and Barrett, 1976). It has even been postulated that spleen elastase could be derived, at least in part, from the neutrophils of the spleen (Starkey, 1977). The enzyme has a molecular weight of about 30 000 daltons and exists in at least three molecular forms (Fig. 1). Its optimum pH, depending on the substrate, is between 7.5 and 8.5 and it is active upon elastin and proteins in general. It has been purified from the granular fraction of PMNs in several laboratories by chromatography (for a review, see Starkey, 1977). In our laboratory, the enzyme is usually separated by gel chromatography on Sephadex G-75, using the soluble proteins extracted from the granular fraction of partially purified human PMNs (Ishikawa and Cimasoni, 1978). As can be seen in Fig. 1, the extract shows the three typical main protein bands in cationic disc gel electrophoresis, which can also be stained by using Naphtol AS-D acetate.

Action on Collagen

Besides elastin, which is a very resistant protein and can only be digested by its specific enzyme, elastase attacks a variety of biologically important substrates, such as proteoglycans, haemoglobin, fibrinogen and collagen. For a long time, it has been thought that collagen could be attacked in its native

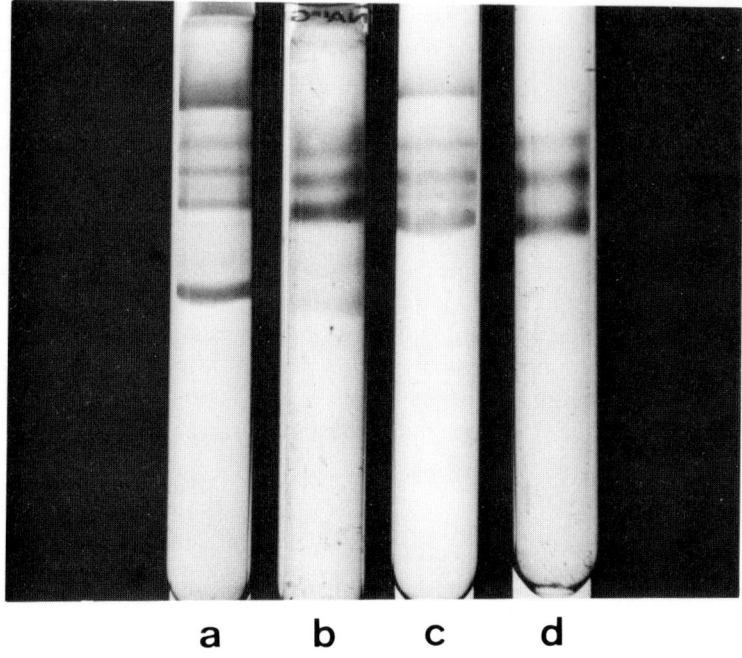

Fig. 1 Polyacrylamide gel electrophoresis of (a) leukocyte granules stained for protein, (b) leukocyte granules stained by AS-D acetate, (c) neutral protease fraction stained for protein and (d) neutral protease fraction stained by AS-D acetate. Cathode is at the bottom.

state only by collagenases, the role of other proteinases being that of further digesting the initial breakdown products. Thanks to the work of Barrett and his group (for a review see Barrett, 1978) we now know that leukocyte elastase (as well as cathepsin G) are able to attack mature collagen fibres. Collagen molecules consist of a helix of three polypeptides, the α (α_1 or α_2) polypeptides. The molecules are held together by cross-links located at their ends, the so-called non-helical regions, where the sequential arrangement of amino acids is different and the helical structure is absent. It is known that mammalian collagenase attacks the collagen molecule in the helical part, and produces fragments of tropocollagen having three-quarters (the "A" fragment) and one-quarter (the "B" fragment) of the original molecular length. Barrett and his colleagues have employed SDS gel electrophoresis to examine the material solubilized from articular cartilage incubated in the presence of PMN elastase or cathepsin G. They found that the solubilized collagen consisted largely of intact α chains and not of the A and B fragments of collagen molecules, typical of collagenase action. They concluded that elastase and cathepsin G cleave the terminal peptides proximally to the cross-link site; the separated modified tropocollagen molecules then tend to become soluble. Once solubilized, the molecules would be more susceptible to the action of collagenase, but would also soon denature at body temperature, with the liberation of the α chains.

We have employed SDS gel electrophoresis to examine the breakdown products of collagen after incubation with the granular extract of human PMNs (Kowashi et al., 1980b). Our patterns will be presented when discussing gingival collagenase (Fig. 5); they confirmed that collagen is attacked by PMN collagenase and elastase, according to the mechanisms described above.

Other Possible Biological Actions of PMN Elastase

Among the biologically important substrates of elastase, one should mention immunoglobulins and complement components. Human IgG is particularly sensitive to the action of the enzyme (Solomon, 1978; Folds et al., 1978; Ishikawa and Cimasoni, 1978); some of the fragments obtained by enzymatic cleavage of IgG retain their antigenic binding properties (Folds et al., 1978).

In vitro, most components of the complement system are affected by the proteases of PMNs (Venge, 1978). Of the three neutral proteases of leukocytes, cathepsin G seems to be the most active in this respect. Formation of biologically active products by this process *in vitro* might be one way by which the neutrophils amplify their function in the inflammatory process.

In view of the well-known participation of immunocompetent cells in gingivitis and periodontitis (Lehner, 1977), a third potentially important action of elastase (and cathepsin G) should be mentioned here, the stimulation of lymphocytes. Both elastase and cathepsin G are able, *in vitro*, to stimulate incorporation of [^{3}H]thymidine by B lymphocytes, together with the appearance of more lymphoblasts and an increased production of immunoglobulins (for a review, see Bretz, 1978).

Finally, one should note that both serine proteinases of PMNs possess bactericidal properties. These are not due to their proteolytic activity, since the latter can be abolished without interference with the antimicrobial action (Olsson et al., 1978).

Gingival Elastase

As reviewed in the previous symposium (Cimasoni et al., 1977), crevicular washings, as well as crevicular fluid, possess proteolytic activity not only at an acid pH but also in the neutral and alkaline range. Although a bacterial origin cannot be excluded, it is probable that most of this neutral proteolytic activity is due to elastase originated from migrating PMNs.

In a recent investigation, we have followed the activity of neutral protease in the washings of eight human volunteers who refrained from tooth brushing during a 21-day period. Using haemoglobin as substrate, the enzyme was

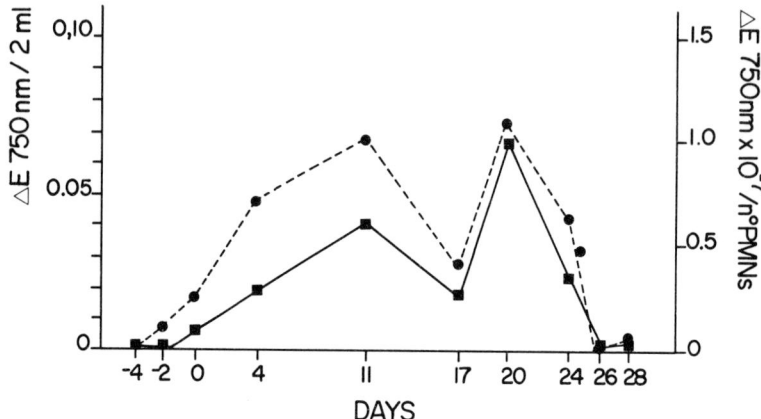

Fig. 2 Neutral protease in the washings of eight volunteers during experimental gingivitis. The mean activities of the enzyme are shown either as differences in extinction between experimental and blank in 2 ml of washing (■———■) or as specific activities (●-----●), i.e. enzyme activities divided by the number of polymorphonuclear leukocytes counted in the same volume.

assayed in the concentrated supernate of the washings, performed at regular intervals before, during and after the period of experimental gingivitis. As shown in Fig. 2, the concentration of free elastase rose significantly during the period of abstention from tooth-brushing and returned to baseline levels after tooth-brushing was resumed. When the free activity of elastase was expressed in relation to the number of PMNs in a given volume of washings, the specific activity also increased during the period of experimental gingivitis which could be due to increased liberation of enzymes from PMNs or from other host and bacterial sources (Kowashi *et al.*, 1980*a*).

As shown in Fig. 2, washings of sound gingiva collected at days 4 and 2 showed very little or no free elastase activity, at least when using haemoglobin as a substrate. As will be discussed later, this could be due to the binding of elastase to physiological inhibitors.

The type of destruction resulting *in vitro* when exposing sections of gingiva to partially purified PMN elastase has been presented in the previous symposium (Cimasoni *et al.*, 1977). We have shown that elastase, when acting upon sections of fresh human gingival biopsies, seems to attack preferentially the epithelial structures, although a general loss of straining could be also found in the connective tissue (Heiniger and Cimasoni, 1980).

More recently, these findings have been reinvestigated and partially confirmed with the aid of the electron microscope (Cergneux *et al.*, 1979).

3. Proteinases of the Gingival Crevice

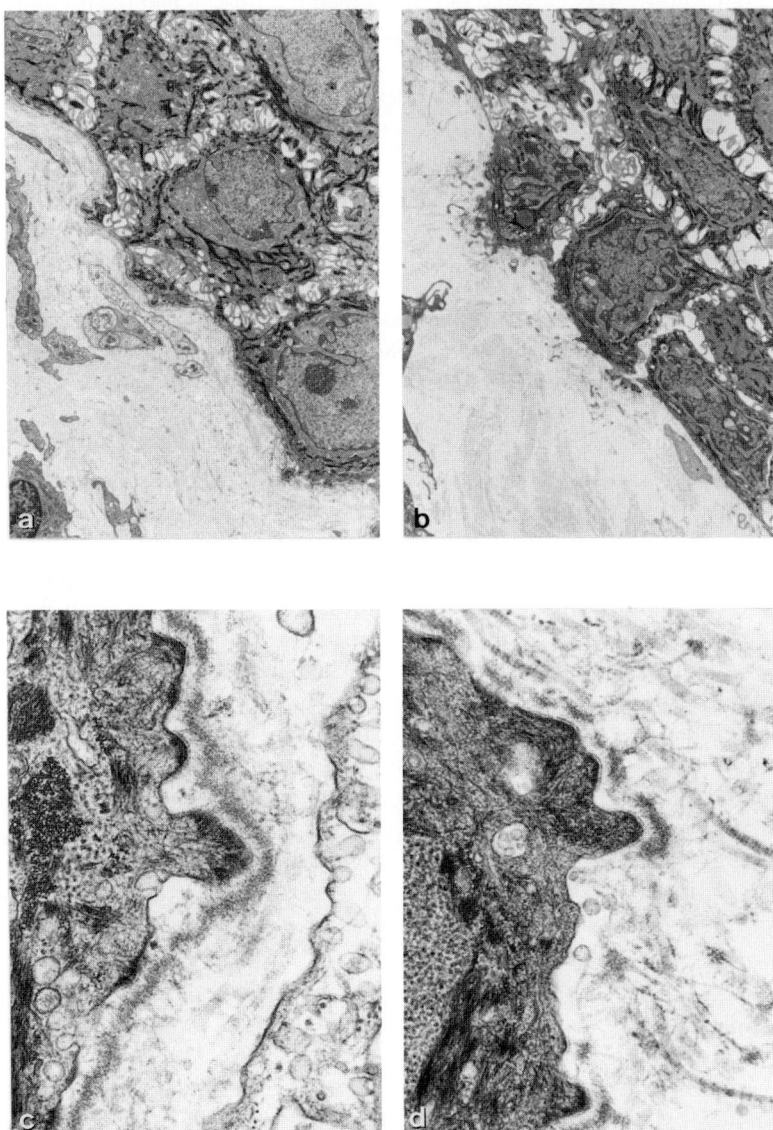

Fig. 3 Effects of elastase from human polymorphonuclear leukocytes on gingival biopsies *in vitro*. High power view of the basal layers of gingival epithelium from a biopsy of human gingiva cultured in Eagle's medium in the absence (a,c) or in the presence (b,d) of elastase. Widening of epithelial intercellular spaces (b) and partial destruction of basal membrane (d) can be observed. (Cergneux *et al.*, 1979).

Carefully dissected explants of human marginal gingiva, having a dimension of about 1 mm^3, were cultured in Eagle's medium for 2–4 h in the presence or in the absence of increasing concentrations of human PMN elastase. After fixation in glutaraldehyde, the blocks were embedded in Epon and semithin as well as ultrathin sections were examined. The observations have been limited to the deep layers of oral epithelium and underlying connective tissue of the marginal gingiva. The enzyme caused a loss of intercellular material in the basal epithelial layers as well as disruption of the basal membrane (Fig. 3). Initial visible changes could be observed with a concentration of elastase as low as 100 μg/ml. For the 1 mm^3 volume occupied by the biopsy, this corresponds to 0.1 g of elastase, which represents the enzyme content of about 25 000 PMNs (Ohlsson and Delshammar, 1975). From our recent studies with gingival washings (Kowashi et al., 1980c) and from the data of Schiött and Löe (1970) it can be shown that 25 000 PMNs roughly represent the average number of PMNs migrating into the oral cavity around one tooth in about 15 min.

The morphological observations are being confirmed by current biochemical investigations (Benoit, unpublished observations). Lyophilized human gingiva was incubated for 24 h in 0.1 M Tris-HCl buffer, pH 7.5, containing 0.15 M NaCl, in the absence or in the presence of increasing concentrations of either whole granular fraction or elastase from human PMNs. Glucuronic acid released in the incubation medium was determined as a measure of proteoglycan solubilization, while hydroxyproline was analysed as an indicator of collagen breakdown.

Preliminary results suggest that the granular fraction of human PMNs was able to solubilize as much as 75% of the total gingival glucuronic acid but only about 5% of the total hydroxyproline. With partially purified PMN elastase up to a protein concentration similar to that used for the granular fraction, 45% of glucuronic acid and about 20% of hydroxyproline could be solubilized. It is possible that, as postulated for cartilage, proteoglycans exert a protective action on collagen fibres against the attack by proteinases (Starkey et al., 1977).

Cathepsin G

Cathepsin G (EC 3.4.21.20) is the second serine endopeptidase contained in the azurophyl granules of human PMNs (Barrett, 1977). It is also called chymotrypsin-like, because it attacks a number of synthetic substrates typical for chymotrypsin and is inhibited by the same inhibitors (Starkey, 1977; Rindler-Ludwig et al., 1978). It has an optimum pH of about 7.5 and a molecular weight of about 30 000 daltons. Similarly to elastase, cathepsin G from spleen is immunologically identical to the enzyme from PMNs (Starkey,

1977). The enzyme has been shown to hydrolyse haemoglobin and fibrinogen, casein and, as mentioned earlier, collagen and proteoglycans, (Starkey, 1977). It is also active upon a variety of low molecular weight substrates which are known substrates of chymotrypsin, the most suitable being the naphtol esters.

Since no data could be found in the literature on the existence of cathepsin G in the gingival sulcus, a few determinations were performed in our laboratory, using gingival washings collected from human volunteers with clinically sound gingiva. Using N-acetyl-D,L-phenylalanine naphthyl ester as substrate and Fast Garnet salt as coupling agent, cathepsin G activity could be shown in the concentrated supernatant of gingival washings. Treatment of aliquots of whole gingival washings with the detergent Triton X100 (0.1%) caused a massive increase in the concentration of free enzyme. These results, however, need confirmation, since low molecular weight substrates of cathepsin G, such as the one used in our laboratory, are susceptible to a variety of esterases (Starkey, 1977).

Plasminogen Activators

The removal of a fibrin clot is accomplished by the fibrinolytic system, following the activation of plasminogen into the active lytic enzyme plasmin.

The amino acid sequence of plasminogen is now known; the transformation of this precursor or zymogen into plasmin is due to two proteolytic cleavages of plasminogen activators. The best characterized plasminogen activator is a serine proteinase called urokinase, but streptokinase and many other proteinases can activate plasminogen. Plasminogen activators are ubiquitous and their presence has clearly been shown in blood, in various tissues, in urine, in leukocytes, and, more recently, in tissue cultures. However, their concentration is extremely low, which makes their study a difficult task. Besides their role in fibrinolysis, plasminogen activators have major roles in inflammation. Plasmin activates the third component of complement, which causes increased vascular permeability and accumulation of PMNs and monocytes. Plasminogen activators are also essential in wound healing and their role in the invasive growth of tumours has also been investigated (for review see Christman *et al.*, 1977).

Inflamed gingiva of dogs showed increased fibrinolytic activity; this was found by placing frozen gingival sections upon films of fibrin clots and observing the areas of fibrin lysis in the presence or the absence of plasminogen (Lucas, 1977). As reviewed earlier (Cimasoni, 1974; Cimasoni *et al.*, 1977), the presence of a fibrinolytic system as well as plasminogen and plasminogen activators in human crevicular exudate was shown by Gustafsson and Nilsson (1961).

Collagenase

The rapid and early breakdown of collagen in inflamed gingiva justifies the attention that many investigators have paid to the presence of collagenase in the gingival environment. As discussed above, other proteinases such as elastase and cathepsin G are active upon mature collagen, but collagenase has been known for many years to be the specific enzyme capable of attacking this fibrous protein. After a brief introduction of the general properties of mammalian collagenases, this section will discuss in detail the recent literature on gingival collagenase, as well as some of the results from our own laboratory.

General Properties of Collagenase

Among mammalian collagenases, a distinction has been made between the so-called vertebrate collagenases, found in many types of mammalian cells, and the enzyme isolated from the specific granules of human PMNs, the granulocyte collagenase (Lazarus et al., 1968; Barrett, 1977; Harris and Cartwright, 1977). The granulocyte enzyme has a higher molecular weight, but both collagenases have the same designation in the international nomenclature (EC 3.4.24.7).

Collagenase has an optimum pH of 8.5. It is a metal-dependent enzyme, active only in the presence of Zn^{2+} and Ca^{2+} and inhibited by chelating agents (for a review see Harris and Cartwright, 1977). It is generally accepted that most of the extracellular collagenases exist in a latent form, but the true nature of this latency is still a subject of controversy. It could be due to the existence of a zymogen or of a complex between the enzyme and an inhibitor (Birkedal-Hansen et al., 1975; Golub et al., 1976; Uitto and Raeste, 1978; Woolley et al., 1978).

Mammalian collagenase makes only one scission per molecule of collagen, as opposed to microbial collagenases, which produce multiple scissions in the same molecule (Robertson and Simpson, 1976). As already pointed out, the two fragments of the collagen molecule obtained by the action of mammalian collagenase are of two different lengths, one representing a 75% fragment (or three-quarter fragment) of the molecule, the A piece, and the second a 25% fragment, the B piece. Fragments A and B can be shown by electrophoresis to be the products of collagen digestion by collagenase (Fig. 5). The original triple helix structure is, however, lost in these preparations, especially with long incubation times, and the fragments shown by electrophoresis represent three-quarter and one-quarter pieces of monomers (αA and αB) or dimers (βA and βB) of the native trimer (γ).

Collagenase of the Gingival Crevice

Collagenase has been identified in the culture fluid of gingival tissue (Fullmer

3. Proteinases of the Gingival Crevice

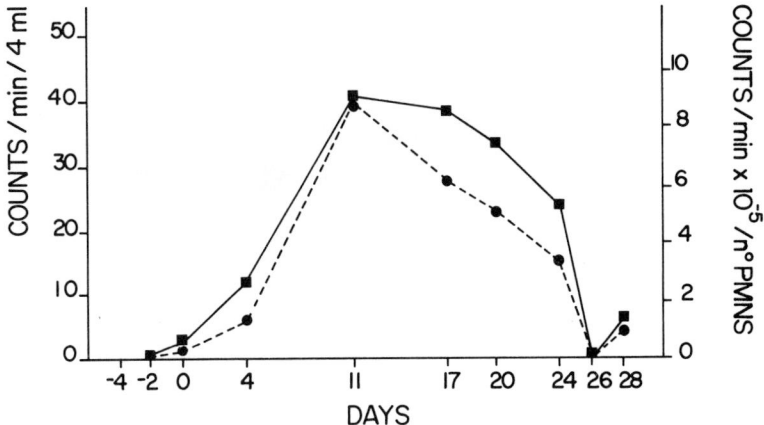

Fig. 4 Collagenase in the washings of eight volunteers. The mean activities of the enzyme are expressed either in counts per minute in 4 ml of washings (■————■) or in counts per minute divided by the number of polymorphonuclear leukocytes (●-------●).

and Gibson, 1966; Woolley et al., 1978), in culture fluid of both epithelial and connective tissue cells of gingiva (Fullmer et al., 1969) and in homogenates of gingival biopsies (Uitto et al., 1978). Collagenolytic activity has been found in gingival fluid (Cimasoni, 1974), where it increases with the severity of the disease (Robertson et al., 1973). Ohlsson et al. (1973) have shown a higher concentration of collagenase and elastase from crevicular material of chronically inflamed gingiva, compared with material from clinically healthy tissue. An increase of collagenase activity in the gingival sulcus during inflammation was also found in our recent investigation (Kowashi et al., 1980a). As shown in Fig. 4, the mean concentration of free collagenase rose significantly in the gingival washings in eight male subjects during a 21-day period of experimental gingivitis. The increase was probably not due to the number of PMNs migrating through the sulcus, since the specific activity of collagenase (free enzyme/number of PMNs) also rose during the period of abstention from tooth-brushing (Fig. 4). Detailed analyses of collagenase in crevicular fluid have been reported by Golub et al. (1976) and Uitto and Raeste (1978); both groups confirmed the presence of mammalian collagenase in human gingival crevices. They studied breakdown products resulting from incubation of collagen with gingival fluid and showed typical αA and αB fragments on acrylamide gel electrophoresis. Uitto and Raeste (1978) used much shorter incubation times, which is an important point, for long incubation periods are known to result in changes of collagenase activity.

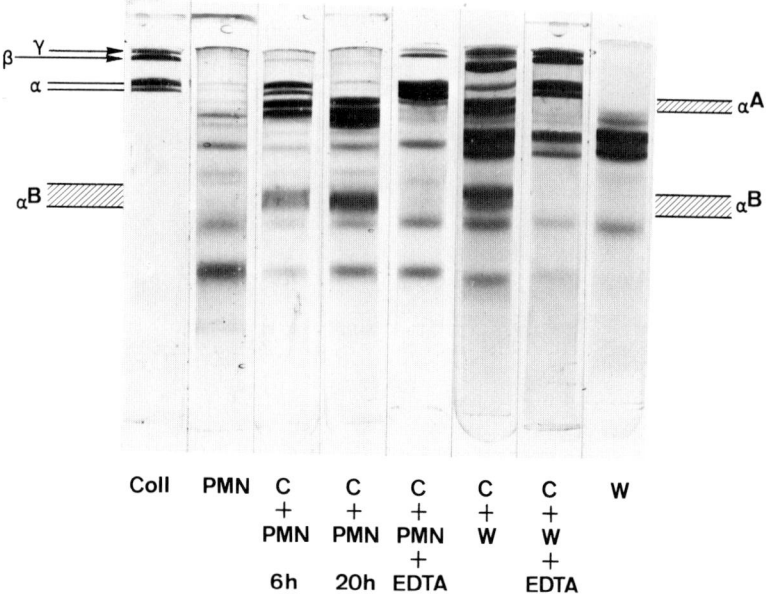

Fig. 5 SDS-polyacrylamide gel electrophoresis of collagen digestion products. Aliquots of polymorphonuclear leukocytes (PMN) granule fractions, alone (C + PMN) or in the presence of EDTA (C + PMN + EDTA) and aliquots of concentrated gingival washings alone (C + W) or in the presence of EDTA (C + W + EDTA) were incubated with rat skin collagen. The incubation time was 20 h, except for one of the assays (6 h). Native collagen (coll), granule fraction of PMN (PMN) and concentrated gingival washings (W) in the absence of collagen are included as references for intact γ, β and α chains of collagen and for bands of foreign proteins.

Figure 5 shows the electrophoretic patterns of collagen digestion products obtained after incubation of gingival washings from clinically sound gingiva with neutral salt-soluble collagen from rat skin (Kowashi et al., 1980b). The breakdown products obtained by incubation of collagen with the granular fraction of human PMNs are also shown. In some instances, ethylenediaminetetraacetic acid (EDTA) was added to the assay medium. Our results confirmed the presence of active collagenase in the gingival sulcus. Typical αA and αB fragments were found after incubation of collagen with both gingival washings and the granular extract. These breakdown products were not formed in the presence of EDTA.

Surprisingly, none of the reports on the collagen breakdown by neutral proteases of the gingival fluid has dealt with the possible attack of collagen by enzymes other than collagenase.

To investigate the activity of elastase, special attention was paid in our electrophoretic patterns to the intensity of the γ and the β bands after different times of incubation. The γ and β bands represent, respectively, trimers and dimers of the α chains; with long incubation times they tend to disappear, due to denaturation of collagen. However, with the granular extract, these bands disappeared with an incubation time as short as 6 h (Fig. 5), which suggests the presence of elastase. When inhibiting collagenase by EDTA, the γ and β bands were weakened while the α band was strongly increased, which is again evidence of elastase activity. After incubation of collagen with concentrated human gingival washings the results were quite different; even after 24 h of incubation (Fig. 5), the γ and β bands persisted, while the α band showed a very moderate increase when inhibiting collagenase with EDTA. This confirms the observation that the concentration of free elastase in the crevice of a clinically sound gingiva is very low.

Serum Proteinase Inhibitors

The activity of proteases in the tissues is probably modulated by the presence of inhibitors either produced locally or circulating in plasma (Davies, 1976; Ohlsson, 1978; Travis et al., 1978). The main plasma protease inhibitors are α_2-macroglobulin and α_1-antitrypsin, accounting for more than 90% of the total protease-inhibiting capacity of serum (Ohlsson, 1978). A third physiological inhibitor, α_1-antichymotrypsin, seems to inactivate only chymotrypsin-like enzymes, for instance cathepsin G, but its precise biological role has not yet fully identified (Ohlsson, 1978; Travis et al., 1978).

α_2-Macroglobulin is a very large molecule, with a molecular weight of about 700 000 daltons; its concentration in serum is 2 mg/ml (Starkey and Barrett, 1977). It is synthesized in the liver and its turnover in man is very rapid. α_2-Macroglobulin inhibits all three neutral proteinases from PMNs by a similar mechanism which consists in the irreversible trapping of the enzyme molecule by the inhibitor. Only active proteases can be bound and the enzymes, after being trapped by the globulin, can still show some activity upon substrates of low molecular weight. Radial immunodiffusion plates (Mancini et al., 1965) for determining α_2-Macroglobulin are available commercially, but this type of determination does not distinguish between free and bound α_2-Macroglobulin. A separation of the complexed from the free inhibitor form is only possible by isoelectric focusing. Indeed, it has been shown that the molecules of complexed macroglobulin become more compact, with an increase in isoelectric point, regardless of the free charge of the proteinase involved (Ohlsson, 1978). As will be shown in detail later (Fig. 6), the procedure of crossed immunoelectrophoresis involves isoelectric focusing followed by immunoelectrophoresis and allows identification of the free and bound globulins.

α_1-Antitrypsin (also called α_1-proteinase inhibitor) inactivates mainly the serine proteinases, elastase and cathepsin G and only partially mammalian collagenase (Ohlsson, 1978). It is a smaller molecule, with a molecular weight of about 50 000 daltons and its concentration in plasma is higher than 200 mg/100 ml (Davies, 1976). In man, it has longer half-life, as compared with α_2-macroglobulin. When inhibited by α_1-antitrypsin, elastase forms a complex which becomes dissociated, with a transfer of the enzyme to α_2-macroglobulin (Ohlsson, 1978).

Proteinase Inhibitors in the Gingival Crevice

The presence of physiological inhibitors of protease activity in the gingival crevice has received very little attention. Ohlsson et al. (1973) reported the presence of α_1-antitrypsin and α_2-macroglobulin in material from human gingival crevices. These investigators studied α_1-antitrypsin in more detail and showed, by crossed immunoelectrophoresis, that all of the inhibitor was in a bound form, both in healthy and inflamed crevices. They concluded that the inhibiting capacity of α_1-antitrypsin seems to be insufficient to saturate the proteolytic activity of the crevice.

Both α_1-antitrypsin and α_2-macroglobulin were found in gingival fluid by Schenkein and Genco (1977), in concentrations representing about 75% of those found in serum. More recently, Uitto and Raeste (1978) confirmed that α_2-macroglobulin is present in human gingival fluid, but could find no correlation between the concentration of the globulin and that of collagenase in a group of nine patients.

In our laboratory, the concentration of serum protease inhibitors in human gingival crevices has been investigated in two studies, firstly in the products of gingival washings during a 21-day period of experimental gingivitis and second in the crevicular fluid, collected with filter paper strips before and after initial periodontal therapy. In the products of gingival washings from eight patients, α_1-antitrypsin and α_2-macroglobulin were determined by radial immunodiffusion (Mancini et al., 1965). The washing collected at the end of the period of abstention from tooth-brushing contained roughly twice the amount of both inhibitors, as compared to the washings obtained when the gingiva was healthy at the beginning of the experiment.

These findings have now been confirmed in our second study, which deals more specifically with α_2-macroglobulin, but has as yet been limited to five patients showing gingivitis and periodontitis. In each patient crevicular fluid was collected by means of filter paper strips from the crevice of one front tooth before and after initial periodontal therapy. The treatment caused a significant decrease of gingival inflammation as measured by the gingival index (Löe and Silness, 1963). For the determination of α_2-macroglobulin, the strips soaked with fluid were placed in microtubes and 40 µl of physiological

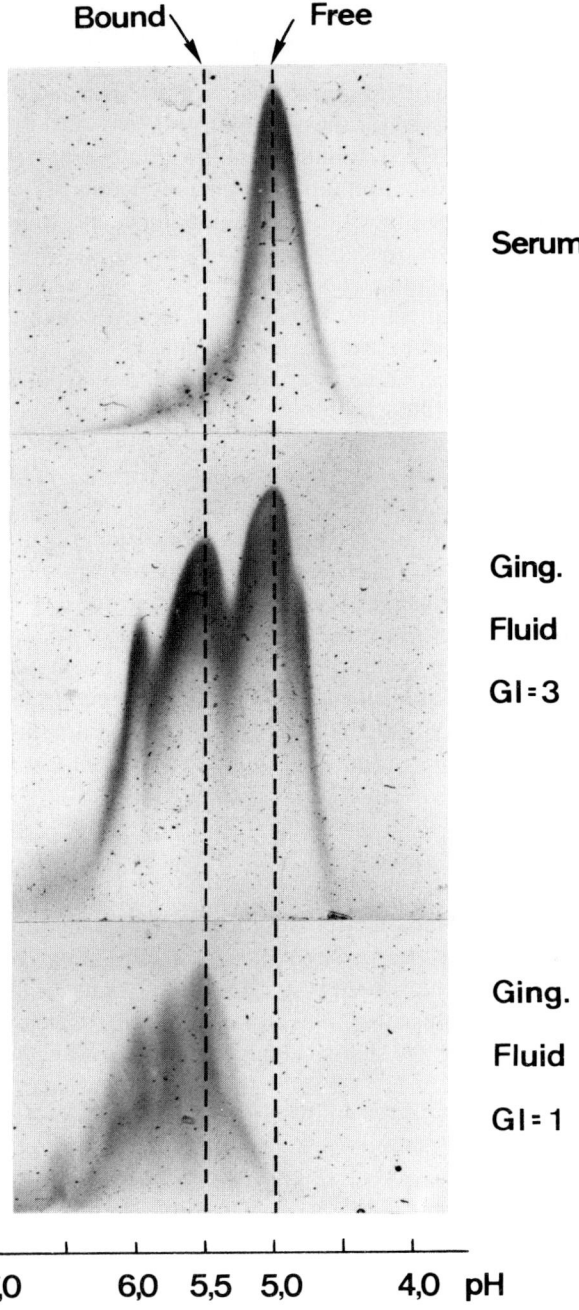

Fig. 6 Patterns of crossed immunoelectrophoresis for α_2-macroglobulin in serum and in the gingival fluid. The fluid was collected with filter paper strips on tooth no. 13, in the same patient, before and after initial periodontal therapy. The gingival index of inflammation decreased from a value of 3 (GI = 3) to a value of 1 (GI = 1).

saline were added. The tubes were shaken, kept for 24 h and centrifuged. The supernatant was then used for the quantitative determination of the total α_2-macroglobulin by an electroimmunoassay (Laurell, 1966). The samples of crevicular fluid collected from inflamed gingiva before periodontal therapy contained about twice as much α_2-macroglobulin as the samples collected in the same area after therapy.

As already pointed out, determinations of α_2-macroglobulin by either immunodiffusion (Mancini *et al.*, 1965) or electroimmunoassay (Laurell, 1966) do not distinguish between free and bound globulin. For this reason, a modification of the technique of crossed immunoelectrophoresis was used (Ohlsson and Skude, 1976), with microamounts of crevicular fluid from the same patients. The strips were soaked with fluid, laid directly on the polyacrylamide gel and submitted to isoelectric focusing. This was followed by crossed immunoelectrophoresis. Our preliminary results seem to indicate that crevicular fluid collected from less inflamed gingiva after periodontal therapy contains no free α_2-macroglobulin. In contrast the fluid collected from the same patients before therapy, in the presence of severe inflammation, invariably showed peaks of both free and complexed α_2-macroglobulin. The degree of complexing could be also estimated; about 40% of the α_2-macroglobulin was found in a bound form in the fluid collected from severely inflamed gingiva. Typical patterns of crossed immunoelectrophoresis obtained for serum and for gingival fluid are shown in Fig 6.

Summary

The information available about the proteinases in the gingival sulcus is limited. There have been no studies on the presence and role of cathepsin G in the gingiva and there have been very few investigations on other important PMN enzymes, such as elastase. This lack of knowledge is even more apparent when one considers the physiological inhibitors of these enzymes. Practically no free elastase seems to be present in the gingival crevice in the absence of inflammation, but we do not know whether this is due to the presence of inhibitors or to other factors, such as minimal liberation of enzymes from PMNs. The concentration of total α_2-macroglobluin and α_1-antitrypsin seems to increase in the sulcus during inflammation, but the relative proportions of bound and free inhibitors have not yet been clearly established. Clearly, studies on the gingival condition of individuals deficient in protease inhibitors could be particularly useful. Specific antisera to PMN proteases and to inhibitors should allow immunohistochemical studies on the distribution of these components within the tissues and therefore a better understanding of their role *in vivo*.

3. Proteinases of the Gingival Crevice

Acknowledgements

Studies mentioned in this review and carried out in the laboratory of the authors were supported by grant 3.604-0.75 of the Swiss National Fund for Scientific Research. We are grateful to Mrs I. Condacci and E. Andersen for their very competent assistance.

References

Baggiolini, M. (1972). *Enzyme* **13**, 132–160
Barrett, A. J. (1977). In *Proteinases in Mammalian Cells and Tissues* (A. J. Barrett ed.), pp. 1–55, North-Holland, Amsterdam.
Barrett, A. J. (1978). In *Neutral Proteases of Human Polymorphonuclear Leukocytes* (K. Havemann and A. Janoff, eds), pp. 385–389, Urban and Schwarzenberg, Baltimore and Munich.
Birkedal-Hansen, H., Cobb, C. M., Taylor, R. E. and Fullmer, H. M. (1975). *Archs oral Biol.* **20**, 681–685.
Bretz, U. (1978). In *Neutral Proteases of Human Polymorphonuclear Leukocytes* (K. Havemann and A. Janoff, eds), pp. 323–327, Urban and Schwarzenberg, Baltimore and Munich.
Cergneux, M., Heiniger, R., Andersen, E., Condacci, I. and Cimasoni, G. (1979). Preprinted abstracts, 16th Annual Meeting of the Continental European Division of IADR, Athens, 1979. Abstract no. 22.
Christman, J. K., Silverstein, S. C. and Acs, G. (1977). In *Proteinases in Mammalian Cells and Tissues* (A. J. Barrett, ed.), pp. 91–149, North-Holland, Amsterdam.
Cimasoni, G. (1974). In *Monographs in Oral Science*, Vol. 3 (H. M. Myers, ed.), Karger, Basel.
Cimasoni, G., Ishikawa, I. and Jaccard, F. (1977). In *Borderland between Caries and Periodontal Disease* (T. Lehner, ed.), pp. 13–41, Academic Press, London.
Davies, Ph. (1976). In *Structure and Function of Plasma Proteins* (A. C. Allison, ed.), pp. 189–238, Plenum, New York.
Dewald, B., Rindler-Ludwig, R., Bretz, U. and Baggiolini, M. (1975). *J. exp. Med.* **141**, 709–723.
Folds, J. D., Prince, H. and Spitznagel, J. K. (1978). *Lab. Invest.* **39**, 313–321.
Fullmer, H. M. and Gibson, W. A. (1966). *Nature, Lond.* **209**, 728–729.
Fullmer, H. M., Gibson, W. A., Lazarus, G. S., Bladen, H. A. and Whedon, K. A. (1969). *J. dent. Res.* **48**, 646–651.
Golub, L. M., Siegel, K., Ramamurthy, N. S. and Mandel, I. D. (1976). *J. dent. Res.* **55**, 1049–1057.
Gustafsson, G. T. and Nilsson, J. M. (1961). *Proc. Soc. exp. Biol. Med.* **106**, 277–280.
Harris, E. D. and Cartwright, E. C. (1977). In *Proteinases in Mammalian Cells and Tissues* (A. J. Barrett, ed.), pp. 249–283, North-Holland, Amsterdam.
Hasegawa, K., Cimasoni, G. and Vuagnat, P. (1975). *Experientia* **31**, 765–766.
Havemann, K. and Janoff, A. (eds) (1978). *Neutral Proteases of Human Polymorphonuclear Leukocytes*, Urban and Schwarzenberg, Baltimore and Munich.
Heiniger, R. and Cimasoni, G. (1980). *J. Biologie buccale* **8**, 3–16.
Ishikawa, I. and Cimasoni, G. (1977). *Biochim. biophys. Acta* **480**, 228–240.
Ishikawa, I. and Cimasoni, G. (1978). *Archs oral Biol.* **23**, 933–940.
Ishikawa, I., Cimasoni, G. and Ahmad-Zadeh, C. (1972). *Archs oral Biol.* **17**, 111–117.
Kowashi, Y., Jaccard, F. and Cimasoni, G. (1980s). *Archs oral Biol.* **24**, 645–650.

Kowashi, Y., Cimasoni, G. and Matter, J. (1980*b*). *Experientia* **36**, 395–397.
Kowashi, Y., Jaccard, F. and Cimasoni, G. (1980*c*). *J. periodont. Res.* **15**, 151–158.
Laurell, C. B. (1966). *Analyt. Biochem.* **15**, 45–52.
Lazarus, G. S., Daniels, J. R., Brown, R. S., Bladen, H. A. and Fullmer, H. M., (1968). *J. clin. Invest.* **47**, 2622–2629.
Lehner, T. (1977). In *Borderland between Caries and Periodontal Disease* (T. Lehner, ed.), pp. 129–144, Academic Press, London.
Löe, H. and Silness, J. (1963). *Acta odont. scand.* **21**, 532–551.
Lucas, O. N. (1977). *J. dent. Res.* **56**, 1533–1538.
Mancini, G., Carbonara, A. D. and Heremans, J. F. (1965). *Immunochemistry* **2**, 235–254.
Ohlsson, K., Olsson, J. and Tynelius-Bratthall, G. (1973). *Acta odont. scan.* **31**, 51–59.
Ohlsson, K. and Delshammar, M. (1975). In *Dynamics of Connective Tissue Macromolecules* (P. M. C. Burleigh and A. R. Poole, eds), pp. 259–275, North-Holland, Amsterdam.
Ohlsson, K. and Skude, G. (1976). *Clin. chim. Acta* **66**, 1–7.
Ohlsson, K. (1978). In *Neutral Proteases of Human Polymorphonuclear Leukocytes* (K. Havemann and A. Janoff, eds), pp. 167–178, Urban and Schwarzenberg, Baltimore and Munich.
Olsson, J., Odeberg, H., Weiss, J. and Elsbach, P. (1978). In *Neutral Proteases of Human Polymorphonuclear Leukocytes* (K. Havemann and A. Janoff, eds), pp. 18–32, Urban and Schwarzenberg, Baltimore and Munich.
Paunio, K. U., Mäkinen, K. K. and Scheinin, A., (1971). *Acta odont. scand.* **29**, 583–590.
Rindler-Ludwig, R., Bretz, U. and Baggiolini, M. (1978). In *Neutral Proteases of Human Polymorphonuclear Leukocytes* (K. Havemann and A. Janoff, eds), pp. 138–149, Urban and Schwarzenberg, Baltimore and Munich.
Robertson, P. B. and Simpson, J. (1976). *J. Periodont.* **47**, 29–33.
Robertson, P. B., Grupe, H. E., Jr., Taylor, R. E., Shyn, K. W. and Fullmer, H. M. (1973). *J. oral Path.* **2**, 28–32.
Schenkein, H. A. and Genco, R. J. (1977). *J. Periodont.* **48**, 772–777.
Schiött, C. R. and Löe, H. (1970). *J. Periodont. Res.* **5**, 36–41.
Solomon, A. (1978). In *Neutral Proteases of Human Polymorphonuclear Leukocytes* (K. Havemann and A. Janoff, eds), pp. 423–436, Urban and Schwarzenberg, Baltimore and Munich.
Starkey, Ph. M. (1977). In *Proteinases in Mammalian Cells and Tissues* (A. J. Barrett, ed.), pp. 57–89, North-Holland, Amsterdam.
Starkey, Ph. M. and Barrett, A. J. (1976). *Biochem. J.* **155**, 265–271.
Starkey, Ph. M. and Barrett, A. J. (1977). In *Proteinases in Mammalian Cells and Tissues* (A. J. Barrett, ed.), pp. 663–696, North-Holland, Amsterdam.
Starkey, Ph. M., Barrett, A. J. and Burleigh, M. C. (1977). *Bioc. biophys. Acta* **483**, 386–397.
Travis, J., Baugh, R., Giles, P. J., Johnson, D., Bowen, J. and Reilly, C. F. (1978). In *Neutral Proteases of Human Polymorphonuclear Leukocytes* (K. Havemann and A. Janoff, eds), pp. 118–128, Urban and Schwarzenberg, Baltimore and Munich.
Tzamouranis, A., Matthys, J., Ishikawa, I. and Cimasoni, G. (1977). *Archs oral Biol.* **22**, 375–378.
Uitto, V. J. and Raeste, A. M. (1978). *J. dent. Res.* **57**, 844–851.
Uitto, V. J., Turto, H. and Saxen, L. (1978) *J. periodont. Res.* **13**, 207–214.
Venge, P. (1978). In *Neutral Proteases of Human Polymorphonuclear Leukocytes* (K.

Havemann and A. Janoff, eds), pp. 264–275, Urban and Schwarzenberg, Baltimore and Munich.
Wolley, D. E., Akroyd, Ch., Evanson, J. M., Soames, J. V. and Davies, R. M. (1978). *Biochim. biophys. Acta* **522**, 205–217.

4. Passage of Serum Immunoglobulins into the Oral Cavity

S. J. CHALLACOMBE

Introduction

Immunoglobulins and other proteins in mixed saliva are derived from three principal sources, the major salivary glands, the minor salivary glands and crevicular fluid. In addition, contributions to the total immunoglobulin content of mixed saliva may be made by direct passage across epithelium, particularly if this is inflamed (Brandtzaeg et al., 1970).

The source and function of immunoglobulins in the oral cavity is currently of great interest, particularly with regard to dental caries. The tooth surface is unique in that it is exposed to both the secretory immune system, as represented by saliva, and the systemic humoral system via antibodies in crevicular fluid which are assumed largely to be derived from serum. Theoretically either or both of these systems may play a role in protection against dental caries. The area of the tooth surface which is exposed primarily to saliva may be different from that exposed to crevicular fluid, and the terms salivary domain and crevicular domain have been proposed to distinguish between these areas (Lehner et al., 1976a).

The role of systemic and secretory humoral systems in protection against caries has been carefully evaluated in different animal models. In rodents it appears that protection against caries can be achieved by inducing salivary antibodies. Immunization with *Streptococcus mutans* or glucosyltransferase preparations in the vicinity of the salivary glands gives rise to high titres of salivary antibodies, and in addition serum antibodies, and a reduction in caries of smooth surfaces (Taubman and Smith, 1974, 1977; McGhee et al., 1976). The role of secretory antibodies in the rodent model has been further demonstrated by the finding that ingestion of *Strep. mutans* cells by gnotobiotic rats may induce antibodies in saliva in the absence of serum antibody, and may lead to protection against caries (Michalek et al., 1976). In addition, passive transfer of IgG and IgA antibodies in colostrum and milk from rat dams to their offspring resulted in protection against caries (Michalek and McGee, 1977).

In contrast to these results in rodents, experiments using the primate model strongly suggest a role for serum antibodies in protection against caries. Subcutaneous (s.c.) immunization with *Strep. mutans* in Freund's incomplete adjuvant in Rhesus monkeys induced serum antibodies and cellular immunity (Lehner *et al.*, 1976*b*), but this route is ineffective at producing salivary antibodies (Challacombe and Lehner, 1980). Such s.c. immunization leads to a significant reduction in caries, suggesting that serum antibodies may reach the tooth surface and be functional. Protection against caries was associated with serum IgG antibodies (Lehner *et al.*, 1978*a*). In the Irus monkey systemic immunization has also been shown to lead to a reduction in caries which was presumably mediated through serum antibodies (Bowen *et al.*, 1975; Cohen *et al.*, 1979). The role of serum IgG antibodies has been convincingly demonstrated by the observation that passive transfer of IgG from immunized donors intravenously into recipients can result in significantly reduced caries in the recipients (Lehner *et al.*, 1978*b*). This clearly suggests that serum antibodies may protect against caries in the absence of salivary antibodies in the primate. The situation in man may be more analogous to the primate model than the rodent model since subjects of low caries experience have high titres of serum IgG antibodies to *Strep. mutans*, but low titres of salivary antibodies (Challacombe and Lehner, 1976; Challacombe, 1978). These findings suggest that in man, as well as in primates, serum IgG may be functional within the oral cavity.

In this paper evidence from work performed in conjunction with Dr M. Russell and Professor T. Lehner is presented to show that the major immunoglobulin isotypes can pass directly from serum to the oral cavity. This pathway has been favoured in the past by indirect evidence, and this will be reviewed.

Materials and Methods

Monkey Immunoglobulins

Rhesus monkey IgG, IgA and IgM were isolated from pooled monkey serum. IgG was purified by a combination of DEAE cellulose chromatography and gel filtration on Biogel P 300 (Russell *et al.*, 1976); IgM by gel filtration and zone electrophoresis; and IgA by gel filtration, DEAE cellulose chromatography, hydrophobic chromatography and zone electrophoresis (Challacombe and Russell, 1979). Each immunoglobulin gave a single precipitation line against rabbit anti-monkey serum. The purified immunoglobulins were radiolabelled with ^{125}I (IMS-3, Radiochemical Centre, Amersham) by a modification of the chloramine-T method (Challacombe *et al.*, 1978*a*) to give an activity of between 0.5 and 1 µCi/µg protein.

4. Immunoglobulin Passage into Oral Cavity

Injection of Labelled Immunoglobulins

Twelve Rhesus monkeys which weighed between 2.3 and 4.7 kg were injected with radiolabelled immunoglobulins into the small saphenous vein. Each isotype was injected into four animals in amounts of approximately 50 µg.

Collection of Samples

Samples of serum, crevicular fluid washings (CFW), mucosal washings, parotid saliva and mixed saliva were taken at 0, 0.5, 1, 2, 4 and 24 h as detailed previously (Challacombe et al., 1978a). The animals were given subcutaneous pilocarpine (0.5 mg/kg) before collection of saliva samples. CFW were taken from the gingival crevice and the approximal spaces of the deciduous molar teeth and the first permanent teeth by the method of Skapski and Lehner (1976). Approximately 5 µl of saline was instilled twice into each approximal space, and up to 40 µl of CFW was recovered from each animal. Mucosal washings were taken of an area in the left buccal sulcus. All the animals had mild gingival inflammation with a mean gingival index of 1.1 (Löe and Silness, 1963).

Immunoglobulin Concentrations

These were assayed by a modification of the single radial diffusion method (Challacombe, 1976) using monospecific antisera raised in rabbits against Rhesus monkey IgG, IgA and IgM and purified monkey immunoglobulins as standards.

Sucrose Density Gradient Rate Zonal Ultracentrifugation

Sucrose density gradients were prepared as described previously (Challacombe et al., 1978b). For IgG samples linear 10–25% w/w gradients were used, for IgA 10–30% and for IgM 10–40%. Samples of serum (20 µl) were made up to 100 µl with saline for analysis. For CFW 20 µl of sample were added to 20 µl of carrier serum and made up to 100 µl with saline, and for saliva, 50 µl samples were made up to 100 µl in the same way. After centrifugation at 65 000 r.p.m. for 16 h at 4 C, fractions were collected and assayed for radioactivity and protein concentration (Challacombe et al., 1978a).

Determination of the Volume of Crevicular Fluid

Ten microlitres of a solution of radiolabelled immunoglobulin of a known number of counts per minute was instilled into each approximal space of four monkeys and four human volunteers and as much as possible recovered. The volume recovered was measured and the number of counts per minute determined. The volume of crevicular fluid is related to the dilution of the number of counts per minute according to the formula $v = (s/r \times w) - 10$, where s is the total number of counts per minute applied at the start, r is the total number of counts per minute recovered, and w is the volume of fluid recovered.

Results

Serum Radioactivity

The mean number of counts per minute in samples of serum taken after 0.5 h was 310 000 counts min^{-1} ml^{-1} in animals given IgA, 290 000 counts min^{-1} ml^{-1} in animals given IgM, and 245 000 counts min^{-1} ml^{-1} in animals given IgG. The mean count by 2 h was approximately the same in all groups at about 220 000 counts min^{-1} ml^{-1}, and at 4 h it was 200 000 counts min^{-1} ml^{-1}. By 24 h the serum radioactivity in IgG animals had decreased by 55% of the value at 0.5 h, and in the IgA and IgM animals by 75%.

Radioactivity was detectable in CFW after 30 min from all animals given IgG or IgA. The activity expressed as a percentage of the serum values increased over the period of study (Fig. 1), although the actual number of counts per minute had fallen in each case at 24 h. Radioactivity was not detectable in CFW from animals given IgM until 2 h after i.v. injection of the labelled immunogobulin. This reached maximum levels at 4 h and had fallen to low levels by 24 h. The values for IgM were significantly lower than for IgG or IgA at all times examined, although the values in serum were similar.

Activity in mucosal washings was significantly less than in CFW at all times. Slight but significant amounts of activity were found with IgG after 1 h and with IgA after 4 h (Fig. 1). Little or no activity was found in animals given IgM.

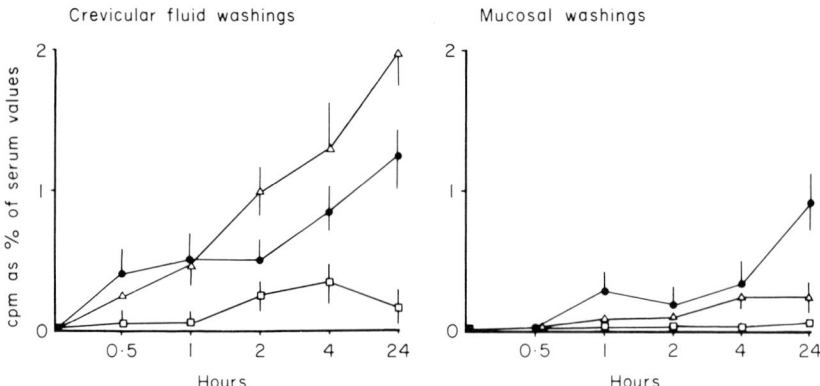

Fig. 1 Radioactivity ($\pm$ S.E.) in sequential samples of crevicular fluid washings and mucosal washings from four Rhesus monkeys after intravenous injection of IgG (●—●), IgA (△—△) and IgM (□—□).

4. Immunoglobulin Passage into Oral Cavity

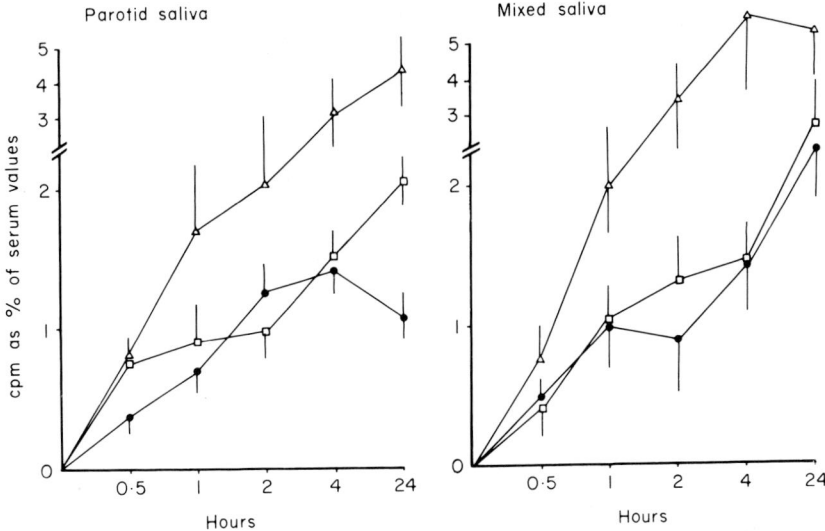

Fig. 2 Radioactivity (± S.E.) in sequential samples of parotid and mixed saliva from four Rhesus monkeys after intravenous injection of IgG (●—●), IgA (△—△) and IgM (□—□).

Similar curves were found with both parotid and mixed saliva (Fig. 2) Radioactivity was found in all samples at 30 min and increased over the experimental period to a maximum of over 5% of the serum values. The activity in mixed saliva was not significantly greater than that in parotid saliva.

Ultracentrifugal Analysis

After injection of labelled IgG, greater than 99% of the serum activity was located in the 7 s zone on sucrose density gradients (Fig. 3). Most of the counts in CFW were associated with 7 s IgG, suggesting that IgG had passed from plasma to the gingival crevice as intact molecules. In contrast, in parotid saliva samples less than 1% of the activity was found in the 7 s region, about 18% in the 4.5 s region and the remainder in a low molecular weight region of approximately 1 s.

In serum samples IgA activity was associated with the 7 s region. In samples of CFW taken 1 or 2 h after injection some 70% of the counts were found in the 7 s region, 15% in the 4.5 s region and the remainder in the 1 s region (Fig. 4). In parotid saliva no activity was found in the 7 s region, indicating that intact IgA had not passed from serum to parotid saliva. All the counts were found in a broad band of salivary protein sedimenting at approximately 1 s.

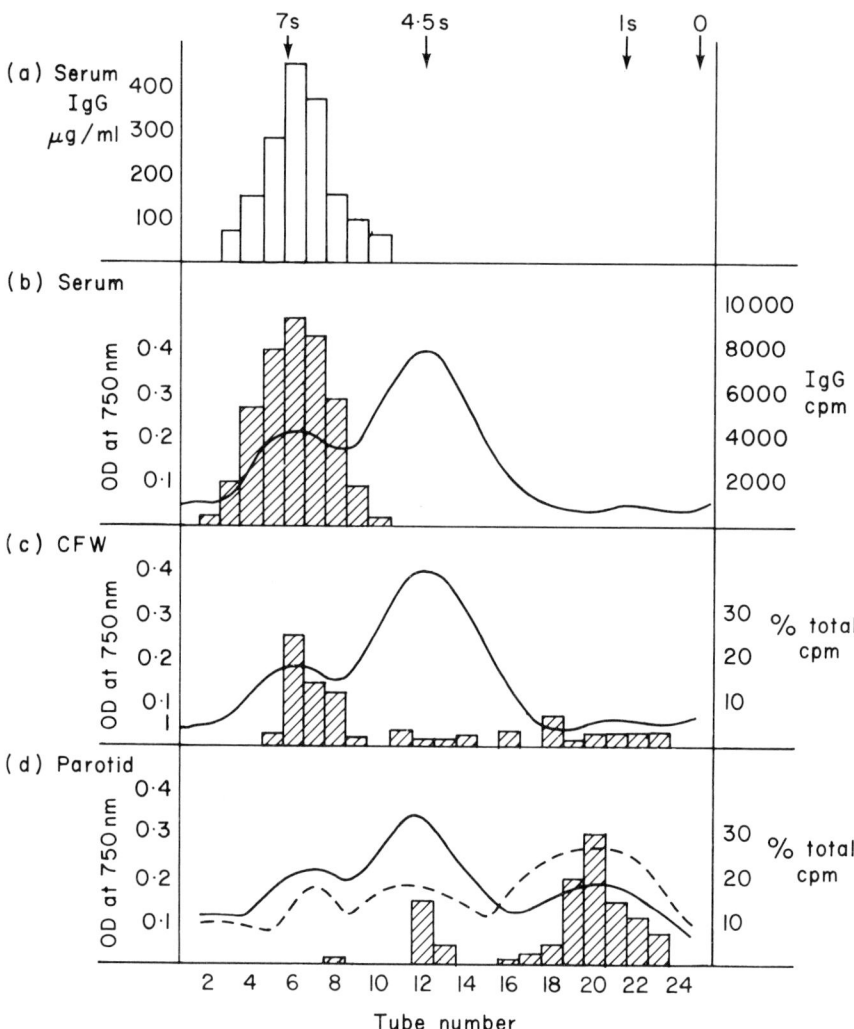

Fig. 3 Sucrose density ultracentrifugation of samples taken 1–2 h after intravenous injection of radiolabelled IgG. (a) Position of IgG assayed by single radial immunodiffusion. Radioactivity shown in samples of (b) serum, (c) crevicular fluid washings, (d) parotid saliva.

In mixed saliva most of the radioactivity was found in the 1 s region, but in contrast to parotid saliva some activity was detectable in the 7 s region and a little in the higher molecular weight region. This suggested that the 7 s IgA in mixed saliva had originated in the gingival crevice.

Serum profiles revealed that most of the IgM radioactivity was present in

4. Immunoglobulin Passage into Oral Cavity

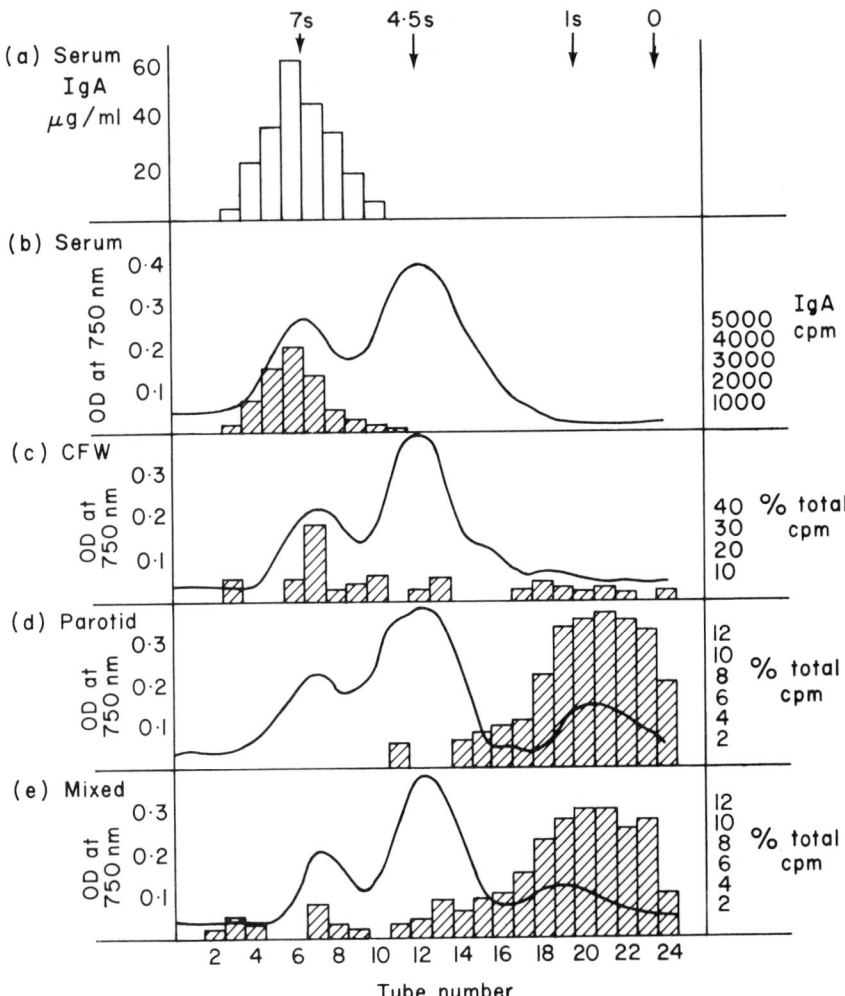

Fig. 4 Sucrose density ultracentrifugation of samples taken 1–2 h after intravenous injection of radiolabelled IgA. (a) Position of IgA assayed by single radial immunodiffusion. Radioactivity shown in samples of (b) serum, (c) crevicular fluid washings, (d) parotid saliva, and (e) mixed saliva.

the 19 s region (Fig. 5) but in addition some activity was found in the 7 s region. In CFW about 55% of the total recoverable radioactivity was found in the 19 s region, with some 35% in the 7 s region. In parotid saliva activity was confined to the low molecular weight regions, suggesting that intact IgM did not pass from plasma to the oral cavity in parotid saliva.

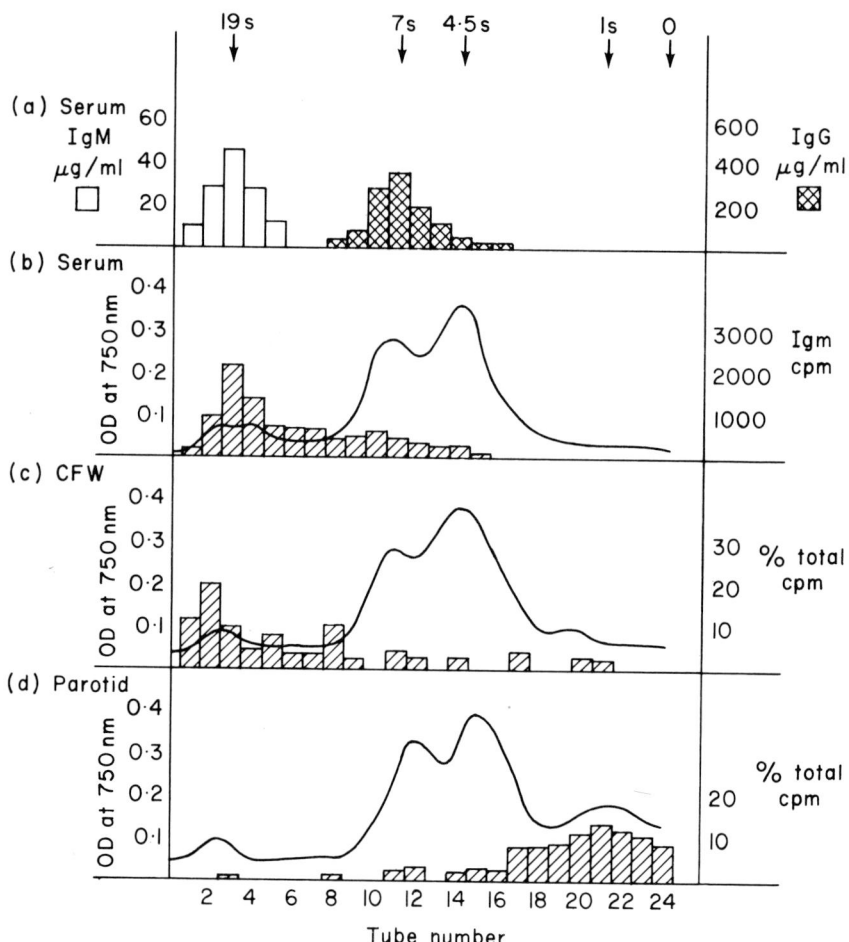

Fig. 5 Sucrose density ultracentrifugation of samples taken 2 h after intravenous injection of radiolabelled IgM. (a) Position of IgM and IgG assayed by single radial immunodiffusion. Radioactivity shown in samples of (b) serum, (c) crevicular fluid washings, and (d) parotid saliva.

Immunoglobulin Concentrations

Serum immunoglobulin concentrations of IgG, IgA and IgM were similar to those reported in man (Table I). All three isotypes were detectable in CFW with mean values of 30 µg/ml IgG, 13.5 µg/ml IgA and 1.9 µg/ml IgM. A striking difference was noted in the ratio of IgA:IgG in parotid saliva (25) compared with a ratio of 3 in mixed saliva, suggesting that extraglandular sources are major contributors of IgG to mixed saliva in the Rhesus monkey.

TABLE I
Immunoglobulin Concentrations in Serum, Crevicular Fluid Washings, Parotid and Mixed Saliva Samples in 12 Rhesus Monkeys

	Mean concentrations ± s.d. (µg/ml)		
	IgG	IgA	IgM
Serum	9360 ± 530	3110 ± 420	490 ± 110
Crevicular fluid washings	29.8 ± 8.7	13.5 ± 3.1	1.9 ± 2.3
Parotid saliva	1.4 ± 1.5	35.1 ± 11.4*	n.d.†
Mixed saliva	17.8 ± 5.6	51.3 ± 15.0*	n.d.‡
Mucosal washings	n.d.	n.d.	n.d.

*Assayed against monomer IgA standard and adjusted by ×3 (Brandtzaeg et al., 1970) to allow for presumed predominance of dimeric form of IgA.
† n.d., not detectable.
‡ Two animals positive at 2 µg/ml and 1 µg/ml.

No immunoglobulins were detected in mucosal washings, and IgM was not detectable in parotid or mixed saliva.

Discussion

Passage of Immunoglobulin to Crevicular Fluid

The results of this study demonstrate that intact IgG, IgA and IgM can pass from plasma to the oral cavity via the gingival crevice. There were differences between the isotypes since IgA and IgG could be found in CFW 30 min after intravenous infusion, whereas IgM was not detected until 2 h after infusion. This differential rate probably reflects the effect of molecular sieving, since the extravascular distribution of immunoglobulins is dependent on the concentration and molecular size. About 75% of IgM is intravascular compared with about 50% of IgG and IgA (Waldmann and Strober, 1969).

Sucrose density ultracentrifugation analysis of CFW showed that the radiolabelled immunoglobulin isotypes were in their expected positions, that is in the 7 s region for IgG and IgA and the 19 s region for IgM. A small amount of activity was found in regions of lower molecular weight. This may have been due to slight contamination by saliva which contained large amounts of iodine in regions of low molecular weight (Figs 3–5) or may have reflected immunoglobulin fragments resulting from degradation by proteolytic enzymes in crevicular fluid (Cimasoni, 1974; Cimasoni et al., 1977) or in plaque (Taubman et al., 1978). Enzymes which can cleave IgG (Taubman et al. 1978) or IgA (Plaut et al., 1974) have been detected in dental plaque.

Nevertheless, the majority of activity was in the higher molecular weight regions, suggesting that the different immunoglobulins pass in an intact form from plasma to crevicular fluid. A similar route has previously been demonstrated with substances of low molecular weight in dogs (Brill and Krass, 1958; Bader and Goldhaber, 1966).

Many investigators have examined the immunoglobulin content of crevicular fluid (CF). In general an immunoglobulin content approaching that of serum has been found (Brandtzaeg, 1965; Holmberg and Killander, 1971; Schenkein and Genco, 1977), although lower values than that have been reported (Shillitoe and Lehner, 1972), and Brandtzaeg (1972) demonstrated a relative deficiency of IgA and IgM compared with serum. It should be borne in mind that the immunoglobulin content of crevicular fluid from patients with periodontal disease may not reflect that in subjects with relatively normal gingiva. In this study in Rhesus monkeys IgG, IgA and IgM were found in CFW in concentrations of 30, 13.5 and 1.9 μg/ml, respectively (Table I). The dilution of crevicular fluid by the washing procedure was calculated as up to 1:100, and thus the immunoglobulin concentrations in neat crevicular fluid would be well below 50% of the serum values. This may reflect a species difference, or may be dependent on age since samples were taken from animals with a mixed dentition. All the animals had a mild gingivitis with a mean gingival index of 1.1 and it is not known in this model whether the immunoglobulin concentration of crevicular fluid is related to the degree of gingival inflammation.

The maximum contribution to crevicular fluid immunoglobulins in man by local synthesis has been calculated to be 17% for IgG and 8% for IgA (Brandtzaeg, 1972). The findings in this study, based on an estimation of specific activity, are similar. The mean specific activity of IgG in CFW was approximately 20% lower than in plasma (27 and 34 counts min^{-1} $μg^{-1}$, respectively), which suggests that up to 20% of the IgG in CFW could have been derived from local synthesis. This may be an over-estimate since the method assumes equilibration between plasma and CFW which might not have been completed at the time of sampling. With IgA and IgM no significant differences in the mean number of counts per minute per microgram of plasma and CFW were found (Challacombe et al., 1978b), suggesting that little if any of the IgA and IgM in CFW was derived from local synthesis. However, measurement of IgA and particularly IgM at very low concentrations was not sufficiently accurate for this to be determined with certainty.

Passage of Immunoglobulins to Saliva

Transfer of immunoglobulins from plasma to parotid saliva was not found in this study. Although radioactivity was detected in samples of parotid saliva within 30 min of intravenous infusion of labelled immunoglobulins, sucrose density gradients revealed that this activity was not bound to IgG, IgA or IgM but was present in regions of low molecular weight. This lack of transfer is consistent with the findings of Tomasi *et al.* (1965), who also found radioactivity associated with low molecular weight proteins in saliva within 15 min of intravenous infusion of radiolabelled IgA. If these observations with parotid fluid also apply to the other major salivary glands, the view that the gingival crevice is a major source of salivary IgG and monomer IgA would be strongly supported.

Such a view has been advocated by the findings that subjects with periodontitis have significantly greater levels of IgG in mixed saliva than normal controls (Brandtzaeg *et al.*, 1970). In addition, a highly significant correlation was found between the salivary IgG concentration and the product of the serum IgG concentration and the extent of gingival inflammation (periodontal index), although not with the serum IgG levels alone (Brandtzaeg *et al.*, 1970). Salivary IgM concentration was related to both the serum IgM concentration and the product of serum concentration and periodontal index. Moreover, Basu *et al.* (1976) showed that the salivary IgG concentration was significantly reduced after periodontal therapy, further indicating the gingival crevice as the source of salivary IgG. The findings in the present study of direct passage of immunoglobulin from plasma to CFW supports and extends these conclusions. Some radioactivity was found, however, in mucosal washings after 4 h in animals given IgG or IgA, and it cannot be excluded that direct passage of small amounts of these immunoglobulins occurs across normal epithelium. The amounts concerned were too small for accurate analysis, but the absence of radioactivity in animals given IgM suggests that it is not due to contamination from saliva.

It is of interest that the third component of complement (C3) is not normally found in the secretions of the major salivary glands (Williams *et al.*, 1975) but is present in mixed saliva. The main source appears to be the gingival crevice, but the finding that C3 could be detected in some edentulous subjects with clinically normal oral epithelium suggests that in some subjects C3 may also pass across the epithelium in small amounts.

Volume of Crevicular Fluid

If immunoglobulin, or more specifically antibodies in CF, play a role in protection against dental caries, then it might be expected that the availability of antibodies will depend on both the volume of crevicular fluid and the flow rate. Both these indices are difficult to measure, and unfortunately the terms have been used interchangeably in the dental literature, but are clearly different. The method outlined in this paper gives an indication of the volume at a given time but does not allow an estimation of the flow rate of crevicular fluid. The mean ($\pm$ S.D.) crevicular fluid volume (CFV) in decidous teeth in

Rhesus monkeys was found to be 0.30 ± 0.44 µl in anterior teeth compared with 0.34 ± 0.46 µl in posterior teeth. In samples from four human volunteers with a mean gingival index of <1.0 the mean CFV in approximal spaces from molar teeth ranged from 0.43 µl to 1.56 µl. In anterior teeth the CFV in three subjects was between 0.24 µl and 0.43 µl per tooth, but in one subject with three porcelain jacket crowns it was 1.15 µl per tooth (Table II).

TABLE II
Calculated Volumes of Crevicular Fluid

	Anterior teeth		Posterior teeth	
	Volume (µl)*	GI†	Volume (µl)*	GI†
Rhesus monkeys				
Deciduous	0.30 ± 0.44 (7)		0.34 ± 0.46 (12)	
Permanent	0.78 ± 0.51 (6)		0.57 ± 0.51 (6)	
Man				
Subject A	0.43 ± 0.46 (4)	0.5	0.65 ± 0.46 (6)	1.0
Subject B	0.33 ± 0.25 (4)	0.5	0.43 ± 0.27 (6)	0.5
Subject C‡	1.15 ± 0.85 (5)	1.0	0.83 ± 0.55 (5)	0.8
Subject D	0.24 ± 0.43 (4)	0.3	1.56 ± 0.88 (6)	0.5

*Mean ±S.D. Volume calculated by isotope dilution method (see Materials and Method section). Number of approximal spaces sampled is given in parentheses.
† GI, gingival index.
‡ Subject C had three anterior crowned teeth.

The volume of CF in man appears to be closely related to the gingival index (Oliver *et al.*, 1969; Rudin *et al.*, 1970; Borden *et al.*, 1977). Using the method of insertion of calibrated filter paper strips, a CFV of approximately 0.2 µl was found to correspond to a gingival index of 1.0 (Borden *et al.*, 1977). The method suffers from the possibility that only those areas accessible to the insertion of strips can be assayed, and that insertion of the strip itself may stimulate fluid flow. An advantage of the method is that the flow rate of CF can be measured, and Alfano *et al.* (1976) have reported a flow rate of 10–13 nl/min in teeth with a gingival index of zero. Application of human serum albumin to the crevice increased the flow rate by 100%. An area of further study is to determine whether individuals of identical clinical gingival inflammation might vary in the fluid volume, and the fluid flow rate, and to see whether this might be related to protection against caries and the development of progressive periodontal disease. Certainly, the composition of CF from inflamed gingiva appears to differ from that from healthy gingiva (Biswas *et al.*, 1977).

It is possible to make an estimate of the total volume of CF secreted into the mouth per day by determining the concentration in saliva of proteins thought to be derived from the gingival crevice. Thus, the concentration of IgG in mixed saliva has been reported as between 1 and 4.8 mg/100 ml (Salmon et al., 1969; Brandtzaeg et al., 1970), and the concentration in CF is about the same as in serum (1200 mg/100 ml). If the volume of saliva secreted per day is about 600 ml (Jenkins, 1978) this would indicate a CF flow of 0.5–2.4 ml/day into the oral cavity. Similarly, the concentration of C3 in saliva has been estimated to be 0.52 µg/ml (Williams et al., 1975) and in CF as 40 mg/100 ml (Shillitoe and Lehner, 1972). This would indicate a total CF fluid flow of 0.8 ml/day, which is consistent with the estimate derived from IgG. Given a dentition of 32 teeth, this figure converts to between 0.7 and 3.1 µl per tooth per hour. This figure is not dissimilar to that obtained by Alfano et al. (1976) of 0.6–0.8 µl per buccal sulcus per hour, assuming that the total fluid flow from all the sulci of a tooth would presumably be three or four times this amount.

TABLE III
Volume of Crevicular Fluid per Day

Based on	Salivary concentration (µg/ml)	Crevicular fluid concentration (mg/ml)	Volume of crevicular fluid per day (ml)	Volume of crevicular fluid per tooth (µl/h)
IgG	10–48	12.0	0.5–2.4	0.7–3.1
C3	0.5	0.4	0.8	1.1
Alfano et al. (1977)	Flow per sulcus = 0.6 µl/h		0.9–1.3	2.7–3.9

Immunoglobulins in Plaque

Indirect evidence for the passage of immunoglobulins through the gingival crevice has been obtained by the examination of immunoglobulins in plaque. The major classes found in supragingival plaque were IgG and IgA with very little IgM (Taubman, 1974; Holt and Mestecky, 1975). According to Taubman most of the IgA was salivary in origin, and associated with secretory component, whereas most of the IgG appeared to be gingival in origin. The third complement component (C3) was also detectable (Holt and Mestecky, 1975), presumably crevicular in origin. Thus, plaque may contain proteins characteristic of either saliva or serum.

The topographical distribution of immunoglobulins in plaque has been studied on extracted teeth by Newman et al. (1979). Using fluoresceinated antisera, 80% of samples were positive for IgG, 50% for IgA and 6% for IgM.

Fluorescence was most apparent at the apical border of plaque, suggesting that crevicular fluid was the principle source of these immunoglobulins, including IgA, since the sub-contact area is relatively inaccessible to saliva. It is not certain that all the IgG and IgA found in plaque is in fact antibody to plaque antigens. Taubman and Smith (1976), using a two-step elution precedure, suggested that only about 20% of the total IgG and IgA in plaque was specific antibody to antigens in plaque, with the remainder being non-specifically bound.

Functional Activity of Immunoglobulins

The presence of bacterial cell ghosts at the apical border of plaque (Newman, 1975, 1977) suggests that specific antibody or antibacterial factors may be effective in this region. Since CF contains complement and IgG, IgM, and large numbers of functional polymorphonuclear leukocytes (Wilton *et al.*, 1977; Scully and Challacombe, 1979), effector mechanisms for antibacterial activity are present. Antibodies have been detected in CF (Wilton, 1977) and are currently being further characterized. It is not known how the presence of proteolytic enzymes specific for IgG and IgA (Plaut *et al.*, 1974; Taubman *et al.*, 1978) might affect the functional activity of antibodies in this area. There are many theoretical mechanisms by which antibodies in CF might function in caries immunity including inhibition of adherence of *Strep. mutans* or other cariogenic organisms (Olson *et al.*, 1972), enhancement of phagocytosis and intra- or extracellular killing (Scully and Lehner, 1979), inhibition of glucosyltransferase activity (Evans and Genco, 1973) or direct bacteriocidal activity.

While passive transfer experiments demonstrate that serum antibodies must function in some way at the tooth surface (Lehner *et al.*, 1978*b*), and while this study demonstrates direct passage of immunoglobulins from serum to the oral cavity, the exact mechanisms of action of these immunoglobulins remains to be elucidated.

Summary

Immunoglobulins in mixed saliva are derived from three major sources, the major salivary glands, the minor salivary glands, and crevicular fluid. Whereas the main immunoglobulin in saliva is secretory IgA, in crevicular fluid it is IgG. Salivary secretions also contain secretory IgM and a trace of IgG. The concentration of IgG in mixed saliva is directly related to the degree of gingival inflammation, indicating a serum source. In the Rhesus monkey direct passage of immunoglobulins to the oral cavity can be demonstrated. Radiolabelled IgG and IgA can be found in crevicular fluid washings and in mixed saliva within 30 min of intravenous administration, and IgM after 2 h;

maximal levels were found after 4 h with each immunoglobulin. Immunoglobulins did not pass from serum to parotid saliva. Ultracentrifugation on sucrose density gradients revealed that the labelled immunoglobulin which had passed into the crevicular fluid from serum was present in the 7 s regions for IgG and IgM, and in the 19 s region for IgM, indicating that the molecules were in an intact form. Determination of specific activity suggested that all of the IgA and IgM found in crevicular fluid was derived from serum, but that up to 20% of the IgG could have been synthesized locally. The volume of crevicular fluid present in each approximal site was estimated by a radioactivity dilution technique and in Rhesus monkeys was 0.33 µl in deciduous teeth and 0.74 µl in permanent teeth. In man the mean volume in anterior teeth was 0.54 µl and in posterior teeth 0.87 µl. The volume of crevicular fluid secretion into the oral cavity was estimated to be between 0.5 and 2.4 ml/day or between 0.7 and 3.1 µl per tooth per hour. Passive transfer experiments in animals suggest that serum IgG may operate at the tooth surface and this study demostrates that serum IgG, IgA and IgM can pass in an intact form from serum to the oral cavity via crevicular fluid. Antibodies induced systemically can therefore reach the oral cavity, they can be found in crevicular fluid and mixed saliva, and they could influence the development of both caries and periodontal disease.

Acknowledgements

The investigation was supported by a project grant from the Medical Research Council to Professor T. Lehner. The skilled technical help of Mrs J. E. Hawkes and Miss L. A. Bergmeier is gratefully acknowledged.

References

Alfano, M. C., Brownstein, C. N., Chasens, A. I. and Kaslick, R. S. (1976). *J. dent. Res.* **55**, 1132.
Bader, N. I. and Goldhaber, P. (1966). *J. oral Ther. Pharmac.* **2**, 324.
Basu, M. K., Glenwright, H. D., Fox, E. C. and Becker, J. F. (1976) *J. periodont. Res.* **11**, 226.
Biswas, S., Duperon, J. F. and Chebib, F. S. (1977). *J. periodont. Res.* **12**, 250.
Bordon, S. M., Golub, C. M. and Kleinberg, I. (1977). *J. periodont. Res.* **12**, 160.
Bowen, W. H., Cohen, B., Cole, M. and Colman, G. (1975). *Br. dent. J.* **139**, 45.
Brandtzaeg, P. (1965). *Archs oral Biol.* **10**, 795.
Brandtzaeg, P. (1972). In *Host Resistance to Commensal Bacteria* (I. T. MacPhee, ed.), p.116, Churchill Livingstone, Edinburgh.
Brandtzaeg, P., Fjellanger, I. and Gjeruldsen, S. T. (1970). *Scand J. Haemat.* Suppl. 12, 1.
Brill, N. and Krasse, B. (1958). *Acta odont scand.* **16**, 233.
Challacombe, S. J. (1976). *Caries Res.* **10**, 165.
Challacombe, S. J. (1978). *Adv. exp. Biol. Med.* **107**, 303.
Challacombe, S. J. and Lehner, T. (1976). *J. dent. Res.* **55**, C139.

Challacombe, S. J. and Lehner, T. (1980). *Archs oral Biol.* **24**, 917.
Challacombe, S. J. and Russell, M. W. (1979). *Immunology* **36**, 331.
Challacombe, S. J., Russell, M. W. and Hawkes, J. (1978a). *Clin. exp. Immunol.* **34**, 417.
Challacombe, S. J., Russell, M. W., Hawkes, J., Bergmeier, L. and Lehner, T. (1978b). *Immunology* **35**, 923.
Cimasoni, G. (1974). In *Monographs in Oral Science*, Vol. 3 (H. M. Myers, ed.), Karger, Basel.
Cimasoni, G., Ishikawa, I. and Jaccard, F. (1977). In *Borderland between Caries and Periodontal Disease* (T. Lehner, ed.), Academic Press, London.
Cohen, B., Colman, G. and Russell, R. R. B. (1979). *Br. dent. J.* **147**.
Evans, R. T. and Genco, R. J. (1973). *Infect. Immun.* **7**, 237.
Holmberg, K. and Killander, J. (1971). *J. periodont. Res.* **6**, 1.
Holt, R. L. and Mestecky, J. (1975). *J. oral Path.* **4**, 86.
Jenkins, G. N. (1978). *The Physiology and Biochemistry of the Mouth*, 3rd edn, Blackwell Scientific Publications, Oxford.
Lehner, T., Challacombe, S. J. and Caldwell, J. (1976a). *J. dent. Res.* **55**, C166.
Lehner, T., Challacombe, S. J. and Caldwell, J. (1976b). *Nature, Lond.* **254**, 517.
Lehner, T., Russell, M. W., Scully, C. M., Challacombe, S. J. and Caldwell, J. (1978a). In *Steptococci and Streptococcal Diseases* (M. T. Parker, ed.), Reed Books, Chertsey, Surrey.
Lehner, T., Russell, M. W., Challacombe, S. J., Wilton, J. M. A., Scully, C. M. and Hawkes, J. E. (1978b). *Lancet* 283.
Löe, H. and Silness, J. (1963). *Acta odont. scand*, **21**, 533.
McGhee, J. R., Michalek, S. M., Navia, J. M. and Nakates, A. J. (1976). *J. dent. Res.* **55**, C206.
Michalek, S. M. and McGhee, J. R. (1977). *Infect. Immun.* **17**, 646.
Michalek, S. M., McGhee, J. R., Arnold, R. R., Mestecky, J. and Bozzo, L. (1976). *Science, N. Y.* **192**, 1238.
Newman, H. N. (1975). *Br. dent. J.* **138**, 355.
Newman, H. N. (1977). In *Borderland between Caries and Periodontal Disease* (T. Lehner, ed.), p. 97, Academic Press, London.
Newman, H. N., Seymour, G. J. and Challacombe, S. J. (1979). *J. periodont. Res.* **14**, 1.
Oliver, R. C., Holm-Petersen, P. and Löe, H. (1969). *J. Periodont.* **40**, 201.
Olson, G. A., Bleiweis, A. J. and Small, P. A. (1972). *Infect. Immun.* **5**, 419.
Plaut, A. G., Genco, R. J. and Tomasi, T. B. (1974). *J. Immunol.* **113**, 289.
Rudin, H. J., Overdiek, H. F. and Rateitschak, K. W. (1970). *Helv. odont Acta.* **14**, 21.
Russell, M. W., Challacombe, S. J. and Lehner, T. (1976). *Immunology.* **30**, 619.
Salmon, S. E., Mackey, G. and Fudenberg, H. H. (1969). *J. Immunol.* **103**, 129.
Schenkein, H. A. and Genco, R. J. (1977). *J. Periodont.* **48**, 772.
Scully, C. M. and Challacombe, S. J. (1979). *J. periodont. Res.* **14**, 475.
Scully, C. M. and Lehner, T. (1979). *Clin. exp. Immunol.* **35**, 128.
Shillitoe, E. J. and Lehner, T. (1972). *Archs oral Biol.* **17**, 241.
Skapski, H. and Lehner, T. (1976). *J. periodont. Res.* **11**, 19.
Taubman, M. A. (1974). *Archs oral Biol.* **19**, 439.
Taubman, M. A. and Smith, D. J. (1974). *Infect. Immun.* **9**, 1079.
Taubman, M. A. and Smith, D. J. (1976). *J. dent. Res.* **55**, C153.
Taubman, M. A. and Smith, D. J. (1977). *J. Immunol.* **118**, 710.
Taubman, M. A., Smith, D. J. and Murray, R. (1978). *Archs oral Biol.* **23**, 949.

Tomasi, T. B., Tan, E. M., Solomon, A. and Prendergast, R. A. (1965). *J. exp. Med.* **121**, 101.
Waldmann, T. A. and Strober, W. (1969). In *Progress in Allergy* (P. Kallos and B. M. Waksman, eds), Karger, Basel.
Williams, B. D., Challacombe, S. J., Slayney, J. M., Lachmann, P. J. and Lehner, T. (1975). *Clin. exp. Immunol.* **19**, 423.
Wilton, J. M. A. (1977). In *Borderland between Caries and Periodontal Disease* (T. Lehner, ed.), p. 223, Academic Press, London.
Wilton, J. M. A., Renggli, H. H. and Lehner, T. (1977). *Clin. exp. Immunol.* **27**, 152.

5. Transport and Function of Polymorphonuclear Leukocytes in Crevicular Fluid

C. M. SCULLY

Introduction

Polymorphonuclear leukocytes (PMNL) are the main oral leukocytes (Klinkhamer, 1963; Attström, 1970; Raeste, 1972a). They appear to originate as blood PMNL and enter the oral cavity by a number of routes, especially through the gingival crevice (Sharry and Krasse, 1960; Schiott and Löe, 1970; Raeste, 1976). Klinkhamer (1963) estimated the rate of appearance of leukocytes in the oral cavity at 103×10^3 cells/s in the dentate patient.

The PMNL infiltrate in the gingiva increases with an increase in the inflammatory response (Attström, 1970, 1971). PMNL migrate through the gingival crevicular epithelium (Schroeder, 1977) and make contact with dental bacterial plaque (Listgarten, 1976). A dense accumulation of PMNL covers the plaque on the tissue side and phagocytosis of bacteria may occur (Garant, 1976a,b; Lange and Schroeder, 1971).

Crevicular PMNL morphologically resemble the blood PMNL from which they are derived, and they are frequently structurally intact (Lange and Schroeder, 1971). The rate of migration of PMNL into the gingival crevice has not, however, been established. Crevicular PMNL are viable cells (Skapski and Lehner, 1976), with a strong reaction for succinic dehydrogenase suggestive of a high metabolic activity (Lange and Schroeder, 1971). Crevicular PMNL may contain microorganisms (Attström, 1970), but the extent of their activity with regard to oral bacteria is unclear.

The viability and functional capabilities of salivary PMNL are less clearly defined. There is evidence that although some degeneration occurs with time (Wright and Jenkins, 1953; Sharry and Krasse, 1960; Friedman and Tonzetich, 1968; Raeste and Calonius, 1971), a substantial proportion of salivary leukocytes may remain intact under favourable conditions (Wright and Jenkins, 1953; Eichel and Lisanti, 1964; Klinkhamer, 1968). Salivary PMNL may also show phagocytic activity *in vivo* (Rovelstad, 1964) and *in vitro* (Orban and Weinmann, 1939a,b; Rovelstad, 1960; Eichel and Lisanti, 1964; Kenney *et al.*, 1977).

It has recently been postulated that the protection of immunized monkeys against dental caries might be mediated by phagocytosis of cariogenic bacteria by oral leukocytes (Lehner et al., 1976). Parenteral immunization of Rhesus monkeys with vaccines of *Streptococcus mutans* in adjuvant elicits protection against caries (Lehner et al., 1975, 1976, 1977). Protection is associated with a reduction in the colonization of plaque by *Strep. mutans* (Lehner et al., 1977) and a rise in serum complement-fixing, but not salivary, specific antibodies to *Strep. mutans* (Lehner et al., 1975, 1976). Immunization is associated within 6 weeks with a significant rise in serum opsonic activity for *Strep. mutans* (Scully and Lehner, 1979a) which resides mainly in the IgG and IgM fractions of serum (Scully and Lehner, 1979b) and can be passively transferred (Scully, 1979). Serum opsonic activity is detectable at concentrations as low as 0.25% (Scully and Lehner, 1979b, suggesting that, if opsonic antibodies were to enter crevicular fluid and saliva, they might still be at concentrations adequate for the opsonization of *Strep. mutans*. However, although opsonic antibodies to *Strep. mutans* have been detected in serum they have not been found in crevicular fluid.

The aims of this study were therefore as follows: (a) to examine the route and rate of migration of blood PMNL into the oral cavity of monkeys; (b) to examine the viability and function of crevicular and salivary PMNL, and the effects of crevicular fluid and mixed saliva on the viability and function of blood PMNL; (c) to examine the crevicular fluid, parotid and mixed saliva of immunized monkeys for opsonic activity towards *Strep. mutans*.

Materials and Methods

Rhesus monkeys (*Macaca mulatta*) aged 11–21 months were caged and maintained as previously described (Lehner et al., 1975). Animals were immunized subcutaneously with a vaccine of *Strep. mutans* serotype c (Ingbritt) in Freund's incomplete adjuvant ("immune group"), or with saline ("controls") and samples obtained at 18 months after immunization.

Examination of the Route and Rate of Migration of PMNL to the Oral Cavity

Blood PMNL isolated by dextran sedimentation (Scully and Lehner, 1978) were radiolabelled with ^{111}In (as indium chloride) and administered intravenously to the donor monkeys. At sequential time intervals from 20 min to 24 h, samples of crevicular fluid washings (CFW), mucosal washings (MW), parotid saliva (PS) and mixed saliva (MS) were obtained.

CFW were obtained by the method of Skapski and Lehner (1976). MW were collected from the vestibule. Salivation was induced with pilocarpine (0.2 mg/kg) and PS collected by parotid cannulation, MS by expectoration. Labelled PMNL were isolated from samples by filtration, and counted on a γ counter (Scully and Challacombe, 1979).

Examination of the Viability and Function of Crevicular and Salivary PMNL

Crevicular and salivary PMNL were obtained from CFW and MS, and viability assessed by trypan blue dye exclusion.

Monolayers of crevicular PMNL were exposed to unlabelled *Strep. mutans* (serotype c, Ingbritt) at a PMNL: bacterial ratio of 1:10, in the presence of serum from monkeys immunized with an homologous strain of *Strep. mutans*. After incubation at 37°C for 30 min, the percentage of cells containing bacteria was counted visually (Scully, 1979).

Blood PMNL were exposed to CFW or MS for up to 60 min, and PMNL viability and phagocytic activity for ^{14}C-labelled *Strep. mutans* assessed as previously described (Scully and Lehner, 1979*a*). ^{51}Cr-labelled blood PMNL were also exposed to MS, and the ^{51}Cr released was assayed at 30 min and 60 min.

Assay for Opsonic Activity in Oral Fluids

^{14}C-labelled *Strep. mutans* were incubated in serum, CFW, MS and PS from immunized or control monkeys for 60 min. Treated bacteria were then washed and exposed to blood PMNL at a PMNL: bacterial ratio of 1:100 for 30 min at 37 °C. The percentage of bacteria phagocytosed was then measured by the PMNL ^{14}C uptake. Results were analysed by a two-way analysis of variance and the Q test.

Results

Route and Rate of Migration of PMNL to the Oral Cavity

The pattern of migration of ^{111}In-labelled PMNL is shown in Fig. 1. The greatest number of labelled PMNL were detected in crevicular fluid washings. Smaller numbers of leukocytes were detected in washings from the vestibular mucosa and in mixed saliva, but parotid saliva consistently contained only a very low number of cells.

Labelled PMNL were not detected at any oral site by 10 min after intravenous administration. However, by 20 min significant numbers of labelled PMNL were detected in crevicular fluid.

Direct microscopic counts of PMNL in oral fluids showed maximum cell numbers in crevicular fluid ($1.9 \pm 0.4 \times 10^6$ PMNL/ml mean $\pm$ standard error) and mixed saliva ($1.3 \pm 0.4 \times 10^5$ PMNL/ml) (Table 1).

Viability and Function of Oral PMNL

The viability of PMNL determined by dye exclusion was $96.1 \pm 2.0\%$ for blood PMNL, $78.3 \pm 6.2\%$ for crevicular PMNL ($p<0.05$) and $49.0 \pm 8.2\%$ for salivary PMNL ($p<0.01$ compared with blood PMNL). The viability of

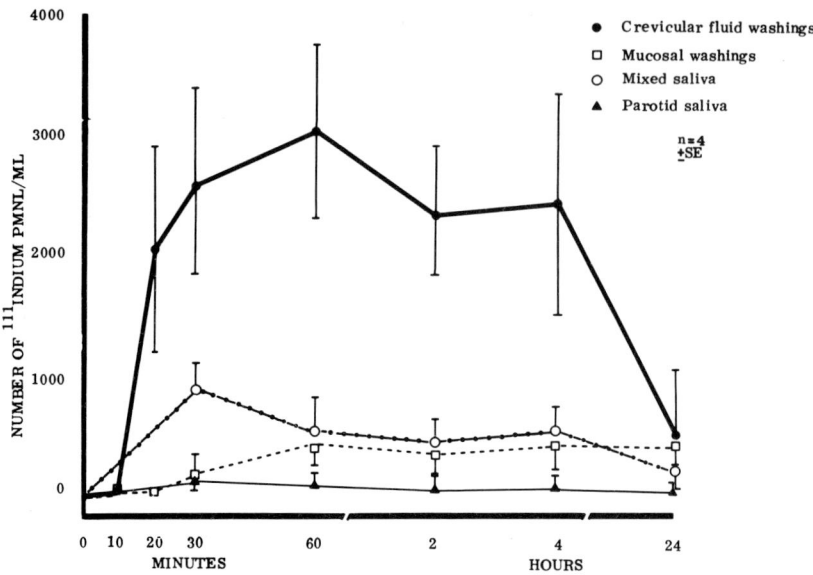

Fig. 1 Migration of ^{111}In-labelled polymorphonuclear leukocytes into the oral cavity of the monkey.

crevicular PMNL collected 30 min after the initial gingival crevicular washing rose to $96.0 \pm 2.7\%$ ($p > 0.05$ compared with blood PMNL).

The phagocytic activity of PMNL was determined by exposure of monolayers of blood PMNL, or of crevicular PMNL, to *Strep. mutans* in the presence of immune serum or Hank's Balanced Salt Solution (HBBS, Wellcome, Kent). After 30 min incubation $69.4 \pm 8.0\%$ blood PMNL, and $68.1 \pm 4.8\%$ of crevicular PMNL contained bacteria if immune serum was

TABLE I
Direct Counts of Polymorphonuclear Leukocytes in Monkey Fluids

Fluid	Mean*	Range
Blood	9.2×10^6	$3–14 \times 10^6$
Crevicular fluid washings	1.9×10^6	$0.8–3 \times 10^6$
Mixed saliva	1.3×10^5	$0.3–2 \times 10^5$
Parotid saliva	8.8×10^3	$0–3 \times 10^4$
Mucosal washings	4.6×10^4	$1–8 \times 10^4$

* Mean of samples from six animals expressed as PMNL/ml.

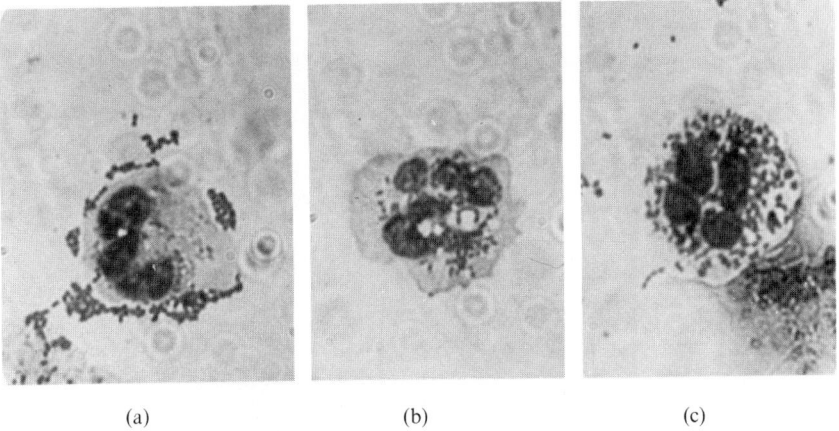

Fig. 2. Phagocytosis of *Strep. mutans* opsonized with immune serum by monkey crevicular polymorphonuclear leukocytes (a) at 0 min, (b) at 30 min, (c) at 60 min.

present (Fig. 2). However, $5.3 \pm 3.3\%$ of the crevicular PMNL collected from a second crevicular washing contained bacteria on collection, so that the phagocytosis was slightly, but not significantly, less than for blood PMNL.

Insufficient numbers of salivary PMNL could be isolated for reliable assay of their phagocytic activity, and therefore the effect of the exposure of blood PMNL to oral fluids was determined. Neither crevicular fluid washings nor mixed saliva had a significant effect by 60 min either on the viability or on the total count of the exposed blood PMNL.

Salivary cytotoxicity for blood PMNL was also assessed by the release of ^{51}Cr from labelled blood PMNL, and showed a release of $30.8 \pm 8.5\%$ ^{51}Cr by 60 min. This was significantly greater than the release from PMNL incubated in HBSS ($13.3 \pm 3.5\%$, $p<0.05$).

The capacity of blood PMNL to phagocytose ^{14}C-labelled *Strep. mutans* was assayed after exposure of the PMNL to crevicular fluid washings or to mixed saliva for up to 60 min (Fig. 3). Crevicular washings failed to impair significantly the activity of blood PMNL ($44.4 \pm 5.0\%$ phagocytosis, compared with $46.1 \pm 4.4\%$ when PMNL were exposed to HBSS). Blood PMNL treated with mixed saliva for 30 min still achieved $46.3 \pm 11.8\%$ phagocytosis, but after treatment for 60 min the phagocytic activity was significantly impaired ($21.4 \pm 12.6\%$ phagocytosis, $p<0.05$).

Opsonic Activity of Oral Fluids

Opsonic activity for *Strep. mutans* was detected in immune serum, crevicular fluid washings and mixed saliva, but not in parotid saliva (Fig. 4). Fluorescent antibodies of IgG, IgA or IgM class were not detected in any of the oral fluids.

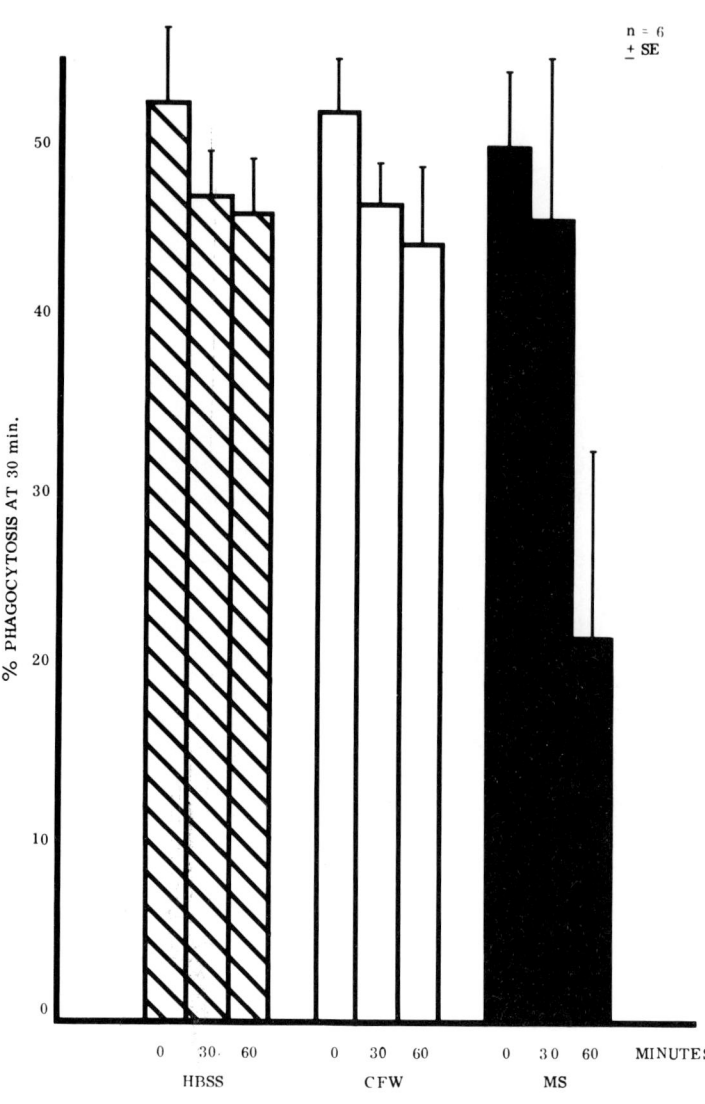

Fig. 3 Effect of exposure of blood polymorphonuclear leukocytes to crevicular fluid washings or mixed saliva, on the phagocytic activity for *Strep. mutans*. Blood PMNL were exposed to Hanks' Balanced Salt Solution (HBSS), crevicular fluid washings (CFW), or mixed saliva (MS) for 0, 30 or 60 min and then assayed for phagocytic capacity for *Strep. mutans* using 0.25% immune serum.

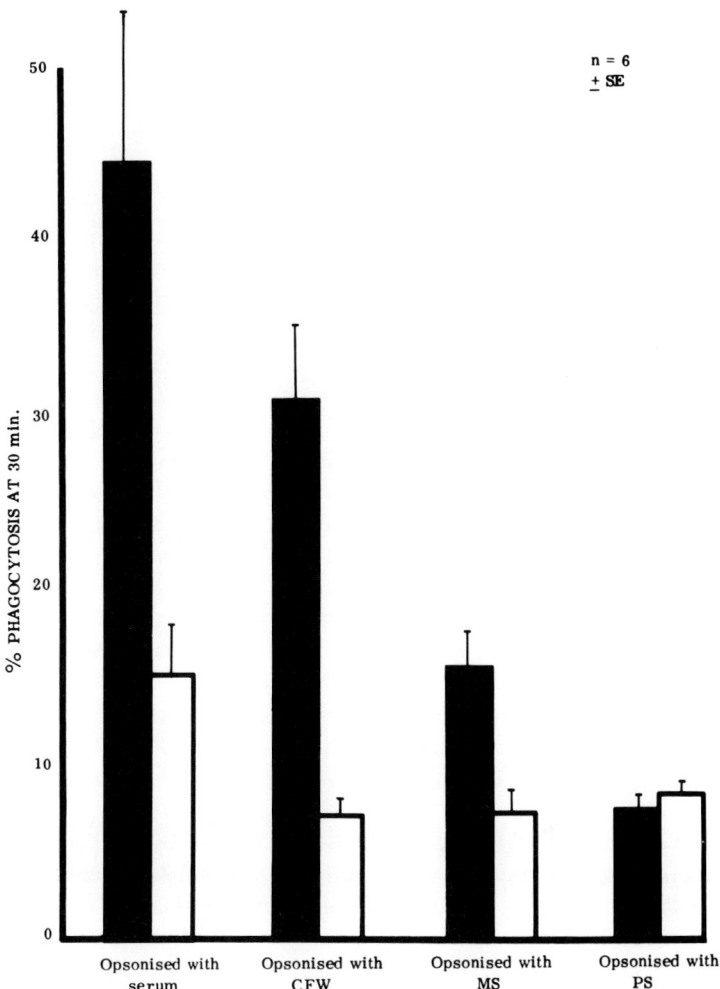

Fig. 4 Opsonic activity for *Strep. mutans* in serum, crevicular fluid washings (CFW) mixed saliva (MS) and parotid saliva (PS) from immunized (solid bars) and control (open bars) monkeys.

The opsonic activity in immune crevicular fluid ($31.2 \pm 4.7\%$ phagocytosis) was less than that in 0.25% immune serum ($44.9 \pm 6.9\%$), but this difference failed to reach the 5% level of significance. The activity was not significantly reduced by heating at 56°C for 30 min ($30.9 \pm 5.2\%$). However, absorption with the immunizing strain of *Strep. mutans* reduced the activity ($18.7 \pm 2.0\%$, $p < 0.05$), although *Strep. sanguis* had no effect ($32.5 \pm 3.1\%$).

The opsonic activity in immune mixed saliva (16.2 ± 3.0%) was significantly less than that in immune serum ($p<0.01$) or crevicular fluid ($p<0.05$). Opsonic activity in all fluids from control monkeys was significantly lower than in those from immune monkeys.

Discussion

Monkey blood PMNL migrated rapidly from the blood mainly into the gingival crevice, and nearly 80% of the crevicular PMNL were viable. Crevicular PMNL appeared as capable as blood PMNL in phagocytosing *Strep. mutans*, and crevicular fluid washings were not significantly cytotoxic to blood PMNL. In excess of 45% of salivary PMNL were viable. Although the function of salivary PMNL has not been assessed directly, mixed saliva was only minimally cytotoxic to blood PMNL over short periods of exposure, but prolonged exposure significantly impaired PMNL viability and function. Immunization of monkeys with *Strep. mutans* elicited serum opsonic antibodies which entered crevicular fluid and retained activity therein.

PMNL migrated from blood into the monkey gingival crevice within 20 min, in agreement with the results reported in dogs (Attström and Egelberg, 1970). The latter workers used an intravenous injection of carbon in an attempt to label phagocytes *in vivo*, when carbon-containing PMNL appeared in the crevice within 30 min. ^{111}In-labelling has little effect on PMNL function; the cells remain viable and follow a normal blood clearance but may show some impairment of PMNL mobility (Segal *et al.*, 1978). It is possible, therefore, that the rate of migration into the oral cavity may exceed that demonstrated here.

PMNL also appeared to migrate across the oral mucosa and enter the pool of saliva, as shown previously (Raeste, 1976). Parotid saliva contained only low numbers of PMNL, confirming reports in man (Isaacs and Daniellian, 1927; Wright, 1959).

Direct assay of the viability of PMNL from blood, gingival crevice and mixed saliva, revealed a progressive decrease in viability which might be accounted for by the exposure to noxious elements in the oral fluids or plaque. Indeed, collection of crevicular PMNL after preliminary washing out of the crevice increased the cell viability from 78 to 96%, suggesting the influx of fresh PMNL. A similar increase in PMNL viability with sequential washings has been noted in man (Skapski and Lehner, 1976).

Crevicular PMNL possessed phagocytic activity for *Strep. mutans* comparable with the activity of blood PMNL. In man these cells are also capable of phagocytosing other microorganisms (*Candida albicans*) and inert particles, e.g. latex beads (Wilton *et al.*, 1977). Crevicular fluid washings failed to impair either the viability or phagocytic activity of blood PMNL for *Strep.*

mutans, further suggesting that these cells can retain activity in the gingival crevice.

About 47% of monkey salivary PMNL were viable by dye exclusion, and similar results have been reported in man (Eichel and Lisanti, 1964; Raeste, 1972*b*; Sonis *et al.*, 1979). Although mixed saliva appeared to be only minimally cytotoxic to blood PMNL over 30 min exposure, prolonged exposure for up to 60 min caused about 20% more ^{51}Cr release from PMNL than did buffer. Lantzmann (1976) found that in man some 48% of blood PMNL were still viable 60 min after exposure to mixed saliva, although her method of viability assessment was not described. The present results indicated that although mixed saliva was cytotoxic to PMNL on prolonged incubation, blood PMNL retained some 50% of their phagocytic activity, suggesting that PMNL may retain activity in saliva. Early observations that salivary PMNL could phagocytose a number of bacteria, including *Strep. viridans* (Orban and Weinmann 1939*a,b*) have been followed by brief reports of phagocytosis by salivary PMNL of other bacteria (Rovelstad, 1960; Eichel and Lisanti, 1964) and latex beads (Kenney *et al.*, 1977). Salivary PMNL are also capable of other functional activity, e.g. antibody-dependent cellular cytotoxicity (Sonis *et al.*, 1979).

It would appear, therefore, that PMNL which enter the gingival crevice and saliva in monkeys may retain viability for sufficient time for these cells to carry out phagocytic activity for *Strep. mutans*. The phagocytic activity of PMNL (from blood) also appears to be unimpaired by moderate changes in pH and oxygen tension, such as might be expected in the vicinity of dental plaque (Scully, 1979). IgG, IgM and IgA have previously been found in crevicular fluid (Brandtzaeg, 1965; Holmberg and Killander, 1971; Shillitoe and Lehner, 1972). The demonstration of opsonic activity in crevicular fluid suggests that intact and functional antibodies persist at that site. The dilution of crevicular fluid by the washing technique and by saliva, as well as possibly some protein degradation, may explain the slightly lower opsonic activity in crevicular washings as compared with serum. The opsonic activity in crevicular fluid from immunized monkeys was higher than in crevicular fluid from controls, it was heat-stable, and it was removed by absorption with the immunizing organism but not with a heterologous organism. This opsonic activity was therefore probably antibody in nature.

The results of this investigation therefore support the hypothesis that opsonization and phagocytosis of *Strep. mutans* is possible in the crevicular domain, where it may mediate immunological protection against dental caries in the Rhesus monkey. However, it is possible that serum antibodies might afford protection by an additional or alternative mechanism in the monkey. In the rodent protection seems to be related to a salivary antibody response (Michalek *et al.*, 1978*a,b*).

PMNL may also constitute an important protective mechanism against periodontal disease, as indicated by the severe periodontal destruction that complicates patients with PMNL defects such as neutropenia (Cohen and Morris, 1961). Similar periodontal damage may affect patients with functional PMNL defects such as leukaemia (Deasy et al., 1976), the lazy leukocyte syndrome (Miller et al., 1971) and the Chediak–Higashi–Steinbrinck syndrome (Lavine et al., 1976). Moreover, PMNL functional defects have been reported in some patients with juvenile periodontitis (Cianciola et al., 1977; Lavine et al., 1979), and in some cases of rapidly progressive periodontitis (Lavine et al., 1979).

However, there is evidence to suggest that the host response to plaque may include destructive PMNL-dependent reactions leading to inflammatory periodontal disease (Taichman, 1970; Taichman and McArthur, 1975). Dogs experimentally rendered neutropenic appear, at least in the short term, to develop less gingivitis (Attström, 1971; Attström et al., 1971; Attström and Schroeder, 1979; Rylander et al., 1975) and there is no tissue bacterial invasion. Many other forms of inflammatory disease appear to be mediated, at least in part, by the release of lysosomal enzymes from PMNL (Janoff, 1972) and it may be significant that PMNL from inflamed gingival tissues or from gingival crevicular fluid show evidence of degranulation, suggesting that some lysosomal enzyme release may have occurred (Freedman et al., 1968; Lange and Schroeder, 1971). Furthermore, the intradermal injection of dental plaque into rabbits is associated with a PMNL accumulation, the release of lysosomal enzymes, and an inflammatory reaction (Taichman et al., 1966; Freedman et al., 1967). Leukopenic animals, however, fail to show the inflammatory responses (Freedman et al., 1967). In addition to this *in vivo* evidence, *in vitro* studies also support the concept that PMNL lysosomal enzyme release is a factor in periodontal disease (Taichman, 1970). Supra- and subgingival dental plaque, and a variety of plaque bacteria, are capable of initiating the release of lysosomal enzymes from PMNL (Taichman and McArthur, 1976; McArthur and Taichman, 1976; McArthur et al., 1976; Taichman et al., 1978). The enzyme release appears to be selective and is induced mainly by those microorganisms that produce extracellular polysaccharides (Taichman and McArthur, 1976). The release of enzymes by PMNL appears to correlate with phagocytosis of the bacteria (Baehni et al., 1977) but may also be induced by a variety of chemotactic factors including denatured proteins and C5a (Wilkinson, 1974). The enzyme release induced by 21-day-old plaque is mainly lactoferrin, rather than lysozyme or myeloperoxidase (Baehni et al., 1979). Lactoferrin is a major component of the secondary or specific PMNL granules which also contain other cationic proteins, proteinases and collagenases (Baggiolini et al., 1978), and these might be released concurrently. The release of collagenase could be responsible for the dissolution of collagen fibrils which is a prominent feature in the initial stages of gingivitis (Schroeder et al., 1975).

Examination of crevicular fluid has revealed high levels of lysosomal enzymes including acid phosphatases, β-glucuronidase, cathepsin D, lysozyme and other enzymes (Cimasoni, 1974, 1977). Many of these crevicular fluid lysosomal enzymes increase in periodontal disease, and the increases probably reflect true enzyme secretion, since the level of lactic dehydrogenase, an enzyme marker of cell death, is not increased (Bang et al., 1972). The findings are consistent with the hypothesis that the enzyme release is associated with the periodontal inflammatory reaction.

In conclusion, it is evident that polymorphonuclear leukocytes may act in a defensive capacity with regard to the immunological protection against dental caries, and clinical evidence at least suggests a similar defensive role in periodontal disease. However, apart from these beneficial results, the leukocyte response may also be harmful to the host—an apparent paradox already evident in other immunological reactions.

Summary

Polymorphonuclear leukocytes (PMNL) radiolabelled with ^{111}In migrated from the blood into the oral cavity of Rhesus monkeys within 20 min. The majority of leukocytes entered the oral cavity through the gingival crevice and only small numbers passed across the oral mucosa. About 80% of crevicular PMNL were viable, and they retained phagocytic activity for *Streptococcus mutans* almost as well as blood PMNL. Slightly less than 50% of salivary PMNL were viable. Neither crevicular fluid washings nor mixed saliva were cytotoxic to blood PMNL on exposure for 30 min, but saliva was cytotoxic to blood PMNL by 60 min.

Opsonic activity to *Strep mutans* was detected not only in the serum from monkeys immunized subcutaneously with a vaccine of formalinized *Strep. mutans* in Freund's incomplete adjuvant, but also in immune crevicular fluid and mixed saliva. This activity was heat-stable and could be absorbed out only with the immunizing organism, and was therefore probably antibody in nature. No such activity was detected in crevicular fluid or mixed saliva from control animals. The immune components essential for the phagocytosis of *Strep. mutans* are therefore present and functional in crevicular fluid, supporting the hypothesis that phagocytosis may be a protective mechanism against caries.

Acknowledgements

My thanks are to Professor T. Lehner for advice and constructive criticisms and to Miss H. Stadler for technical assistance.

References

Attström, R. (1970). *J. periodont. Res.* **5**, 42–47.
Attström, R. (1971). *J. periodont. Res.* **8**, 7–15.
Attström, R. and Egelberg, J. (1970). *J. periodont. Res.* **5**, 48–55.
Attström, R. and Schroeder, H. E. (1979). *Scand. J. dent. Res.* **87**, 7–23.
Attström, R. Tynelius-Bratthal, G. and Egelberg, J. (1971). *J. periodont. Res.* **6**, 200–210.
Baehni, P., Listgarten, M. A., Taichman, N. S. and McArthur, W. P. (1977). *Archs oral Biol.* **22**, 685–692.
Baehni, P. C., Tasi, C. C., Norman, M. E., Stoller, N., McArthur, W. P. and Taichman, N. S. (1979). *J. periodont. Res.* **14**, 279–288.
Baggiolini, M., Bretz, U. Dewald, B. and Feigenson, M. (1978). *Agents Actions* **8**, 1–10.
Bang, J. S., Rosenbusch, C., Ahmad-Zadeh, C. and Cimasoni, G. (1972). *Helv. odont. Acta* **16**, 89–93.
Brandtzaeg, P. (1965). *Archs oral biol.* **10**, 795–803.
Cianciola, L. J., Genco, R. J., Patterson, M. R., McKenna, J. and Van Oss, C. J. (1977). *Nature, Lond.* **265**, 445–447.
Cimasoni, G. (1974). In *Monographs in Oral Science*, Vol. 3 (H. M. Myers, ed.), Karger, Basel.
Cimasoni, G. (1977) In *Borderland between Caries and Periodontal Disease* (T. Lehner, ed.), pp. 13–42, Academic Press, London.
Cohen, W. D. and Morris, A. T. (1961). *J. Periodont.* **32**, 154–168.
Deasy, M. J., Vogel, R. I., Annes, I. K. and Simon, B. I. (1976). *J. Periodont.* **47**, 41–45.
Egelberg, J. (1963). *Acta odont. Scand.* **21**, 283–287.
Eichel, B. and Lisanti, V. F. (1964). *Archs oral Biol.* **9**, 299–314.
Freedman, H. L., Listgarten, M. A. and Taichman, N. S. (1968). *J. periodont. Res.* **3**, 313–327.
Freedman, H. L., Taichman, N. S. and Keystone, J. (1967). *Proc. Soc. exp. Biol. Med.* **125**, 1209–1213.
Friedman, S. D. and Tonzetich, J. (1968). *Archs oral Biol.* **13**, 647–659.
Garant, P. R. (1976a). *J. Periodont.* **47**, 132–139.
Garant, P. R. (1976b) *J. periodont. Res. Suppl.* **15**, 1–79.
Holmberg, K. and Killander, J. (1971). *J. periodont. Res.* **6**, 1–8.
Isaacs, R. and Daniellian, A. C. (1927). *Am. J. Med. Sci.* **174**, 70–87.
Janoff, A. (1972). *Am. J. Path.* **68**, 539–623.
Kenney, E. B., Kraal, J. H., Saxe, S. R. and Jones, J. (1977). *J. periodont. Res.* **12**, 227–234.
Klinkhamer, J. M. (1963). *Periodontics* **1**, 109–117.
Klinkhamer, J. M. (1968). *Periodontics* **6**, 207–211.
Lange, D. and Schroeder, H. E. (1971).*Helv. odont. Acta Suppl.* **6**, 65–86.
Lantzman, E. (1976). *J. Periodont.* **47**, 72–78.
Lavine, W. S., Page, R. C. and Padgett, G. A. (1976). *J. Periodont.* **47**, 621–635.
Lavine, W. S., Maderazo, E. G., Stolman, J., Ward, P. A., Cogen, R. B., Greenblatt, I. and Robertson, P. B. (1979). *J. periodont. Res.* **14**, 10–19.

Lehner, T., Caldwell, J. and Challacombe, S. J. (1977). *Archs oral Biol.* **22**, 393–397.
Lehner, T., Challacombe, S. J. and Caldwell, J. (1975). *Nature, Lond.* **254**, 517–520.
Lehner, T., Challacombe, S. J. and Caldwell, J. (1976). *J. dent. Res.* **55**, C166–C180.
Listgarten, M. A. (1976). *J. Periodont.* **47**, 1–18.
McArthur, W. P. and Taichman, N. S. (1976). *Infect. Immun.* **14**, 1309–1314.
McArthur, W. P., Baehni, P. and Taichman, N. S. (1976). *Infect. Immun.* **14**, 1315–1321.
Michalek, S. M., McGhee, J. R. and Babb, J. L. (1978a). *Infect. Immun.* **19**, 217–224.
Michalek, S. M., McGhee, J. R. Arnold, L. R. and Mestecky, J. (1978b) *Adv. exp. Biol. Med.* **107**, 261–270.
Miller, M. E., Oski, F. A. and Harris, M.B. (1971). *Lancet i*, 665–669.
Orban, B. and Weinmann, J. P. (1939a). *J. dent. Res.* **18**, 258.
Orban, B. and Weinmann, J. P. (1939b). *J. Am. dent. Assoc.* **26**, 2008–2017.
Raeste, A. M. (1972a). *Scand. J. dent. Res.* **80**, 285–291.
Raeste, A. M. (1972b). *Scand. J. dent. Res.* **80**, 63–67.
Raeste, A. M. (1976). *Scand. J. dent. Res.* **84**, 423–425.
Raeste, A. M. and Calonius, P. E. B. (1971). *Scand. J. dent. Res.* **79**, 327–332.
Rovelstad, G. H. (1960). Ph.D. thesis, Northwestern University, Chicago, Ill.
Rovelstad, G. H. (1964). *J. Am. dent. Assoc.* **68**, 364–373.
Rylander, M., Attström R. and Lindhe, J. (1975). *J. periodont. Res.* **10**, 315–323.
Schiott, C. R. and Löe, H. (1970). *J. periodont. Res.* **5**, 36–41.
Schroeder, H. E. (1977). In *Borderland between Caries and Periodontal Disease* (T. Lehner, ed.), pp. 43–67, Academic Press, London.
Schroeder, H. E., Graf De Beer, M. and Attström, R. (1975). *J. periodont. Res.* **10**, 128–142.
Scully, C. (1979). Ph.D. thesis, University of London.
Scully, C. and Challacombe, S. J. (1979). *J. periodont. Res.* **14**, 475–481.
Scully, C. and Lehner, T. (1978). *Clin. exp. Immunol.* **35**, 128–132.
Scully, C. and Lehner, T. (1979a). *Archs oral Biol.* **24**, 307–312.
Scully, C. and Lehner, T. (1979b). In *Pathogenic Streptococci* (M. T. Parker, ed.), pp. 219–220, Reedbooks, Chertsey, Surrey.
Segal, A. W. Deteix, P., Garcia, R., Tooth, P., Zanelli, G. D. and Allison, A. C. (1978). *J. nucl. Med.* **19**, 1238–1244.
Sharry, J. J. and Krasse, B. (1960). *Acta odont. scand.* **18**, 347–358.
Shillitoe, E. J. and Lehner, T. (1972). *Archs oral Biol.* **17**, 241–247.
Skapski, H. and Lehner, T. (1976). *J. periodont. Res.* **11**, 19–24.
Sonis, S. T., Mirando, D., Stelos, P. and Lamster, I. B. (1979). *Archs oral Biol.* **24**, 235–237.
Taichman, N. S. (1970). *J. Periodont.* **41**, 228–231.
Taichman, N. S., and McArthur, W. P. (1975). *A. Rep. med. Chem.* **10**, 228–239.
Taichman, N. S. and McArthur, W. P. (1976). *Archs oral Biol.* **21**, 257–263.
Taichman, N. S., Freedman, H. L. and Uriuhara, T. (1966). *Archs oral Biol.* **11**, 1385–1392.
Taichman, N. S., Hammond, B. F., Tsai, C. C., Baehni, P. C. and McArthur, W. P. (1978). *Infect. Immun.* **21**, 594–604.
Wilkinson, P. C. (1974) *Chemotaxis and Inflammation*, Livingstone, Edinburgh.
Wilton, J. M. A., Renggli, H. H. and Lehner, T. (1977). *Clin. exp. Immunol.* **27**, 152–158.
Wright, D. E. (1959). *Br. dent. J.* **106**, 278–280.
Wright, D. E. and Jenkins, G. N. (1953). *J. dent. Res.* **32**, 511–523.

6. The Comparative Inflammatory Effect of Dental Plaque, Lipopolysaccharide, Lipoteichoic acid, Dextran and Levan on Leukocytes in the Mouse Peritoneal Cavity

J. M. A. WILTON and O. P. DE ALMEIDA

Introduction

The association of bacterial plaque with human gingival and periodontal disease has been well established (Löe et al., 1965; Lehner et al., 1974; Syed and Loesche, 1978). The precise basis for the pathogenicity of dental plaque is, however, not understood. Although the present evidence suggests that there is no single causative microorganism for human periodontal disease, the use of recent techniques of anaerobiosis in the study of pocket and plaque bacteria has identified previously undescribed bacteria (Socransky, 1977). It is possible, therefore, that further studies may provide evidence for the association of specific bacteria or groups of bacteria with different forms or stages of periodontal disease. One disadvantage of current research is the lack of an appropriate animal model of naturally developing disease. Although some information has been gained from rodents, especially the gnotobiotic rat (Johnson et al., 1978), and from some primate studies (Slots and Hausmann, 1979) regarding the ability of individual plaque bacteria to cause periodontal disease, the form of the disease is acute and atypical and its relevance to human infection remains uncertain.

Mixtures of plaque bacteria will cause acute abscess formation when injected into the skin of rabbits and guinea-pigs (MacDonald et al., 1960) and these studies incriminated Gram-negative bacteria as being essential to the formation of these lesions, especially *Bacteroides melaninogenicus* (reviewed by Gibbons, 1974). Gram-positive bacteria are also pathogenic, particularly *Actinomyces* species producing bone loss in gnotobiotic rats and hamsters (Jordan et al., 1972). Lipids extracted from *A. naeslundii* gave an acute inflammatory reaction with accompanying bone loss (Irving et al., 1979). In vitro, *A. viscosus* can release enzymes from macrophages (MØ) (Page et al., 1973) and polymorphonuclear leukocytes (PMN) (Taichman et al., 1978).

This organism is also capable of activating the alternative pathway of complement (Wilton, 1977).

One important mechanism by which plaque could induce inflammation would be by attracting PMN and MØ into the gingival tissue and the crevicular space. Although these cells are necessary for the integrity of the tissues against bacterial invasion and should be regarded as protective under most circumstances, the continuous emigration of inflammatory cells and fluid components could also lead to tissue damage. The PMN is the principal cell of the gingival crevicular and pocket exudate but there are also significant numbers of MØ, especially within the tissues (Attström 1970; Wilton et al., 1976). The enzymes of PMN and MØ are capable of causing tissue damage and such enzymes can be released from these cells by plaque and plaque bacteria, without accompanying phagocytosis (by binding to the cell membrane) and during phagocytosis (Page et al., 1973; Baehni et al., 1977). Plaque contains both chemotaxins for rabbit and mouse PMN in vitro and in vivo (Tempel et al., 1970; Kraal and Loesche, 1979; Miller et al., 1975; Engel et al., 1976) and chemotaxinogens such as lipopolysaccharide (LPS) which are capable of activating complement via the alternative pathway and producing the chemotactic fragment C5a (Snyderman et al., 1968). LPS from oral bacteria has been extensively investigated and is capable of attracting inflammatory cells in animals both in vivo (Jensen et al., 1964) and in vitro using rabbit PMN (Sveen, 1977). LPS from Veillonella species will attract PMN when placed on human skin, using the skin window technique (Jensen et al., 1966). The topical application of dog serum containing activated complement will enhance migration of PMN into the normal dog gingiva (Kraal and Bowles, 1977) and human plaque filtrate applied to the normal dog and monkey gingival crevice causes an increased number of PMN to accumulate (Hellden and Lindhe, 1973).

Although there are bacteria and bacterial components which are capable of causing inflammatory reactions in experimental animals, some components have not yet been investigated for their inflammatory potential and there are no published studies comparing the properties of the different agents which may be found in dental plaque. The present study was designed to use the peritoneal cavity of the mouse to investigate the ability of plaque and the products of plaque bacteria to cause the accumulation of inflammatory cells, both PMN and MØ, particularly the kinetics of cell accumulation in the exudate, and to examine some properties of these cells. In addition, since inflammation is accompanied by the leakage of plasma proteins, we have examined the exudate for the presence of immunoglobulins, complement and albumin, to find out if there is a relationship between these proteins and the cellular components of the inflammatory response. To induce the peritoneal exudate we have used extracts of dental plaque, LPS from V. alcalescens, lipoteichoic acid, dextran and levan. In this way it was hoped to establish the properties of plaque constituents which can induce inflammation and cellular emigration.

Materials and Methods

Animals

Male CD-1 mice weighing between 25 and 30 g were used in groups of six to eight animals. Control animals received an injection of 0.1 ml sterile pyrogen-free saline (PFS) intraperitoneally and each agent under test was dissolved or suspended in the same volume of PFS. This volume was used in all experiments, since the injection of larger volumes of PFS gave a significant inflammatory response in the control animals. Mice were killed by decapitation and the peritoneal cavity was washed out with 4.0 ml of ice-cold, sterile Hank's Buffered Salt Solution (HBSS, Wellcome Reagents, Beckenham, U.K.) and the washings placed on ice until used. Groups of animals were killed 6, 25, 48 and 72 h after injection and both control and test suspensions were kept as individual samples for cell counting and identification.

Viable cell counts were performed using dye exclusion with 0.1% trypan blue and the results were expressed as the mean viable cells ($\times 10^6$) per millilitre. Differential cell counts were performed on cytocentrifuge preparations stained with Giemsa stain. At least 200 cells were counted for each preparation and the results were expressed as the absolute number of each cell type ($\times 10^6$) of the original viable count. In some experiments the cells were stained with acridine orange to identify their nuclear morphology and to check the Giemsa-stained preparations.

Dental Plaque

This was obtained from 15 patients with periodontal disease at routine prophylaxis, both supragingival and subgingival plaque being collected and placed in PFS. The samples were pooled and centrifuged. The pellet was resuspended in PFS and ultrasonicated whole cells and debris were removed by centrifugation at 2000**g** and the supernatant was used for the experiment. The protein concentration of this material determined by the method of Lowry *et al.* (1951) was 120 µg/ml and 10-fold dilutions were made in PFS immediately before injection. In some experiments plaque extract (12 µg/ml) was heated to 100°C for 15 min to differentiate LPS from other heat-labile toxins. Plaque extract (120 µg/ml) was deacetylated using 0.02 N NaOH at 37°C for 18 h, then neutralized with 1 N HCl and used for injection.

Lipopolysaccharide (LPS)

This was prepared by hot phenol extraction from a human strain of *V. alcalescens* and further purified by treatment with Cetavlon and RNAase (Sigma, London, U.K.). After extensive dialysis against distilled water, the material was lyophilized. Deacetylation of *V. alcalescens* was performed using 0.02 N NaOH at 37°C for 18 h. After neutralizing with 1 N HCl, the deacetylated LPS was resuspended in PFS and used for injection.

Lipoteichoic Acid (LTA)

This was prepared from *Lactobacillus fermentii* (NCTC 6991), using phenol extraction, extraction with chloroform–methanol and molecular sieve chromatography and was kindly donated by Professor Tony Wicken, University of Adelaide, Australia.

Dextran

Dextran T250 (molecular weight 250 000 daltons) was purchased from Pharmacia, Uxbridge, U.K. Dextran sulphate was prepared from Dextran T250 using chlorosulphonic acid and contained an average of 2.1 sulphate groups per glucose unit.

Levan

This was prepared from *Corynebacterium levaniformis*. It was generously donated by Dr Lida Ivanyi, Institute of Dental Surgery, London, U.K.

Measurement of Proteins in Peritoneal Exudate Fluid

IgG, C3 and albumin were estimated using radial immunodiffusion with a pool of normal mouse serum as a standard. IgG and albumin were measured using monospecific rabbit antisera (Miles Laboratories, Stoke Poges, U.K.) and C3 by means of a monospecific rabbit anti-mouse C3 serum, kindly donated by Dr Brian Williams, Hammersmith Hospital, London, U.K. The results were expressed as the percentage of each constituent found in the corresponding normal serum pool assayed simultaneously in the same gel.

Intracellular Immunoglobulins and Complement

Peritoneal exudate cells were cytocentrifuged and fixed in buffered formol acetone (pH 7.2). They were then stained directly with deaggregated (90 000g for 90 min) fluorescein isothiocyanate (FITC)–conjugated monospecific rabbit anti-mouse IgG, IgA, and IgM (Miles Laboratories, Stoke Poges, U.K.). C3 was detected using unlabelled rabbit anti-mouse C3, followed by FITC-conjugated goat anti-rabbit IgG (Wellcome Reagents, Beckenham, U.K.). The slides were counterstained with acridine orange to identify the nuclear morphology and examined using Ploem epi-illumination and a Leitz Ortholux II fluorescent microscope. Some 200 cells were counted in each preparation and the results were expressed as the percentage of fluorescent cells.

Results

In mice injected with 0.1 ml of PFS, the total cell count did not increase significantly during the experiment period. Virtually all the cells were mononuclear and the numbers of PMN never exceeded 4×10^5 cells per animal.

Dental plaque extract induced a cellular infiltrate at doses as low as 1.2 µg protein per animal (Table I). When 120 µg of protein was used there appeared to be an initial toxic effect on mononuclear cells and the peak number of cells was reached at 72 h and consisted of increased numbers of both PMN and MØ. The optimal dose for maximal cell accumulation appeared to be 12.0 µg, and in contrast to the 120 µg dose this response was maximal at 24 h; the increase at this time was due largely to an increase of PMN, although the numbers of MØ also increased slightly. The response at 24 h given by 12.0 µg of plaque extract was unaffected by heating at 100°C but was reduced from 17.9×10^6 to 7.2×10^6, when the extract was deacetylated, which suggested that at least part of the chemotactic effect of plaque extract was due to lipid A. This substance is not the only inflammatory agent in plaque, since there was a residual effect after deacetylation. In addition, the kinetics of the response showed that there was a substance or substances which caused a peak of cell accumulation at 72 h which is clearly different from that shown by purified LPS (see below) and lower concentrations of plaque extract.

In mice injected with *V. alcalescens* LPS, there was a clear, dose-related inflammatory cell response which commenced 6 h after injection (Table II). A dose of 0.05 µg caused a slight rise in total cells at 6 h which was due to an increase of PMN. In animals injected with 0.5 and 5.0 µg there was again a small rise at 6 h, but with these higher doses a much larger increase at 24 h was found, 70% of the cells being PMN. The cell numbers fell over the next 48 h but were still elevated at 72 h. After 24 h, the number of PMN declined sharply, although they still remained above control values after 72 h. MØ also increased after 24 h but then showed a further increase until 72 h, when they accounted for over 90% of the cell population.

In an attempt to find out if the response to *V. alcalescens* LPS depended on the lipid A moiety of the molecule, mice were injected with deacetylated LPS. This material was without any detectable effect at any time, eliciting no cellular response above control values at doses of 0.5 and 5.0 µg, in contrast to the native untreated LPS. For example, at 24 h 5.0 µg of LPS yielded

TABLE I

The Peritoneal Cell Response to the Intraperitoneal Injection of a Soluble Extract of Pooled Human Dental Plaque

Time of sampling (h)	Total cells ($\times 10^6$) elicited by			Mononuclear cells ($\times 10^6$) elicited by			Polymorphonuclear cells ($\times 10^6$) elicited by		
	120 µg	12.0 µg	1.2 µg	120 µg	12.0 µg	1.2 µg	120 µg	12.0 µg	1.2 µg
0*	4.8 ± 0.4†	4.7 ± 0.5	4.7 ± 0.45	4.3 ± 0.3	4.2 ± 04.	4.3 ± 0.3	0.15 ± 0.02	0.18 ± 0.3	0.13 ± 0.05
6	7.5 ± 0.8	6.8 ± 0.8	7.4 ± 0.9	3.2 ± 0.8	3.8 ± 0.6	3.4 ± 0.4	4.0 ± 0.6	4.4 ± 0.3	3.8 ± 0.9
24	7.9 ± 0.7	17.9 ± 1.6	10.0 ± 1.0	3.0 ± 0.7	5.6 ± 0.8	5.1 ± 0.6	5.9 ± 0.55	12.1 ± 1.1	4.1 ± 0.8
48	11.0 ± 0.8	13.2 ± 1.2	6.1 ± 1.1	4.8 ± 0.5	8.0 ± 1.2	5.1 ± 0.6	6.2 ± 0.34	4.9 ± 0.9	0.8 ± 0.3
72	15.1 ± 1.2	10.6 ± 1.3	7.9 ± 0.85	7.9 ± 1.1	8.4 ± 0.9	5.8 ± 0.8	7.6 ± 0.6	2.3 ± 0.8	0.2 ± 0.06

* Sample from mice without injection.
† ± Standard error.

TABLE II

The Peritoneal Cell Response to the Intraperitoneal Injection of Veillonella alcalescens *Lipopolysaccharide*

Time of sampling (h)	Total cells ($\times 10^6$) elicited by			Mononuclear cells ($\times 10^6$) elicited by			Polymorphonuclear leukocytes ($\times 10^6$) elicited by		
	0.05 µg	0.5 µg	5.0 µg	0.05 µg	0.5 µg	5.0 µg	0.05 µg	0.5 µg	5.0 µg
0*	4.5 ± 0.4†	4.3 ± 0.2	4.3 ± 0.4	4.2 ± 0.3	4.1 ± 0.4	4.2 ± 0.3	0.12 ± 0.03	0.16 ± 0.06	0.14 ± 0.01
6	7.2 ± 0.5	7.0 ± 1.2	7.2 ± 0.6	4.4 ± 0.4	4.0 ± 0.4	4.4 ± 0.4	2.6 ± 0.5	3.1 ± 0.6	3.2 ± 0.6
24	6.8 ± 0.3	18.6 ± 1.4	25.4 ± 1.8	6.0 ± 0.3	9.4 ± 1.0	7.6 ± 1.0	0.7 ± 0.15	9.4 ± 0.4	17.4 ± 1.6
48	5.0 ± 0.2	13.6 ± 1.6	19.4 ± 1.6	5.0 ± 0.6	9.8 ± 1.6	4.8 ± 0.8	0.4 ± 0.08	3.9 ± 0.8	9.5 ± 0.8
72	6.0 ± 1.0	14.1 ± 1.4	16.8 ± 1.2	5.9 ± 0.9	12.4 ± 1.1	13.0 ± 1.1	0.2 ± 0.06	1.8 ± 0.4	3.4 ± 1.0

* Sample from mice without injection.
† ± Standard error.

TABLE III
The Peritoneal Cell Response to the Intraperitoneal Injection of Lipoteichoic Acid from Lactobacillus fermentii NCTC 6991

Time of sampling (h)	Total cells (×10⁶) elicited by			Mononuclear cells (×10⁶) elicited by			Polymorphonuclear leukocytes (×10⁶) elicited by		
	0.5 µg	5.0 µg	50 µg	0.5 µg	5.0 µg	50 µg	0.5 µg	5.0 µg	50 µg
0*	3.4±0.4†	3.3±0.4	3.5±0.4	3.3±0.4	3.3±0.4	3.2±0.5	0.2±0.06	0.2±0.1	0.15±0.03
6	3.0±0.4	4.2±0.8	10.1±1.3	2.2±0.5	2.5±0.5	4.0±0.3	0.8±0.03	2.5±0.4	6.0±0.6
24	3.4±0.3	3.6±0.4	5.0±0.4	3.0±0.4	2.6±0.3	4.1±0.4	0.4±0.06	0.5±0.03	1.0±0.3
48	4.0±0.6	4.5±0.6	5.8±0.3	3.3±0.6	3.6±0.6	5.0±0.2	0.3±0.07	0.3±0.06	0.4±0.03
72	4.3±0.6	4.4±0.5	4.8±0.4	4.0±0.3	3.4±0.4	4.5±0.5	0.2±0.07	0.25±0.1	0.2±0.06

* Sample from mice without injection.
† ±Standard error.

TABLE IV
The Peritoneal Cell Response to the Intraperitoneal Injection of Levan from Corynebacterium levaniformis

Time of sampling (h)	Total cell count (×10⁶) elicited by		Mononuclear cells (×10⁶) elicited by		Polymorphonuclear leukocytes (×10⁶) elicited by	
	50 µg	500 µg	50 µg	500 µg	50 µg	500 µg
0*	4.3±0.4†	4.5±0.3	4.2±0.4	4.3±0.4	0.25±0.09	0.18±0.06
6	4.9±0.3	3.6±0.4	4.3±0.5	2.1±0.6	0.5±0.13	1.6±0.6
24	4.6±0.4	4.6±0.6	4.4±0.6	3.9±1.0	0.3±0.10	0.7±0.3
48	4.4±0.5	4.3±0.3	4.3±0.4	3.9±0.8	0.2±0.06	0.2±0.15
72	4.2±0.6	4.6±0.8	4.3±0.6	4.3±0.6	0.14±0.1	0.1±0.15

* Sample from mice without injection.
† ±Standard error.

$15.8 \pm 1.2 \times 10^6$ total cells and 5.0 µg of deacetylated LPS gave $4.1 \pm 0.15 \times 10^6$ cells. Heating LPS at 100 °C had no effect on the inflammatory capacity of the material. Thus a purified LPS from an oral bacterium depends on the presence of lipid A for its chemotactic properties. The similarity of the kinetics and susceptibility of the plaque chemotactic effects to that of purified LPS supports the hypothesis that LPS is a major chemotaxinogen in dental plaque.

LTA injected into mice gave little response at doses of 0.5 and 5.0 µg but a dose of 50.0 µg gave an increase of total cells to 10.1×10^6, due entirely to an increase in PMN, 6 h after injection (Table III). There was a very moderate increase of MØ when 50.0 µg was used, and PMN returned to normal levels after 72 h. It is unlikely that LTA is a potent agent *in vivo* for the attraction of inflammatory cells, and the failure to attract large numbers of MØ and the fact that the maximum PMN response occurred at 6 h clearly distinguishes this material from LPS. Although plaque gave a good 6 h PMN response, this

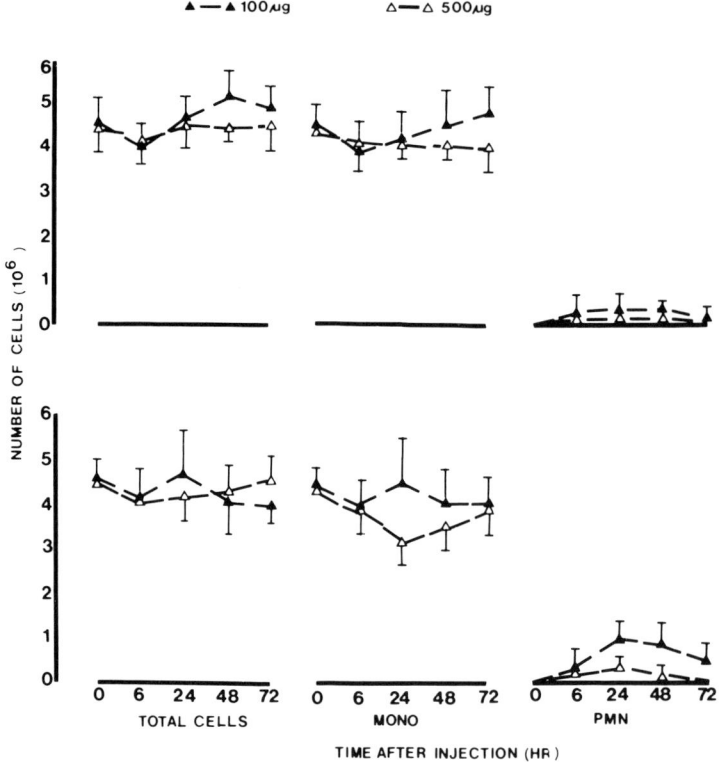

Fig. 1 The peritoneal cell response to the intraperitoneal injection of dextran (molecular weight 2.5×10^4 daltons) and sulphated dextran.

was also shown by a very low dose of LPS (0.05 µg), so that it is unlikely that LTA in plaque contributes to the 6 h response shown by the plaque extract.

Dextran T250 gave no detectable increase in total cell numbers at any time of sampling and neither PMN nor MØ increased during the experiment (Fig. 1). Sulphation of this dextran caused no substantial increase in total cell numbers. Although a small increase in the proportion of PMN was noted at a dose of 100 µg, the mononuclear cell number remained constant.

Levan injected into mice gave no detectable change in cell numbers at doses of 5 and 50 µg (data not shown) but at 500 µg a slight decrease in total cells were found at 6 h (Table IV). This was accounted for by a decrease in MØ, although the numbers of PMN at that time increased. The total number of cells had returned to normal values after 72 h and mononuclear cells accounted for this increase, the PMN having returned to their normal low values.

IgG, C3 and Albumin

The injection of various substances into the peritoneal cavity also gave increased levels of IgG, C3 and albumin. There appeared to be an association with the ability of a substance to attract PMN and the levels of C3 in the exudate fluid at 24 h. These are preliminary observations and a further study must be made to test the validity of this observation. The results are shown in Table V and it can be seen that 500 µg of levan, a poor inducer of inflammatory cells, elicited levels of C3, IgG and albumin which did not exceed the control values. In contrast, *V. alcalescens* LPS and dental plaque extract induced elevated levels of all three proteins 24 h after injection, and the increase was greatest for C3. These results suggest that at least part of the chemotactic ability of LPS and dental plaque depends upon complement activation, and it is known that both these substances can activate the alternative complement pathway (Wilton, 1977).

Since there was an increase in the levels of IgG and C3 in the peritoneal fluid it was possible that these would combine with the inflammatory agent and lead to phagocytosis of the complex by the PMN and MØ. Phagocytosis could proceed via the IgG Fc receptor on both cell types and this possibility was examined in animals treated with 5.0 µg of *V. alcalescens* LPS. It was found in control animals that less than 10% of MØ stained for intracellular IgG and IgM and neither cell type stained for C3. At 6 h after injection, about 40% of PMN and MØ contained IgG, 15% of MØ contained IgM and 40% of PMN stained for C3. At 24 h some 75% of PMN and MØ contained IgG and 86% of PMN contained C3 but the numbers of MØ containing IgM remained at about 15% until the end of the experiment. The percentage of cells staining for IgG and C3 fell to normal by 72 h, except that C3 was present in the few residual PMN at this time. These results are preliminary and must be confirmed in further

TABLE V

The Levels of IgG, C3 and Albumin in the Peritoneal Exudate Fluid from Normal Mice and Mice Injected Intraperitoneally with Veillonella alcalescens LPS, Human Dental Plaque Soluble Extract and Levan from Corynebacterium levaniformis

Time after injection (h)	Veillonella alcalescens LPS (5.0 μg)			Dental plaque (12.0 μg)			Levan (500 μg)		
	IgG	C3	Albumin	IgG	C3	Albumin	IgG	C3	Albumin
0*	15.6†	16.4	18.8	15.6	16.4	18.8	15.6	16.4	18.2
6	16.0	14.2	21.5	41.2	32.1	29.3	10.0	12.1	12.4
24	57.0	79.4	46.2	40.5	98.4	68.1	17.9	19.1	21.2
48	22.1	36.0	23.0	33.0	33.0	20.0	16.8	12.6	19.0
72	20.1	27.2	17.9	29.6	22.1	21.4	20.0	14.5	17.4

* Normal mouse peritoneal washings without stimulation.
† Percentage of standard pooled mouse serum.

investigations, but they suggest that there is an uptake of immunoglobulins and complement by inflammatory cells at least in mice treated with LPS. It is not known whether LPS is present within the same cells as have taken up immunoglobulins and complement, but LPS can bind to PMN (Brunning *et al.*, 1964) and can also be phagocytosed (Schrader *et al.*, 1964), so that it is reasonable to assume that this process would be facilitated by complement and naturally occurring antibodies of both isotypes. The LPS would then be inactivated by the cells and any toxic effect lost (Collins and Wood, 1964).

Discussion

The results presented in this study show that substances which may be found in human dental plaque vary in their capacity to attract inflammatory cells in a murine model of inflammation. Some are powerful inducers such as LPS; others such as levan are virtually unable to attract leukocytes, even at very high doses.

We have confirmed that LPS is a potent mediator of inflammation in animals, causing a rapid increase of PMN, with an initial fall and subsequent rise in the numbers of mononuclear cells (Cohn and Benson, 1965; Shands *et al.*, 1974; Moeller *et al.*, 1978). We have extended these studies by using LPS from an organism present in dental plaque and shown that the lipid A portion of the LPS seems to be responsible for the attraction of both cell types. Our results differ from those of Shands *et al.* (1974), who found larger numbers of PMN at 48 h, and those of Moeller *et al.* (1978), who found the maximum numbers of PMN 12 h after injection, but such differences may be ascribed to the use of different mouse strains and different LPS preparations used at much higher doses than in this study.

It is of interest that plaque extracts were able to mediate inflammation at low doses, and the heat stability and lability to alkaline hydrolysis of the majority of the inflammatory potential indicated that LPS was probably responsible for the capacity to attract inflammatory cells. It should be noted that deacetylated plaque was able to cause some inflammation, suggesting that other non-LPS inflammatory substances were also present. Further support for the concept of a mixture of inflammatory agents in plaque comes from the observation that, at the highest dose tested, the kinetics of the response to plaque was different from that given by the lower doses and did not resemble those given by high concentrations of LPS.

Lipoteichoic acid was not a potent inflammatory agent and the only effects were noted at a very high dose. The only cells attracted were PMN, which were present in greatest numbers at 6 h, in contrast to LPS. It is perhaps relevant that doses of 300 µg of LTA injected into rat gingiva caused an infiltration of

PMN (Bab et al., 1979), but this concentration of LTA is unlikely to be found within plaque or human gingival tissue. PMN hydrolases and lysozyme can release LTA from the surface of bacteria (Sela et al., 1977); it is thus possible that this substance might exert an inflammatory effect mediated by the PMN found in the gingival crevicular fluid.

Levan, dextran and dextran sulphate were all somewhat ineffective. Levan induced a slight PMN response at 6 h but was toxic for MØ. There is little information regarding the inflammatory capacity of any of these substances, but it is known that levan in very high doses (15–150 mg) can suppress the tuberculin reaction in guinea-pigs (Shezen et al., 1978) and inhibit the formation of granulation tissue (Wolman and Wolman, 1956). It is conceivable that such effects are mediated by toxicity for mononuclear cells, but there is also evidence that levan can activate murine peritoneal macrophages at high doses (Robertson et al., 1977). Whatever the basis for the anti-inflammatory effect of doses three or four orders of magnitude greater than those used in our study, it is unlikely that levan exerts a significant inflammatory effect in the gingival tissues.

Dextran was without effect, and sulphation of the molecule which renders a potent B lymphocyte polyclonal stimulator (Diamanstein et al., 1974) produced only a very slight increase in cell numbers at 24 h. Although plaque contains 8.5% soluble $\alpha(1-6)$-linked dextrans (Wood, 1967), there was no effect in the present study at doses as high as 500 µg, so it is unlikely that this substance is involved directly in gingival inflammation.

Our experiments suggest that the capacity of a substance to induce migration of PMN and MØ is associated with the ability to increase vascular permeability, with an increase in immunoglobulins and complement levels in the inflammatory exudate fluid. Immunoglobulins and complement are both present in human gingival exudate fluid (Shillitoe and Lehner, 1972) and are both bound to crevicular PMN (Wilton et al., 1977) and can both be ingested (Wilton, 1980). The association of chemotactic ability with the increased levels of C3 in the exudate fluid could provide an increased opsonic capacity to the fluid, which might enhance the uptake and destruction of bacteria containing LPS via the alternative and classical complement pathways. Activated C3 is known to bind directly to cell wall polysaccharide from *Salmonella abortus* and polysaccharides isolated from IgG (Capel et al., 1978), and LPS can also activate the classical complement pathway (Morrison and Kline, 1977). The MØ and PMN in mice challenged with LPS in this study contained IgG and C3, and such a mechanism could also operate in the human gingival crevice or pocket. It is also possible that this would result in increased tissue damage due to enzyme release by the cells, especially the MØ. LPS causes enhanced synthesis and secretion of lysosomal enzymes both by MØ and PMN (McGivney and Bradley, 1977; Thorne et al., 1977; Morland and Morland, 1978).

It is known that some of the substances used in this study may modulate the immune response, acting either as adjuvant or suppressive agents (Lehner, 1977; Wilton and Lehner, 1980). Although PMN are not known to be important for the induction of the immune response, the macrophage is an essential cell in this process (Unanue, 1972). PMN are, however, the predominant cells in the gingival crevice and these cells could be protective by phagocytosis of bacteria and immune complexes (Wilton, 1980) or cause tissue damage due to the release of enzymes (Taichman *et al.*, 1978; Attström and Schroeder, 1979). The complement system has an important regulatory effect on the function of both PMN and MØ (for reviews see Wilton, 1977; Wilton and Lehner, 1980) and this study has substantiated the importance of C3 in chemotaxis and cellular function.

Since some of the substances we have used induce migration of inflammatory cells, both PMN and mononuclear cells, further studies will be needed to distinguish between their direct effect on the inflammatory reaction and any modulation of the immune response. Gingival inflammation is a destructive process and it is more likely that gingival damage is due to a combination of humoral and cellular factors which can interact in many different ways. The attraction of inflammatory cells and increased vascular permeability can be achieved by non-immune-specific mechanisms, as shown in this study, but antigen–antibody complexes and cell-mediated immunity can also cause inflammation. Complement activation plays a central role in each of these mechanisms as a chemotaxin, opsonin and inducer of enzyme release. Whatever the relative importance of the different mechanisms, whether inducing or sustaining inflammation, the end result will be tissue destruction of chronic periodontal disease.

Summary

Plaque contains bacterial components and extracellular metabolites, which may induce inflammation. A model using the murine peritoneal cavity has permitted us to study the kinetics of cellular inflammatory responses induced by plaque and individual plaque components.

Soluble plaque extract, derived from a dialysed ultrasonicate, induced a brisk polymorphonuclear leukocyte (PMN) infiltrate which started after 6 h and was maximal at 24 h. Elevated cell numbers were still present at 72 h. Plaque also induced a mononuclear cell (MØ) response starting at 24 h which was maximal at 72 h. *Veillonella alcalescens* lipopolysaccharide (LPS) induced a dose-related, progressive infiltration of PMN starting 6 h after injection which reached a maximum at 24 h and declined sharply by 72 h. MØ started to increase at 24 h and continued to increase to 72 h. Lipoteichoic acid (LTA) from *Lactobacillus fermentii* gave a PMN inflammatory response that was maximal at 6 h but returned to normal values after 24 h. There was essentially no MØ response to this material at any time up to 72 h. Dextran from *Leuconostoc mesenteroides* failed to elicit either a PMN or MØ response at any time studies and sulphation of dextran caused it to give slight increase in PMN at 24 h, but it still did not produce a MØ response. Levan from *Corynebacterium levaniformis* caused a small increase of PMN at 6 h but did not cause MØ accumulation at any time studied.

The results indicate that dental plaque contains a substance or substances which elicit an inflammatory response comprising both PMN and MØ. LPS is also a powerful inducer of inflammatory cells of both types with the same kinetics as plaque. LTA differs from LPS and plaque since the maximal PMN response occurred at 6 h and no MØ were attracted. Dextran and levan do not appear to have the capacity to attract inflammatory cells in this model.

Acknowledgements

Dr Almeida was on study leave from the Department of Oral Biology, Dental School, Sao Paolo, Brazil and supported by FASPESP Grant No. 771 066V during the time this research was undertaken.

References

Attström, R. (1970). *J. periodont. Res.* **5**, 42–47.
Attström, R. and Schroeder, H. E. (1979). *Scand. J. dent. Res.* **87**, 7–23.
Bab, I. A., Sela, M. N., Ginsberg, I. and Dishon, T. (1979). *Inflammation* **3**, 345–358.
Baehni, P., Listgarten, M. A., Taichman, N. S. and McArthur, W. P. (1977). *Archs oral Biol.* **22**, 685–692.
Brunning, R. A., Woolfrey, B. F. and Schrader, W. H. (1964). *Am. J. Path.* **44**, 401–409.
Capel, P. J. A., Groenboer, O., Grosveld, G. and Pondman, K. W. (1978). *J. Immunol.* **121**, 2566–2572.
Cohn, Z. A. and Benson, B. (1965). *J. exp. Med.* **121**, 153–170.
Collins, R. D. and Wood, J. B., Jr (1964). *J. exp. Med.* **110**, 1005–1016.
Diamanstein, T., Blitstein-Willinger, T. and Schulz, G. (1974). *Nature, Lond.* **250**, 546–547.
Engel, D., Van Epps, D. and Clagett, J. (1976). *Infect. Immun.* **14**, 548–554.
Gibbons, R. J. (1974). In *Anaerobic Bacteria: Role in Disease* (A. Barlow, R. D. Deliann, V. R. Dowall and L. B. Gaze, eds), pp. 168–285, Charles C. Thomas, Springfield, Ill.
Hellden, L. and Lindhe, J. (1973). *Scand. J. dent. Res.* **81**, 123–129.
Irving, J. T., Heeley, J. D., Amdur, B. H. and Socransky, S. S. (1979). *J. periodont. Res.* **14**, 160–166.
Jensen, S. B., Theilade, E. and Jensen, J. S. (1966). *J. periodont. Res.* **1**, 129–140.
Jensen, S. B., Jackson, F. V. and Mergenhagen, S. E. (1964). *Acta odont. scand.* **22**, 71–93.

Johnson, D. A., Behling, V. H., Listgarten, M and Nowotny, A. (1978). *Infect. Immun.* **22**, 382–386.
Jordan, D. A., Keyes, P. H. and Bellack, S. (1972). *J. periodont. Res.* **7**, 21–28.
Kraal, J. and Bowles, R. D. (1977). *J. periodont. Res.* **16**, 235–241.
Kraal, J. H. and Loesche, W. V. (1979). *J. periodont. Res.* **45**, 780–785.
Lehner, T., Wilton, J. M. A., Challacombe, S. J. and Ivanyi, L. (1974). *Clin. exp. Immunol.* **16**, 481–492.
Lehner, T. (1977). In *Immunology of the Gut*, Ciba Foundation Symposium no. 46, pp. 135–159, Elsevier, Amsterdam.
Löe, H., Theilade, E. and Jensen, S. B. (1965). *J. Periodont.* **36**, 177–187.
Lowry, O. H., Rosebrough, N. J., Farr, A. L. and Randall, J. (1951). *J. biol. Chem.* **193**, 265–270.
MacDonald, J. B., Gibbons, R. J. and Socransky, S. S. (1960). *Ann. N.Y. Acad. Sci.* **85**, 467–482.
McGivney, A. and Bradley, S. G. (1977). *Proc. Soc. exp. Biol. Med.* **155**, 390–394.
Miller R. L., Folke, L. G. A. and Umana, C. R. (1975). *J. Periodont.* **46**, 409–414.
Moeller, G. R., Terry, L. and Snyderman, R. (1978). *J. Immunol.* **120**, 116–123.
Morland, B. and Morland J. (1978). *J. reticuloendothial Soc.* **23**, 469–477.
Morrison. D. C. and Kline, L. F. (1977). *J. Immunol.* **118**, 362–368.
Page, R. C., Davies, P. and Allison, A. C. (1973). *Archs oral Biol.* **18**, 1481–1495.
Robertson, R. A., Papadimitriou, M., Walters, N. M. and Wolman, M. (1977). *J. Path.* **123**, 157–164.
Sela, M. N. Lahav, M. and Ginsberg, I. (1977). *Inflammation* **3**, 59–80.
Schrader, N. H., Woolfrey, B. F. and Brunning, R. D. (1964). *Am. J. Path.* **44**, 597–611.
Shands, J. W., Peavy, D. L. Gormus, B. J. and McGraw, J. (1974). *Infect. Immun.* **9**, 106–112.
Shezen, E., Leibovici, J. and Wolman, M. (1978). *Br. J. exp. Path.* **59**, 454–458.
Shillitoe, E. J. and Lehner, T. (1972). *Archs oral Biol.* **17**, 241–247.
Slots, J. and Hausman, E. (1979). *Infect. Immun.* **23**, 260–267.
Snyderman, R., Gewurz, H. and Mergenhagen, S. E. (1968). *J. exp. Med.* **128**, 259–275.
Socransky, S. S. (1977). *J. Periodont.* **48**, 497–504.
Sveen, K. (1977). *J. periodont. Res.* **12**, 340–350.
Syed, S. A. and Loesche, W. J. (1978). *Infect. Immun.* **21**, 821–829.
Taichman, N. S., Hammond, B. F., Tsai, G. C., Baehni, P. C. and McArthur, W. P. (1978). *Infect. Immun.* **21**, 594–604.
Tempel, T. R. Snyderman, R., Jordan, H. O. and Mergenhagen, S. E. (1970). *J. Periodont.* **41**, 71–80.
Thorne, K. I., Oliver, R. C. and Lackie, J. (1977). *J. Cell Sci.* **27**, 213–225.
Unanue, E. R. (1972). *Adv. Immunol.* **15**, 95–165.
Wilton, J. M. A. and Lehner, T. (1980). In *Recent Advances in Clinical Immunology* (R. A. Thompson, ed.), in press, Churchill Livingstone, Edinburgh.
Wilton, J. M. A. (1980). Submitted for publication.
Wilton, J. M. A. and Lehner, T. (1980). In *Recent Advances in Clinical Immunology* (R. A. Thompson, ed.), in press, Churchill Livingstone, Edinburgh.
Wilton, J. M. A., Renggli, H. H. and Lehner, T. (1956). *J. periodont. Res.* **11**, 262–268.
Wilton, J. M. A., Renggli, H. H. and Lehner, T. (1977). *Immunology* **32**, 955–961.
Wolman, M. and Wolman, B. (1956). *Am. med. Assoc. Archs Path.* **62**, 74–79.
Wood, J. M. (1967). *Archs oral Biol.* **12**, 849–858.

7. Pocket Formation: An Hypothesis

HUBERT E. SCHROEDER and ROLF ATTSTRÖM

Introduction

The formation of gingival and periodontal pockets is the cardinal feature of progressive periodontal disease. There is firm evidence that pocket formation and the progression of periodontitis is related to the colonization of bacteria at subgingival tooth surfaces (Listgarten, 1976; Socransky, 1977; Listgarten and Helldén, 1978; Waerhaug, 1978a,b; Slots, 1979). However, experiments related to the mechanisms of pocket formation are lacking.

In a previous experiment using dogs, we attempted to evaluate the capacity of neutrophilic granulocytes to mediate collagen degradation in the course of early gingivitis (Attström and Schroeder, 1979). We found that an extensive subgingival plaque was formed during a 4-day period of experimental neutropenia. Supragingival plaque control did not prevent subgingival plaque formation (Schroeder and Attström, 1979). Therefore, this experiment offered unique possibilities for studying the histopathological features both of the newly formed subgingival plaque and of the changes at the dento-gingival junction which occurred in neutropenic dogs. Furthermore, this material, and observations derived from it, permitted us to formulate an hypothesis explaining how gingival and periodontal pockets may develop.

Material and Methods

Three 1-year-old Beagle dogs were used. The initially inflamed gingival tissues were freed from inflamation by regular tooth brushing during a period of 90 days before the experiment. Gingivitis was provoked by abolishing oral hygiene procedures and feeding the animals a soft diet. Antineutrophil serum was raised in rabbits. The antiserum was absorbed with dog erythrocytes, liver, kidney and spleen cells. The experiment lasted for 4 days. The antiserum was injected intravenously daily and the effects were monitored by blood cell counts. On day 4 of the experiment, block biopsies were taken from maxillary and mandibular premolars. Details concerning the methods employed have been described elsewhere (Attström and Schroeder, 1979). Random sections (about 1–2 μm thick) of the Epon-embedded tissues were stained with PAS-methylene blue/azure II (Schroeder, 1973) and photographed, using a Leitz orthoplan microscope. Series of up to 200 consecutive sections were used for reconstructing three-dimensional images of subgingival plaque distribution as follows. (1) The cross-sectional features were projected on paper and the profiles of subgingival plaque were redrawn, using a Leitz SM-Lux microscope equipped with a S-tube. (2) The first drawing was enlarged by a factor of two using an epidiascope (Liesegang, Racher, Zürich, Switzerland). (3) The enlarged plaque profiles were redrawn and the consecutive profiles adjusted in their proper topographical relationship.(4) The enlarged profiles were translated into a two-dimensional array of equidistant, parallel-perspectively shortened lines, using the Perspectomat P-40 (Forster, Schaffhausen, Switzerland). (5) The line arrays were connected and shadowed in order to generate an image conveying three-dimensional features.

Ultrathin sections comprising the entire dento-gingival region including the subgingival plaque were cut with a diamond knife (Rawiler, Switzerland), using the LKB Ultrotome III. These sections were contrasted with uranyl acetate and lead citrate (Reynolds, 1963; Fraska and Parks, 1965), and collected on R-150 (Veco) copper grids covered with carbon film. Electron micrographs were recorded with a Philipps 201 electron microscope.

The periodontal and histopathological nomenclature used in the present paper adheres to the recommendations adopted by WHO (1978).

Observations and Results

After 4 days of relatively severe neutropenia, the gingival sulcus and a variable portion of the adjacent dento-gingival junction were severely altered. In each of the dogs used, the coronal part of the junctional epithelium of all teeth had been undermined by subgingival plaque which, to a variable distance, extended in an apical direction. This distance varied between 0.4 and 0.8 mm. In many specimens, the subgingival plaque was continuous with supragingival deposits. In all instances the gingival tissues were moderately inflamed clinically and spontaneous bleeding occurred frequently.

The distribution of subgingival plaque as well as the inflammatory response varied greatly between the various teeth. This is shown in Figs 1–3, which represent three different biopsies taken from a dog. In its cross-sectional profile, the subgingival plaque appeared either as a continuous bacterial integument (Figs 1(a), (b) and 4(a), (b)) or in the form of a succession of discontinuous, discrete colonies of varying size (Figs 2(b) and (c), 4(c) and 5(a), (b)). In some gingival regions, this plaque was close to the junctional epithelium (Figs 2(a), (b) and (c)), while in others inflammatory cells, mononuclear leukocytes, formed a band separating the epithelial cells from the plaque surface, at least in its coronal portions (Figs 1(a) and (b)). Frequently, this band of cellular exudate extended further apically, separating

7. Pocket Formation

Fig. 1 Clinically moderately inflamed buccal gingiva of a lower third premolar (a). The marginal dento-gingival region outlined in (a) is shown at higher magnification in (b) and (c). Note that the supragingival plaque (P) is continuous with subgingival deposits (a) and (b), terminating close to cells of the junctional epithelium (JE), attached to the enamel surface (E). Magnification: (a) ×35; (b) and (c) ×210.

Fig. 2 Clinically moderately inflamed buccal gingiva of an upper third premolar (a). The marginal dento-gingival region outlined in (a) is shown at higher magnification in (b) and (c). Note the subgingival plaque (P) which extends apically in the form of discontinuous islands (c, inset). A short distance apical to the most apically advanced subginival plaque, the junctional epithelium (JE) and the epithelial attachment are still intact. Magnification: (a) ×35; (b) and (c) ×210, inset ×505.

Fig. 3 Clinically moderatly inflamed buccal gingiva of a lower fourth premolar (a). The marginal dento-gingival region outlined in (a) is shown at higher magnification in (b) and (c). Note that the subgingival plaque (P) terminates at some distance coronal to the intact junctional epithelium (JE). Inflammatory cells, mostly mononuclears, separate both the subgingival plaque and the enamel surface (E) from the epithelium and form a band extending apically along the enamel surface ((b) and (c)). Observe that the epithelium facing the band of inflammatory cells resembles a pocket epithelium. Magnification: (a) ×35; (b) and (c) ×210.

Fig. 4 Clinically moderately inflamed gingiva of the lower second premolar. The marginal dento-gingival region outlined in (a) is shown at the higher magnification in (b) and (c). Note that the thin subgingival plaque is continuous with the supragingival plaque. The subgingival plaque is in direct contact with the junctional epithelium (JE) which is still attached to the enamel surface apical to the subgingival plaque (c). Magnification: (a) ×35; (b) and (c) ×210.

Fig. 5 Electron micrographs of the dento-gingival junction as shown in Fig. 4(c) (open brackets). Note discontinuous islands of subgingival plaque consisting of cocci only. Most of the dividing planes are parallel to the enamel surface (E). Note fibrin (F) and exudate between the plaque and degenerated epithelial cells (EP). The most apical termination of subgingival plaque consists of a monolayer of cocci, with the dividing planes perpendicular to the enamel surface (inset in (b)). Magnification: (a) and (b) ×2780; inset ×13 310.

Fig. 6 Cross-section of moderately inflamed gingiva of a lower second premolar, taken from a block adjacent to that shown in Fig. 4. Note the intense mononuclear infiltration along the enamel surface (E), obscuring the junctional epithelium (JE). The supragingival plaque (P, in (a)) extends subgingivally in the form of discontinuous plaque islands ((b) and (c)). Magnification: (a) ×35; (b) and (c) ×210.

Fig. 7 Clinically moderately inflamed gingiva of a lower third premolar (a). The dento-gingival region outlined in (a) is shown at higher magnification in (b) and (c). Note the supragingival plaque (P) extending subgingivally (b), the most apical plaque forming discontinuous islands of variable size (c). These islands are in contact with epithelial cells (JE). Intraepithelial leukocytes are few in number. E, enamel. Magnification: (a) ×35; (b) and (c) ×210.

Fig. 8 Cross-section of the same gingival tissues but observed in a block adjacent to that shown in Fig. 7. Note the supragingival plaque (P in (a)) extending for a long distance subgingivally, in the form of an extremely thin, rather continuous layer ((b), (c) and (d)). Some leukocytes have accumulated in the former junctional epithelium (JE) close to the enamel surface (E). The junctional epithelium covering subgingival plaque resembles a pocket epithelium (a). Magnification: (a) ×35; (b), (c) and (d) ×210.

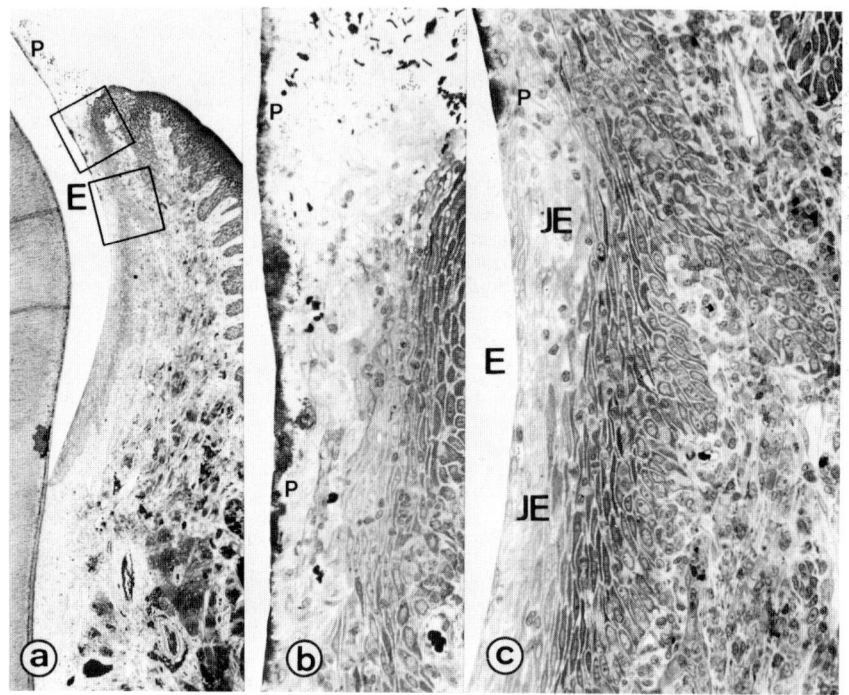

Fig. 1

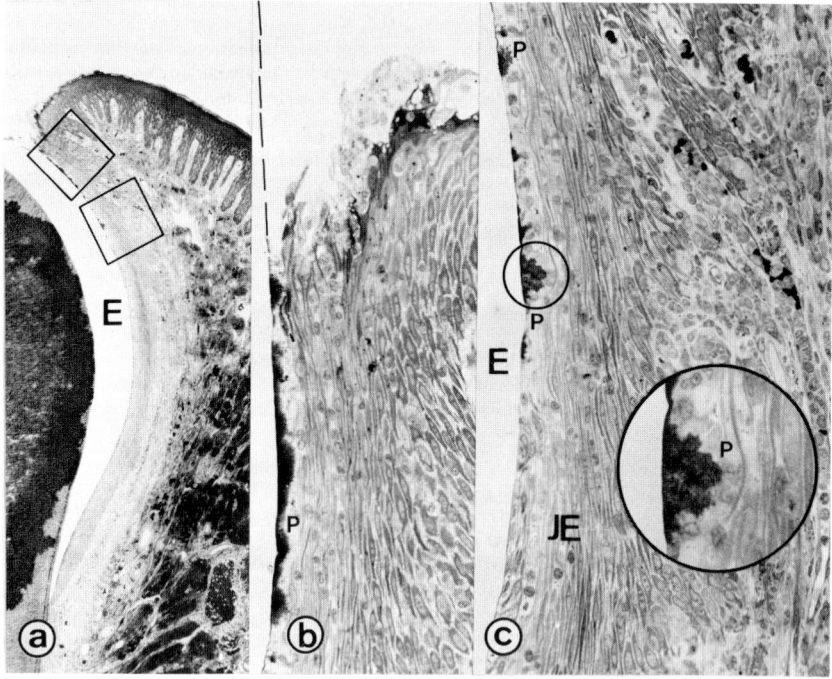

Fig. 2

7. Pocket Formation

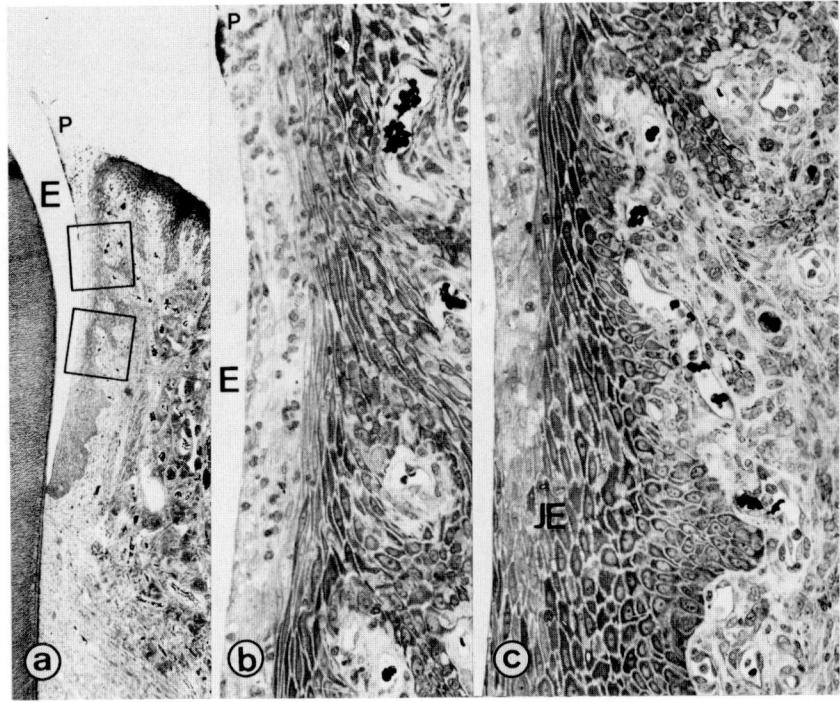

Fig. 3

Fig. 9 Electron micrographs of the dento-gingival junction as shown in Figs 8(b)–(d). Note uniformity and even thickness of the most coronal portion of subgingival plaque comprising cocci along the enamel surface (E), covered by rods and, occasionally flagellated bacteria ((a), inset), filaments and yeasts (b). Adjacent to the plaque there is (1) a zone of rather electron lucent spaces in which groups (inset in (b), arrow) of single bacteria unrelated to the plaque are found, (2) an additional zone of fibrin and exudative material, with degenerating epithelial cells. Magnification: (a) and (b) ×2780; inset in (a) ×13 220; inset in (b) ×1650.

Fig. 10 Continuation in an apical direction of the electron micrographs of the dento-gingival junction as shown in Figs 8(b)–(d), continuous with the portion illustrated in Fig. 9(b). In this region, the rods implanted on a layer of cocci ((a), inset) terminate (b), and the coccoid plaque extends more apically, forming a monolayer ((b), inset). Occasionally, bacteria can be observed inside cross-sectional profiles of phagocytes (b). A few leukocytes and degenerated epithelial cells are seen in the vicinity of plaque. Magnification: (a) and (b) ×2780; insets in (a) and (b) ×13 320.

Fig. 11 Continuation in an apical direction of the electron micrographs on the dento-gingival junction as shown in Figs 8(b)–(d), continuous with the portion illustrated in Fig. 10(b). Note discontinuous plaque comprising monolayers and interposed islands of cocci ((a), (b), (c)). Degenerated epithelial cells (EP) border a structureless zone of moderate electron density, which may represent exudative proteins overlying the subgingival plaque. E, enamel. Magnification: (a), (b) and (c) ×2780.

Fig. 12 Continuation in an apical direction and termination of the electron micrographs of the dento-gingival junction as shown in Figs 8(b)–(d), continuous with the portion illustrated in Fig. 11(c). Note the discontinuous coccoid plaque. In the monolayers of coccoid bacteria the dividing planes are perpendicular, while in the multilayers they are parallel to the enamel surface ((a), inset). The majority of epithelial cells (EP) in the vicinity of the bacteria are degenerated. Note the most apical termination of subgingival plaque in the form of a monolayer of cocci ((a), inset, (b)). Magnification: (a) and (b) ×2780; insets ×13 320.

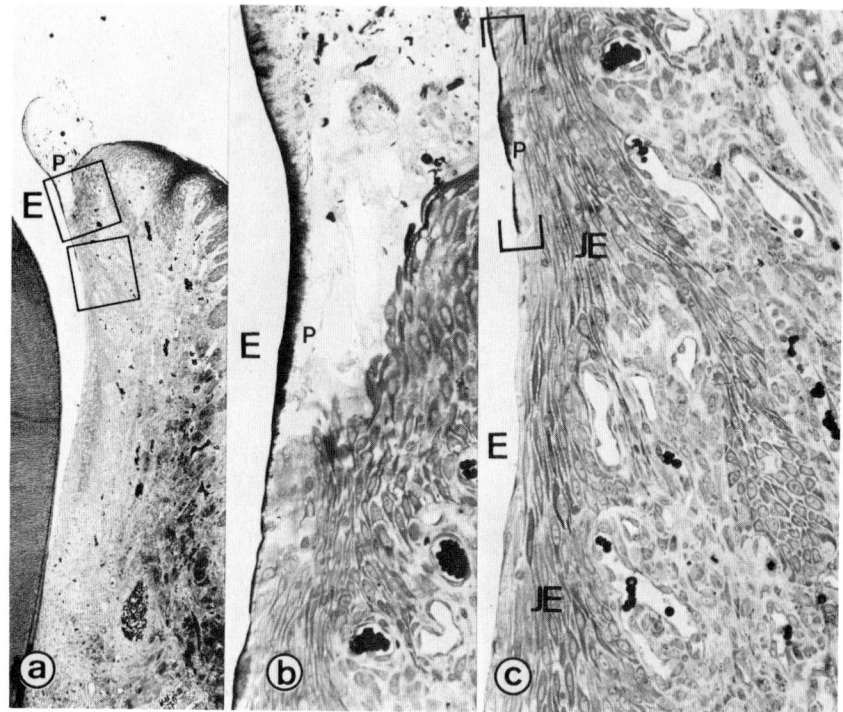

Fig. 4

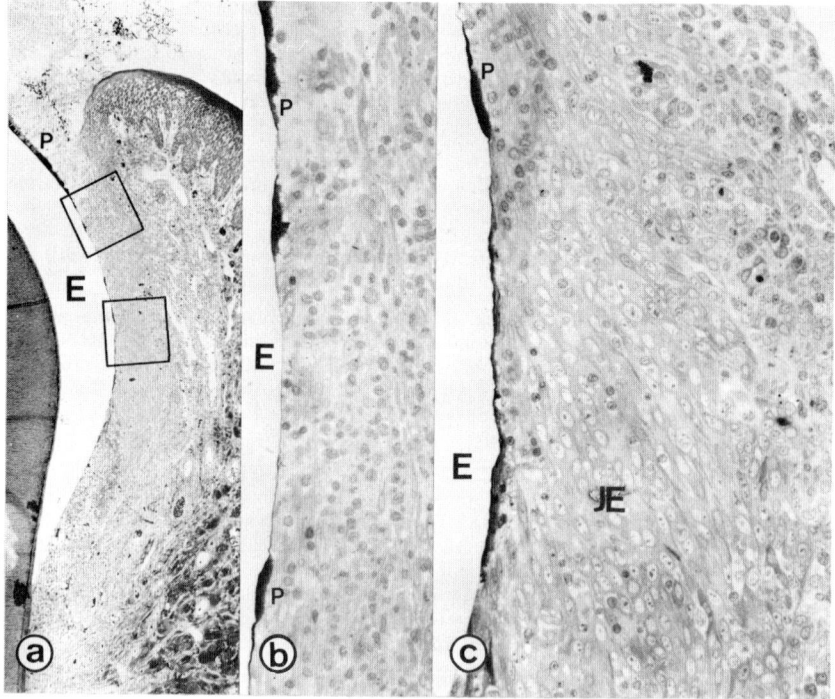

Fig. 6

7. Pocket Formation

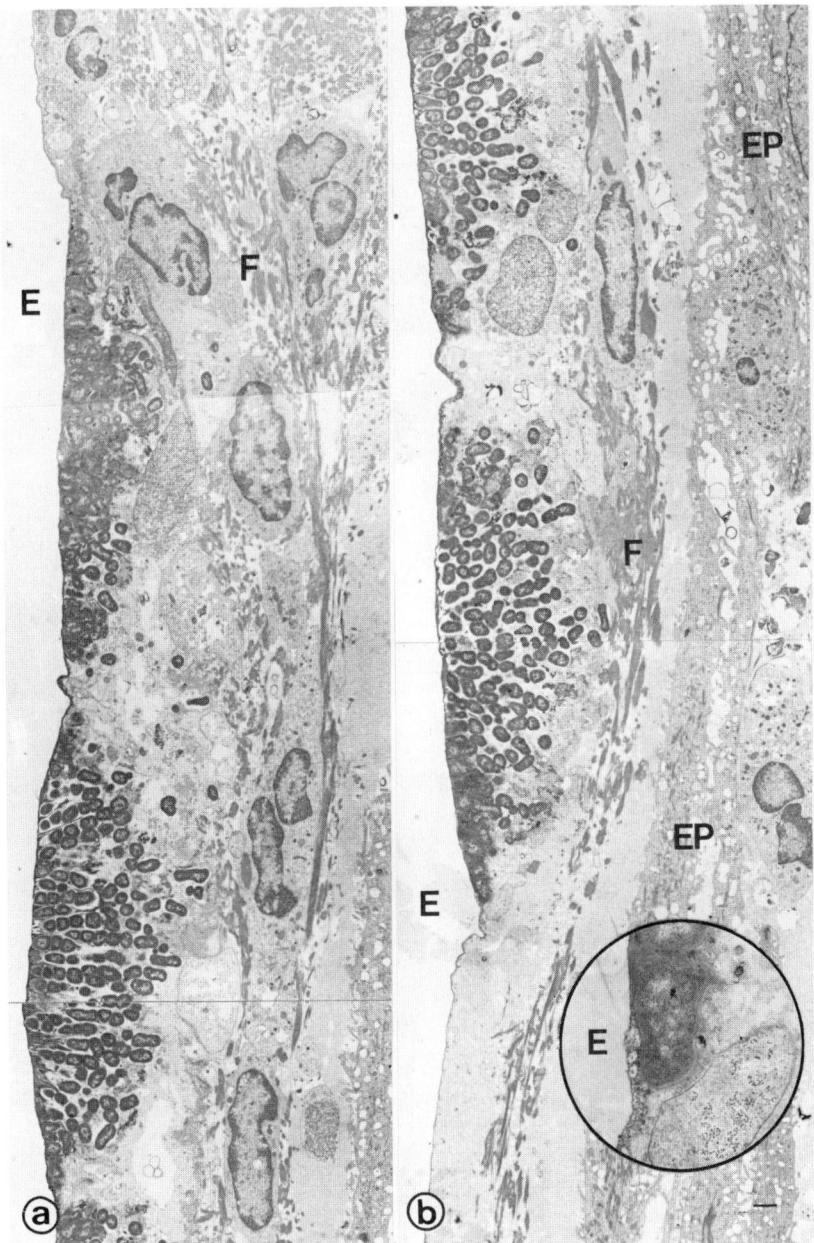

Fig. 5

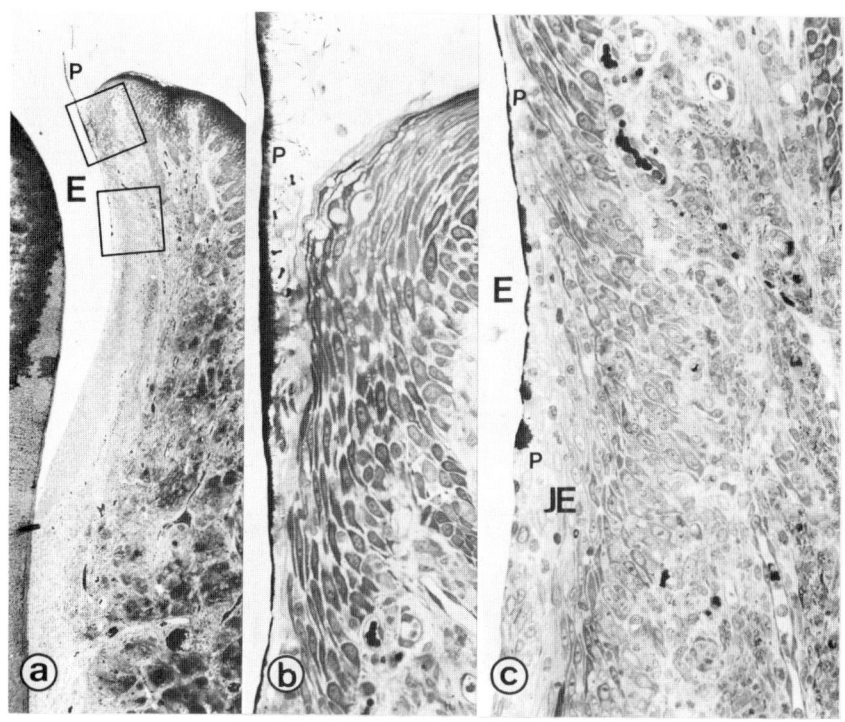

Fig. 7

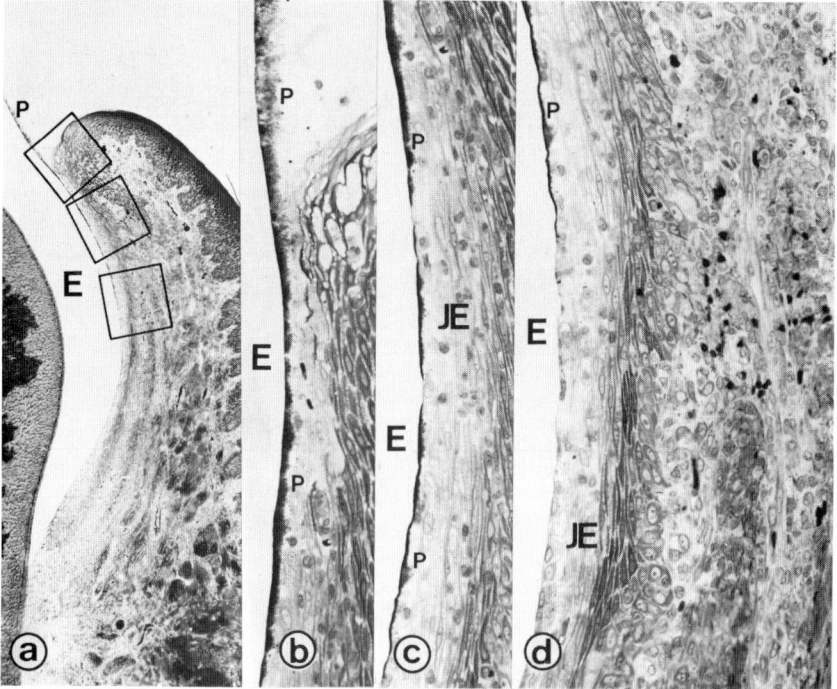

Fig. 8

7. Pocket Formation

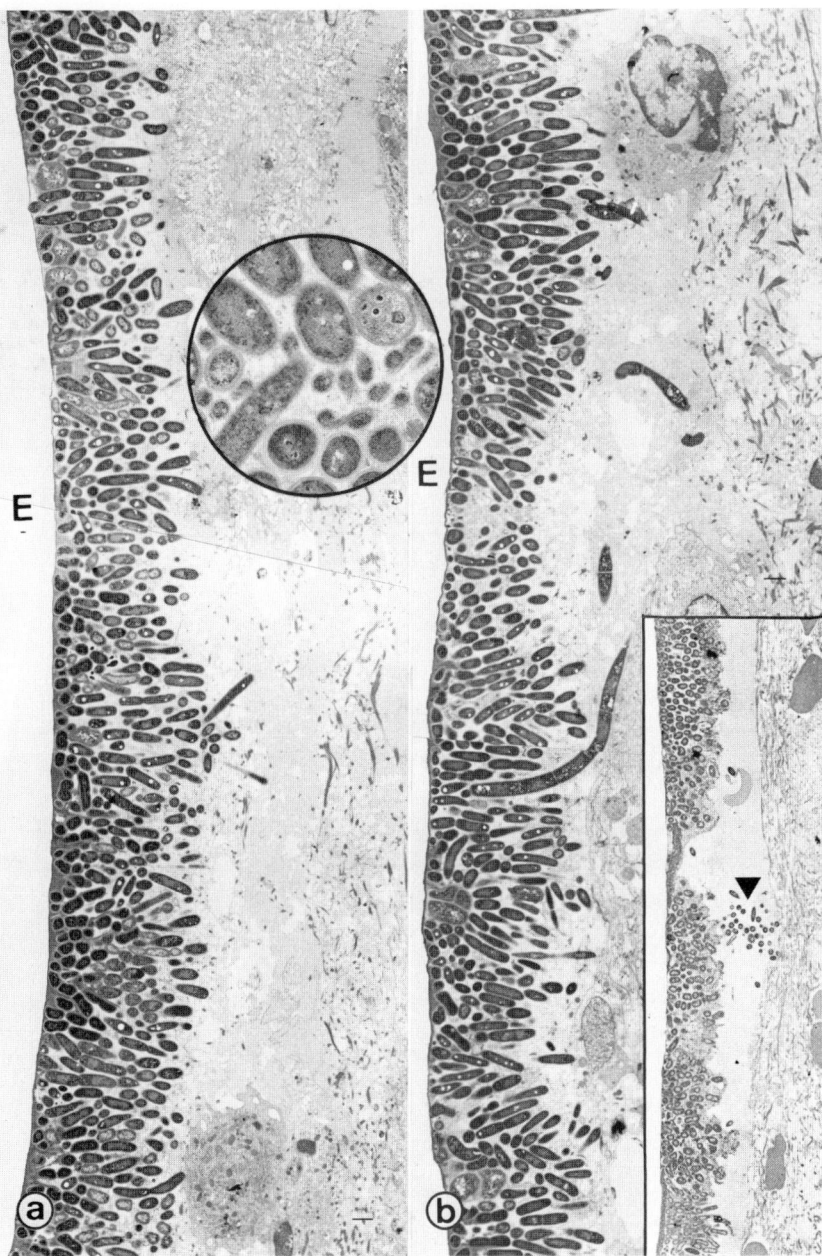

Fig. 9

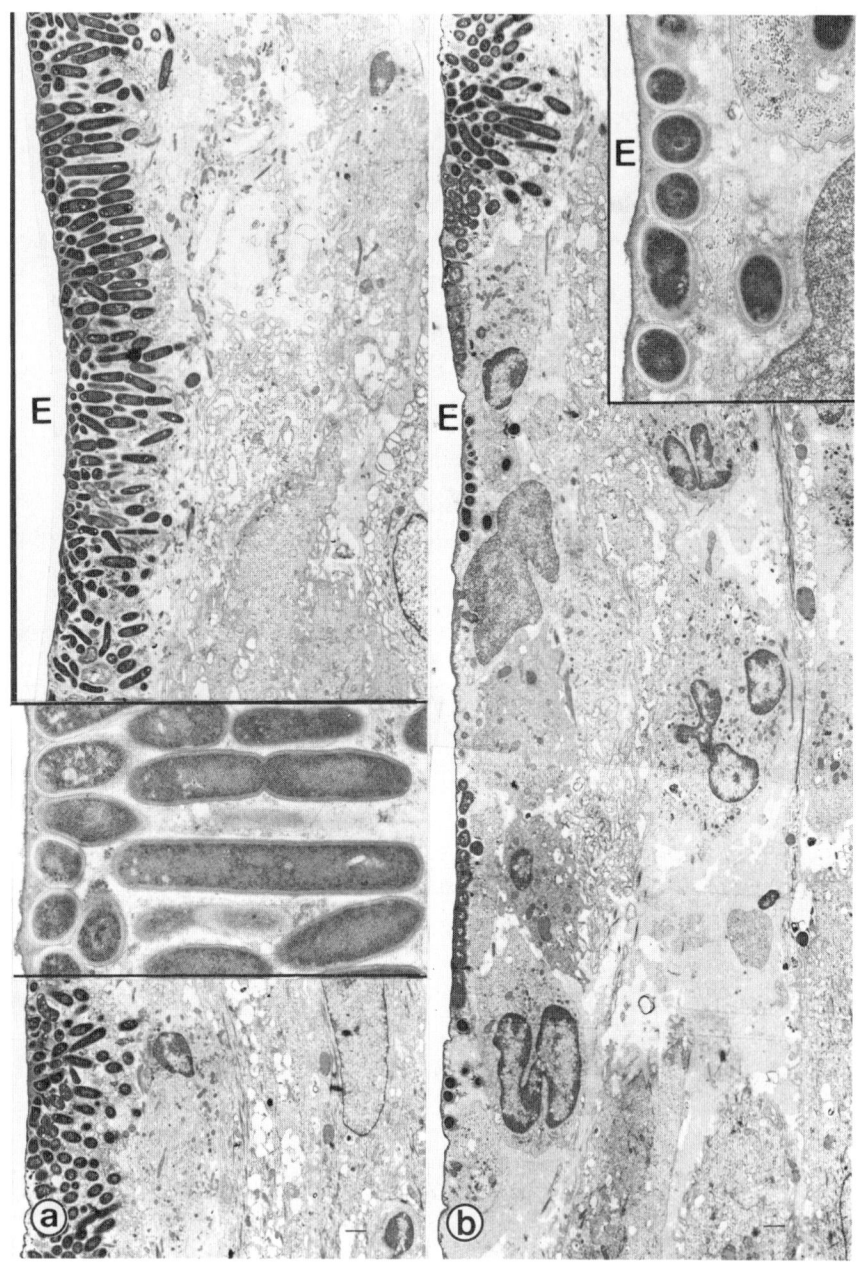

Fig. 10

7. Pocket Formation

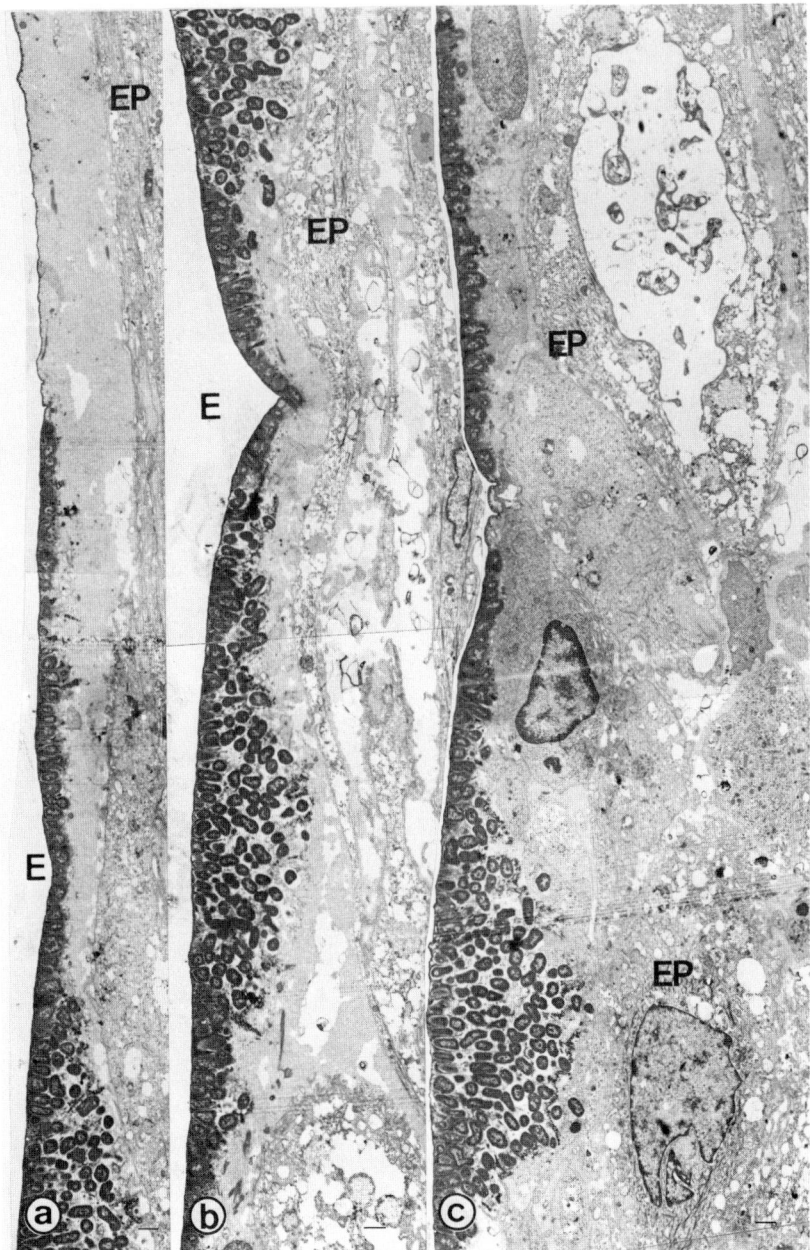

Fig. 11

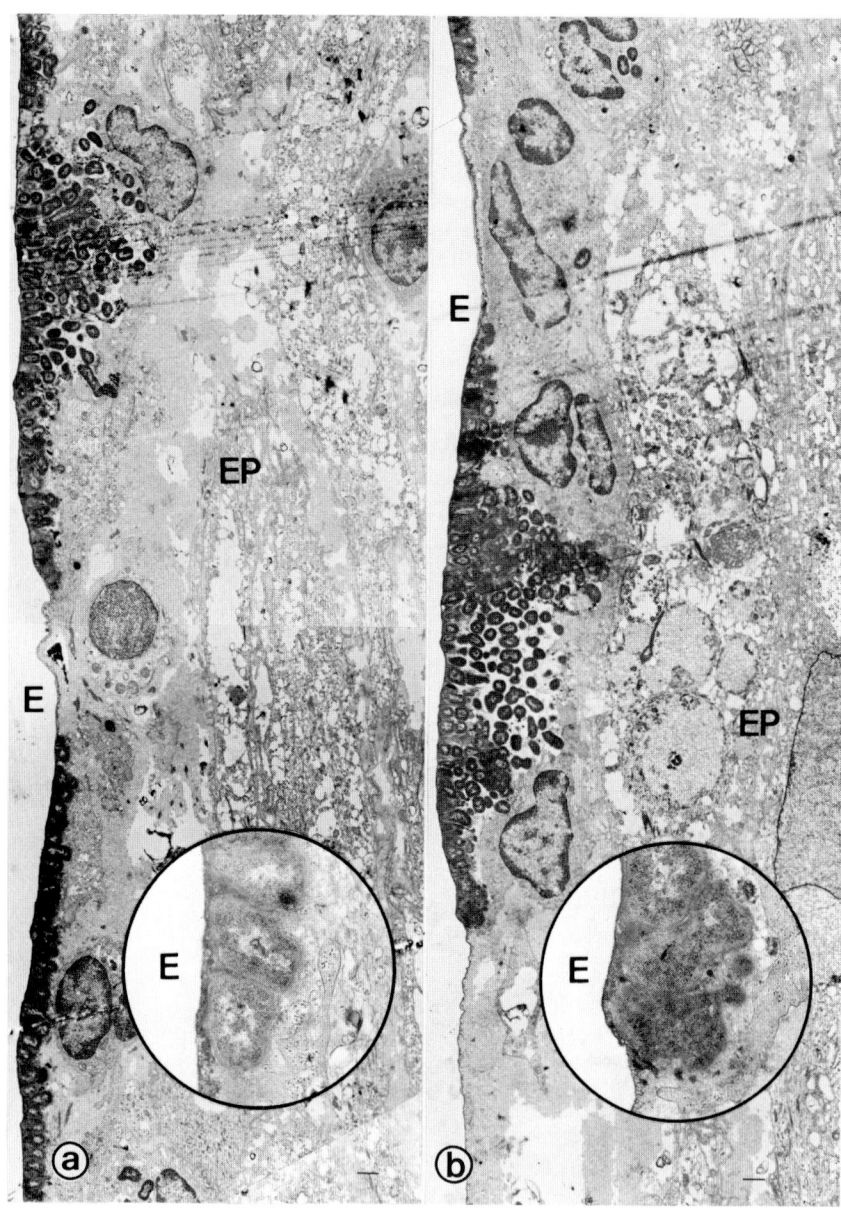

Fig. 12

the epithelium from the enamel surface, even apically to the termination of the subgingival plaque (Figs. 1(c), 3(b) and (c)). In both instances, the junctional epithelium, when separated from its attachment to the tooth surface, resembled a pocket epithelium, i.e. revealed ridge- or finger-like epithelial proliferation into the underlying inflamed connective tissues (Figs 1, 3 and 4).

In general, the supragingival plaque was slightly thicker than its subgingival continuation (Figs. 4(a), (b), and 6(a)); plaque thickness gradually decreased in an apical direction. When seen by electron microscopy, the basal layer of subgingival plaque, facing the enamel surface, consisted predominantly of a monolayer or multilayer of cocci (Figs 5, 9, 10, 11 and 12). Frequently, these cocci were attached to and embedded in an extracellular electron-dense material which also covered some of the enamel (Figs 10(a) and (b), insets). In the coronal part of the subgingival region, the basal layer of cocci was covered by rods, with an occasional presence of filamentous organisms and a few yeasts cells (Fig. 9). Further apically, the subgingival plaque appeared to comprise cocci only, occurring as variably dense monolayers and in the form of larger focal colonies (Figs 5(a), (b) and 7(c)). At its most apical termination, the subgingival plaque ended always in the form of a monolayer of Gram-positive cocci (Figs 5(b) inset, 12(b) and 14(a), (b)). In the monolayers of cocci, the dividing planes appeared to be mostly oriented perpendicular to the enamel surface (Figs 11(a), (c), 12(a)). On the other hand, in multilayers of cocci and rods the dividing planes occurred parallel to the enamel surface (Figs 5(a) and (b), 10(a), 12(a) and (b)).

Laterally to the subgingival plaque an inflammatory exudate, including strands of fibrin and various leukocytes, extended along the entire bacterial layer (Figs 5(a) and (b), 9(a) and (b), 10(a) and (b), 11(a)–(c), 12(a) and (b)). Between discontinuous bacterial colonies, there were plaque-free portions of enamel, covered by remnants of disintegrated epithelial cells and exudate. Occasionally single bacteria, varying in morphology, were found within the exudate at some distance lateral to the plaque surface (Figs 5(a) and 9(b), inset). Many inflammatory cells revealed signs of degeneration but phagocytosis was rarely observed (Figs 5(a), 10(a) and (b), 12(a) and (b)).

The extension of subgingival plaque, as well as the type and degree of inflammatory response, varied greatly, even from block to block within the same gingival biopsy. This is demonstrated by comparing Figs 4 and 6, the latter representing a block adjacent to that of the former. In the block shown in Fig. 6, subgingival plaque was discontinuous, its apical portions consisting of isolated focal patches of bacterial microcolonies. The inflammatory response consisted of a very dense mononuclear infiltrate situated not only in a broad zone of the underlying connective tissue, but also within the junctional epithelium, the latter being almost totally obscured (Figs 6(a)–(c)).

In another tooth taken from the same dog (see Figs 4–6), there was also great variability of subgingival plaque extension (Figs 7(a) and 8(a)), but in contrast to the block shown in Fig. 6, the inflammatory response was minimal. In the block shown in Fig. 7(a), a thin supragingival plaque extended subgingivally, its most apical portion being slightly discontinuous and the focal bacterial islands rather large (Figs 7(b) and(c)). Within a very short distance from this block, the subgingival plaque extended apically, the total subgingival plaque extension amounting close to 1 mm (Fig. 8(a)). In the latter block, the subgingival plaque was rather thin and almost continuous, covered by either degenerated epithelial cells or inflammatory cells (Figs 8(b), (c) and (d)). At the electron microscopic level (Figs 9–12), the entire dento-gingival junction, as shown in Figs 8(b), (c) and (d), is depicted in the form of continuous overlapping series of electron micrographs. In the most coronal portion (Figs 9(a) and (b)), the subgingival plaque consisted of a basal layer of cocci, occasionally interrupted by rods and yeast cells, on which multilayers of additional cocci and rods were implanted. Occasionally, flagellated microoganisms, possibly spirochetes, were seen (Fig. 9(a), inset). These organisms became more numerous as the plaque layer increased in thickness, i.e. at the transition from the sub- to the supragingival deposits. Further apically (Fig. 10), the rod-cocci plaque (Fig. 10(a), inset) became thinner and the rods disappeared (Fig. 10(b)). A monolayer of cocci of variable density continued to extend, albeit discontinuously, in an apical direction (Fig. 10(b) inset). Further apically (Fig. 11), the coccoid monolayer terminated but reappeared again after a short strand of plaque-free enamel (Fig. 11(a)). Still further apically the extending basal monolayer of cocci widened into several multilayered coccoid colonies, following each other at various intervals (Figs 11(a)–(c), 12(a) and (b)).

This pattern of monolayered and multilayered foci of cocci continued until, at its most apical termination, the subgingival plaque ended in the form of a short monolayer of cocci (Fig. 12(b)). In many instances, the basal monolayer of cocci continued along the enamel surface, even underneath the multilayered patches (Figs 11 and 12). Most of the dividing planes in this coccoid monolayer were perpendicular to the enamel surface, the morphology of these bacteria being rather uniform. Lateral to the subgingival plaque (Figs 9–12) there was a broad zone of exudative material, fibrin and inflammatory cells, with the junctional epithelial cells showing signs of degeneration. None of these epithelial cells revealed desmosomal junctions (Figs. 11(a)–(c), 12(a)).

The discontinuity of subgingival plaque observed in random sections cut perpendicular to the enamel was further investigated by means of reconstructions derived from consecutive serial sections over distances of up to 200 μm (Fig. 13). These reconstructions revealed that, within the area of the enamel surface covered by subgingival plaque, there were irregularly shaped plaque-free islands. These islands extended in a mesio-distal direction and, in

7. Pocket Formation 113

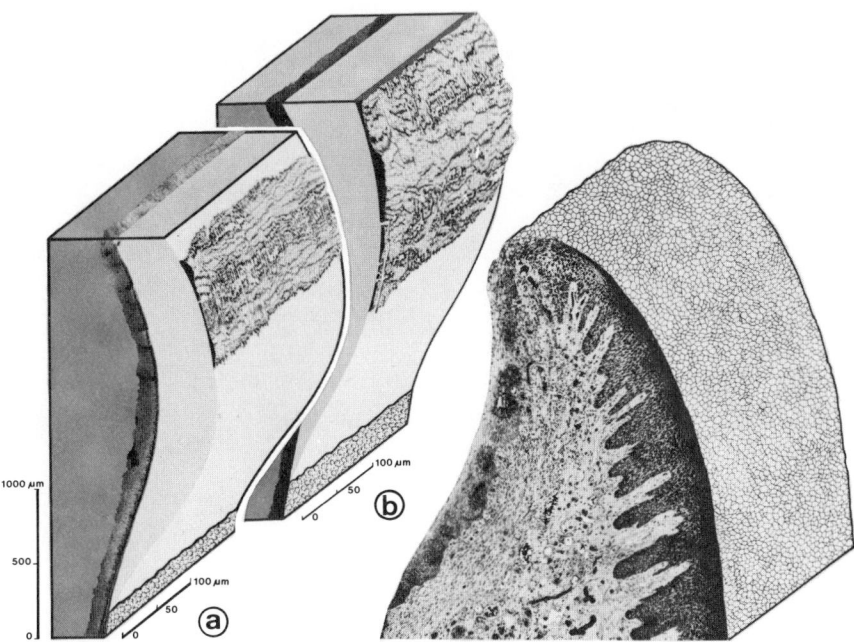

Fig. 13 Reconstruction of the dental plaque incorporated into a three dimensional view of two gingival portions adjacent to either purely subginival plaque (a) or supra- and subginival plaque (b). Note small irregular plaque-free zones within the region covered by subgingival plaque.

part, were either connected to each other or interrupted by continuous portions of subgingival plaque (Figs 13(a) and (b)).

The apical termination of subgingival plaque followed an irregular course in a mesio-distal direction (Fig. 13). It consisted of a monolayer of cocci and was related to the surrounding tissue in either of two principle ways. First, the terminal layer of cocci (Fig. 14(a)) was close to the intact cells of the junctional epithelium, forming an epithelial attachment within a short distance apically to the plaque border. In these cases, the epithelial portion lateral to the subgingival plaque was structurally intact and unimpaired by inflammatory exudate. Second, the apical termination of subgingival plaque and its more coronal protion were separated from the junctional epithelium by a relatively wide zone, comprising single, detached and degenerated epithelial cells, as well as exudative material, such as fibrin and leukocytes (Fig. 14(b)). This zone extended for various distances apically to the plaque border, i.e. the junctional epithelium was separated from the enamel surface in front of the subgingival plaque. Both patterns appeared within the same biopsy.

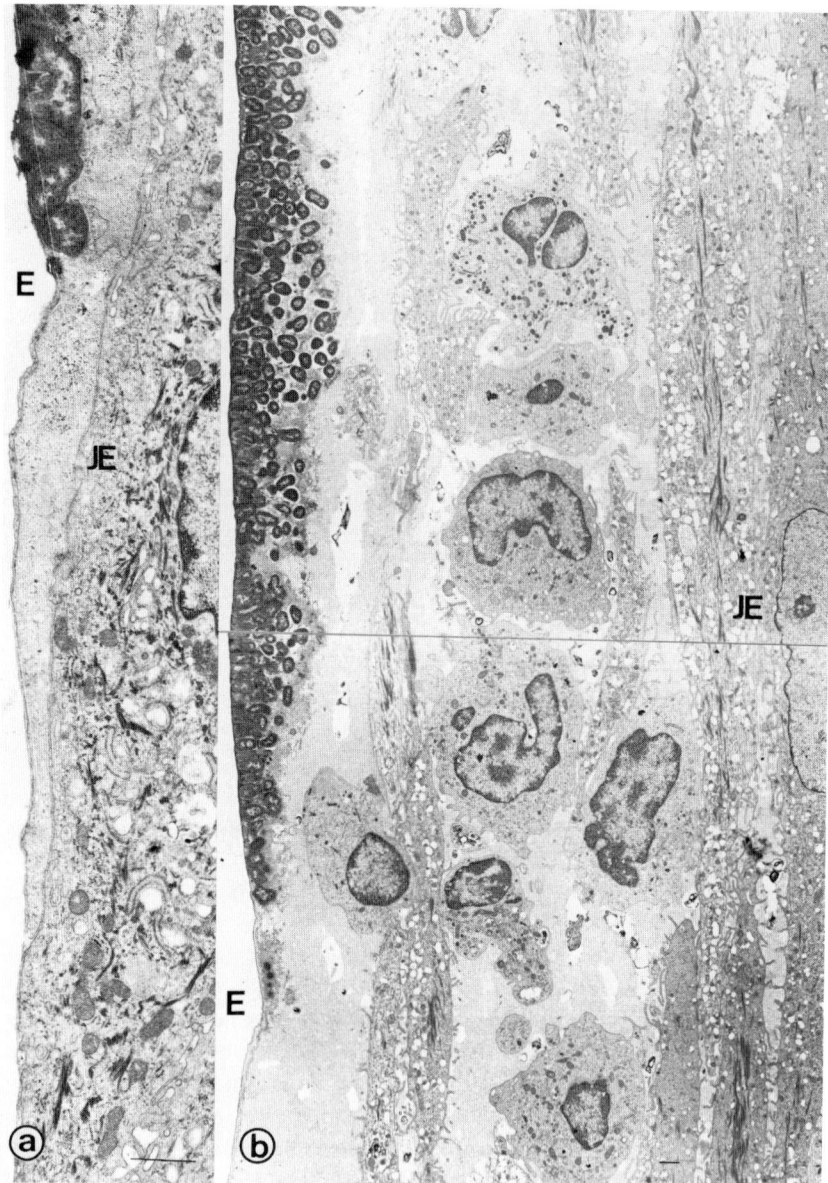

Fig. 14 Electron micrographs of the apical termination of subginival plaque (monolayer of cocci), in close relationship either to the most coronal cells of the junctional epithelium (JE in (a)) or to a band of leukocytes and single degenerated epithelial cells (b) separating the JE from the plaque-covered enamel surface (E). Magnification: (a) ×9180; (b) ×2620.

Discussion

The histopathological material presented in this paper, for the first time, provides information about the tissue changes along the dento-gingival junction after a very short period (4 days) of *de novo* subgingival plaque formation. This material, therefore, offers an opportunity to formulate a new hypothesis of the development of gingival pockets.

Many theories on the mode of formation of gingival and periodontal pockets claimed that apical migration of the junctional epithelium is the main event, leading to pocket formation; this may or may not be preceded by a destruction of the underlying collagen fibre attachment to the root surface (Goldman, 1944; Aisenberg and Aisenberg, 1948, 1951; Fish, 1948). Other authors held the view that pocket formation is initiated by the dissolution of epithelial attachment (junctional epithelium); this dissolution may be due to trauma, infection or to the degeneration of the enamel epithelium (Becks, 1929; Skillen, 1930). They implied that the accumulation of debris and bacteria are secondary to the formation of pockets. Wilkinson (1935) argued that epithelial proliferation and subsequent degeneration of epithelial cells facing the tooth surface would lead to pocket formation and that inflammatory changes are secondary to epithelial changes. A contrary view was held by Nuckolls *et al.* (1950), who claimed that vascular and inflammatory changes in the periodontal tissues were the initial events resulting in epithelial proliferation, keratinization and an increased rate of desquamation which eventually would lead to separation of the epithelium from the tooth surface. These authors also claimed that the epithelium would secondarily cover the primary inflammatory lesion of the connective tissue. Furthermore, Orban (1926, 1927, 1947) and Orban and Weinmann (1942) proposed impaired cementum formation to be the primary cause of pocket formation, resulting in a dissolution of the collagen fibre attachment and subsequent downgrowth of the junctional epithelium. A common feature of these hypotheses is that they all consider subgingival bacterial growth to be secondary to the opening of the pocket.

It is surprising that so much emphasis has been placed on theories around epithelial changes, while almost none of the authors, with two exceptions, related pocket formation to the presence of bacterial deposits. These two exceptions were Box (1941) and Waerhaug (1952). The former proposed that the periodontal pocket is initiated by invasion of bacteria from the base of the sulcus, leading to inflammation, ulceration and loss of epithelial and connective tissue attachment. The latter argued, and later extended his argument (Waerhaug, 1976, 1978*a,b*, 1979), that "the progressive deposition in an apical direction of subgingival calculus appears in most cases to be the immediate cause of the deepening of the pocket" (Waerhaug, 1952).

The present material and the interpretation derived from it is in line with the latter views. In reviewing the essential features detected in this material a number of conclusions can be drawn. (a) In the relative absence of neutrophilic granulocytes, subgingival plaque formed and extended up to 1 mm subgingivally, within a period of 4 days. (b) This subgingival bacterial spread did not meet with an efficient alternative cellular defence, as in spite of numerous mononuclear leukocytes being present, phagocytosis was rarely observed. (c) There was a consistent pattern of subgingival plaque composition. Mostly, Gram-positive cocci formed the basal layer of plaque which was attached to the enamel surface. To a very large extent, the basal layer appeared to be continuous from the supragingival to the subgingival deposits. Apparently discontinuous focal patches of coccoid colonies in the depth of the subgingival space were continuous laterally with strands of deposits which in turn were continuous with more superficial and apical plaque. (d) Basal layers of colonies of cocci were mixed with and overgrown by rods, some yeast cells, and, in more coronal regions, even by flagellated bacteria, possibly spirochetes. (e) The most apical termination of subgingival plaque consisted of cocci only, with their dividing planes perpendicular to the enamel surface. (f) At the apical front of the subgingival plaque, Gram-positive cocci were either surrounded by largely intact cells of the junctional epithelium or covered by a zone of exudate, extending apically to the plaque front. (g) When separated from its attachment to the enamel by subgingival plaque the former junctional epithelium often resembled a pocket epithelium.

In general terms pocket formation can be visualized as the result of successful bacterial strategies adopted to allow invasion of a tissue. The first requirement of the bacterium is to be able to attach and multiply on tissue or cell surfaces (Gibbons and van Houte, 1975). Second, the bacterium must overcome the defence mechanisms. This is done by a variety of options such as resisting phagocytosis by the production of surface slime (polysaccharide capsule) or by other means to avoid opsonization, killing the phagocytes by producing "toxins" (streptolysin), or, when being engulfed by a phagocyte, resisting digestion and inhibiting lysosomal fusion (Mims, 1977). In addition to this, certain bacteria have the ability to inhibit chemotactic movements of neutrophil granulocytes (Mims, 1977). Furthermore, various forms of bacterial locomotion appear to be necessary. There are several ways in which bacteria may be translocated or spread on surfaces or within tissues. If a solid substrate is available, the attached bacteria may spread simply by growth in a lateral direction or by gliding. Provided there is a liquid medium enabling locomotive movements, bacteria may be gliding, propelling, bending by contraction or move by wave-like action of flagella (Smith, 1976; Mims, 1977).

These bacterial strategies have been tested and investigated only to a limited

7. Pocket Formation

degree, as they may relate to the infection of the dento-gingival region (Gibbons and van Houte, 1975). However, the present material allows bacterial behaviour to be interpreted in the relative absence of normal cellular and humoral defences, within a short period of time. Pocket formation was initiated by Gram-positive cocci which attached to the tooth surface and spread by lateral growth, both in a corono-apical as well as in a horizontal direction. Owing to this, the junctional epithelium was split from its attachment to the tooth surface. Second, once this split had been established, other bacteria such as rods, filaments and spirochetes moved into the area, using various forms of locomotion in the liquid phase covering the coccoid plaque. These organisms then colonized and grew perpendicular to the tooth surface. The primary spread of cocci may have occurred unimpaired by any inflammatory response. Some of the secondary bacteria may have elicited a weak abnormal inflammatory response with little phagocytosis. This response resulted in a zone of exudation which helped to separate the former junctional epithelium from the subgingival plaque, as well as from the enamel, apical to the plaque front not yet attacked by bacteria. This in turn offered new surface space for further spread and colonization of bacteria more apically.

If this sequence of events is true for the present experiment, it may also occur in the presence of a competent or a temporarily impaired defence reaction, i.e. under "normal" conditions. Under such circumstances it would be of advantage to bacteria if the initial subgingival spread could be performed by cocci of minimal pathogenic potentiality, i.e. provoking as little acute inflammatory response as possible. Thus, bacterial spread and colonization would proceed unimpeded at the beginning of pocket formation. Furthermore, bacterial locomotion and colonization would be successful only if bacteria had means to evade phagocytosis while approaching the site of subgingival colonization. In fact, a spread by growing bacteria attached to the tooth surface and superficially protected by polysaccharides is probably one of the safest mechanisms to exclude phagocytosis by leukocytes.

Based on these observations and assumptions, an hypothesis can be formulated which, in general terms, attempts to explain pocket formation.

In contrast to most of the previous theories claiming or implying that pocket formation occurs before bacterial colonization in the subgingival area, our hypothesis is that pocket formation is the result of bacteria spreading subgingivally. This general notion is consistent with the views of Waerhaug (1952, 1976, 1978a,b, 1979). Assuming that cocci, possibly "non-pathogenic", are able to split the junctional epithelium from its attachment to the tooth surface and that other bacteria of varying pathogenic potential follow into the established defect, pocket formation and the accompanying shift of pathophysiological and defending host reactions can be summarized as shown in Figs 15, 16 and 17. If not mechanically removed, the supragingival plaque,

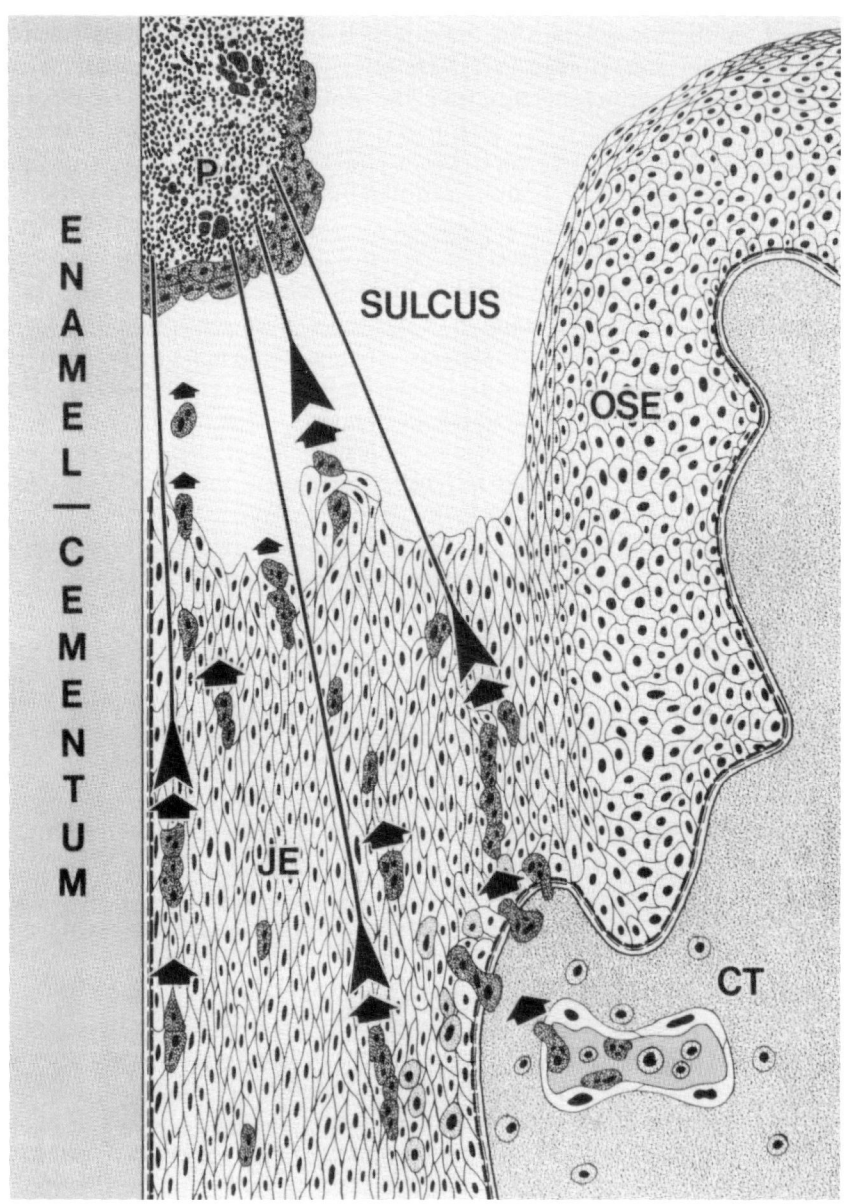

Fig. 15

terminating at a certain distance coronal to the sulcus bottom, may exist in a stable environment for unknown periods of time (Schroeder, 1977). In this situation, there is a balance between bacterial multiplication and metabolism on the one hand and the host defence on the other. The latter includes a continuous cellular exudation with neutrophil granulocytes being chemotactically attracted and moving in an apico-coronal direction (Fig. 15).

Using a variety of strategies, in particular during a period of low or partially impaired host defence bacteria, most probably cocci first, start to grow and translocate in an apical direction. This results in permanent separation of the coronal and deeper portions of the junctional epithelium from the tooth surface (Fig. 16). The separation may be aided by inflammatory exudative factors which result from the bacterial metabolites being produced. Having reached a subgingival site, the bacteria form various types of complex, multilayered deposits. The direction of the defence, i.e. exudation, is shifted horizontally and the former junctional epithelium, being exposed to various degrees of chronic exudation, becomes transformed into a pocket epithelium. In an apical direction, the latter remains continuous with a junctional epithelium of reduced height (Fig. 17). In such a manner, a pocket of varying depth may be formed. Once the bacteria approach a critical distance to the apical termination of the junctional epithelium, the latter begins to proliferate apically in order to maintain an epithelial attachment. In fact, such apical strands of junctional epithelium can always be observed at the bottom of gingival and periodontal pockets in man.

This hypothesis can be tested. Indeed, Slots and Gibbons (1978) have provided data suggesting that colonization of the periodontitis-associated *Bacteroides melaninogenicus* subsp. *asaccharolyticus* is through attachment to Gram-positive bacteria, such as various species of actinomyces and streptococci, rather than to the tooth surface. In other words, the data of these authors imply that the presence of a Gram-positive plaque in the subgingival area is an essential prerequisite for secondary colonization of other particularly pathogenic organisms. These data are in accord with and support the hypothesis presented. Furthermore, experiments can be designed, which would (1) help to determine the means of bacterial spread and the sequence of bacterial colonization in the subgingival area; (2) evaluate the types of bacterial strategies used in order to overcome the defence system; (3) test the potential of various plaque-forming and other subgingival bacteria to elicit

Figs 15–17 Schematic drawings illustrating a possible mechanism of formation of gingival and periodontal pockets, including the pocket epithelium (PE): Fig. 15 shows a balanced situation within the gingival sulcus; Fig. 16 illustrates the progressing front of subgingivally extending plaque, splitting the junctional epithelium (JE) from the tooth surface; Fig. 17 shows an established pocket. Large triangular arrows indicate chemotactic forces attracting neutrophil granulocytes. CT, connective tissue; OSE, oral sulcular epithelium; P, plaque.

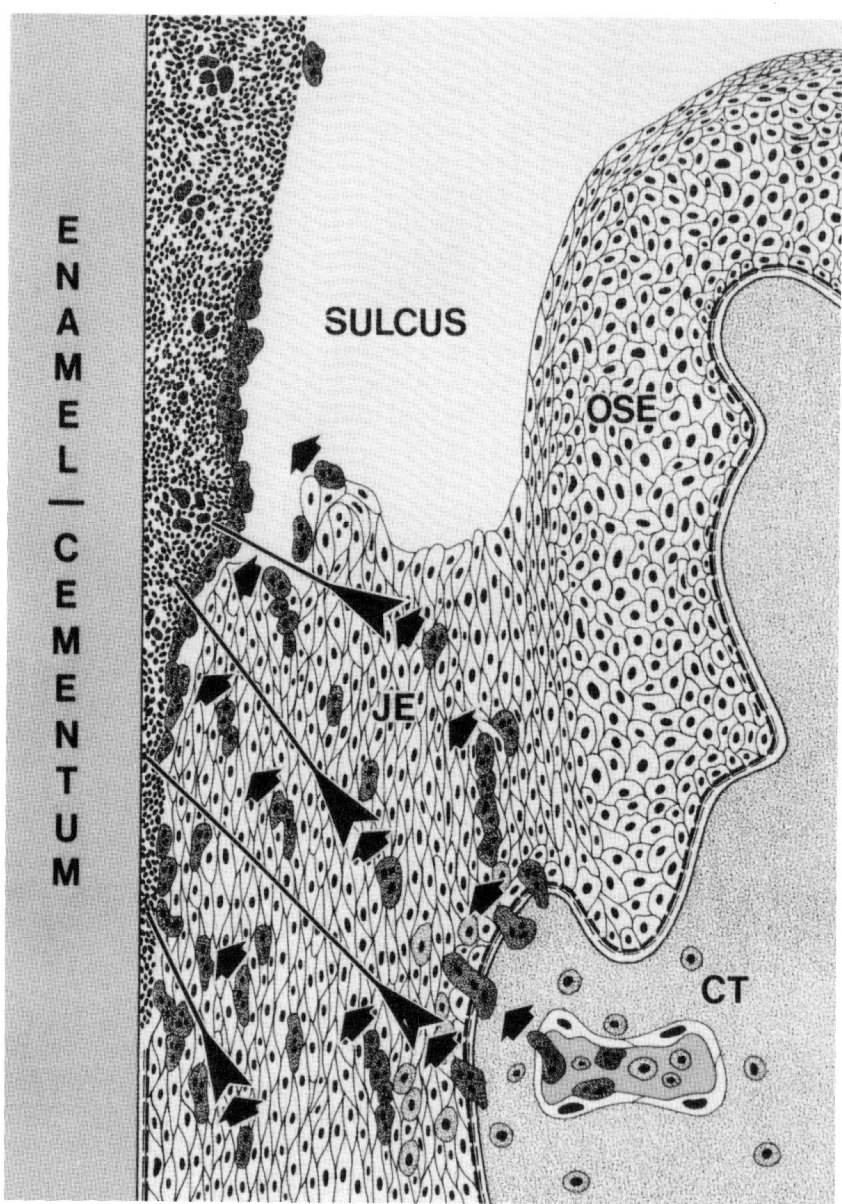

Fig. 16

7. Pocket Formation

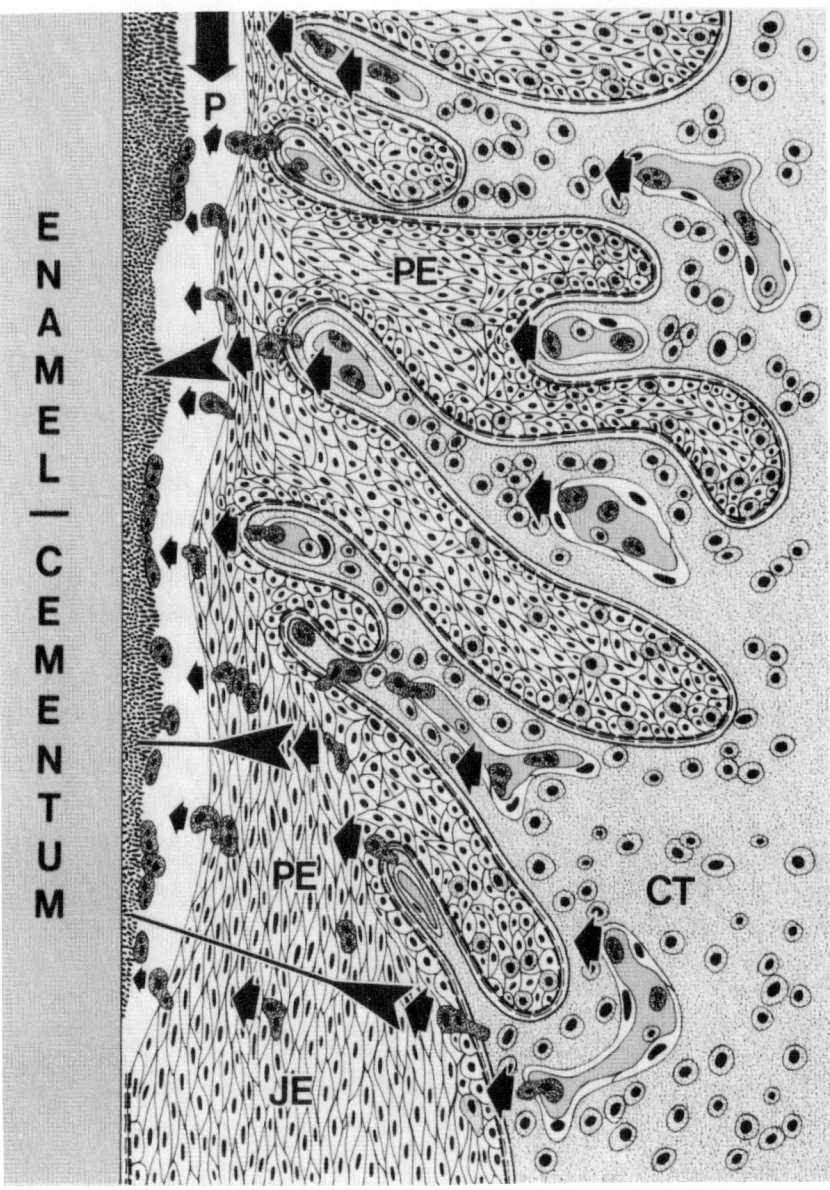

Fig. 17

maximal or minimal inflammatory reactions in the gingivo-dental region. Such experiments, however, cannot be done in rodents as a great number of past experiments in rats has shown that periodontal destruction in these animals occur in the absence of narrow and deep pockets typically seen in monkeys, dogs or man.

Summary

The role of neutrophil granulocytes in initial gingivitis was evaluated by experimental neutropenia in dogs, under clinical conditions known to allow formation of dental plaque. The dogs were kept neutropenic for a period of 4 days by repeated injections of anti-neutrophil serum. On day 4, block biopsies of the gingival tissues were harvested and prepared for light and electron microscopy. Deep subgingival plaque was found to have formed in all gingival biopsies. In the present paper, the histopathology of the newly formed subgingival plaque and the adjacent gingival lesion are presented. The subgingival plaque consisted of a variably thick layer of Gram-positive microorganisms, which also occurred in the form of a monolayer. The bacteria facing the enamel surface were cocci, which were always the only monolayer-forming organism, in particular at the advancing apical front of the subgingival plaque. In more coronal regions there were rods, filaments, and occasionally motile organisms implanted on the coccoid layers. The adjacent epithelial tissue was often but not always separated from the bacteria by an exudate which extended apically to the plaque. Occasionally, the subgingival plaque was in close contact with cells of the former junctional epithelium, which mostly exhibited a morphology resembling that of a pocket epithelium. The histopathology of the dento-gingival region and the formation of subgingival plaque in neutropenic animals during initial gingivitis allowed us to formulate a new and testable hypothesis, attempting to explain the formation of gingival and periodontal pockets. This hypothesis suggests that pathological pockets are formed by microbial invasion of the subgingival tooth areas destroying the coronal epithelial attachment. Inflammatory changes separating the junctional epithelium from the tooth surface appear to be secondary phenomena. The hypothesis is based on considerations of the strategies used by bacteria when they successfully cause infection in higher organisms and is discussed in relation to previous theories on the formation of gingival periodontal pockets.

Acknowledgement

We are greatly indebted to Mrs K. Rossinsky and Mrs A. Schwarzenbach for their skilfull technical assistance. In particular, we wish to thank and acknowledge the help of Miss Marie-Claude Moreillon, who provided the reconstruction of subgingival plaque distribution.

References

Aisenberg, M. S. and Aisenberg, A. D. (1948). *Oral Surg.* **1**, 1047–1055.
Aisenberg, M. S. and Aisenberg, A. D. (1951). *Oral Surg.* **4**, 317–320.
Attström, R. and Schroeder, H. E. (1979). *Scand. J. dent. Res.* **87**, 7–23.
Becks, H. (1929). *J. Am. dent. Assoc.* **16**, 2167–2188.
Box, H. K. (1941). *J. Can. dent. Assoc.* **13**, 3.
Fish, E. W. (1948). *Surgical Pathology of the Mouth*, Isaac Pitman and Sons, London, p. 316.
Fraska, J. M. and Parks, V. R. (1965). *J. Cell Biol.* **25**, 157–161.
Gibbons, R. J. and van Houte, J. (1975). *A. Rev. Microbiol.* **29**, 19–44.
Goldman, H. M. (1944). *J. dent. Res.* **23**, 177–180.
Listergarten, M. A. (1976). *J. Periodont.* **47**, 1–18.
Listergarten, M. A. and Helldén, L. (1978). *J. clin. Periodont.* **5**, 115–132.
Mims, C. A. (1977). *The Pathogenesis of Infectious Disease*, Academic Press, London.
Nuckolls, J., Dienstein, B., Bell, D. G. and Rule, R. W., Jr (1950). *J. Periodont.* **21**, 7–18.
Orban, B. (1926). *Z. Stomat.* **24**, 515–525.
Orban, B. (1927). *Z. Stomat.* **25**, 827–835.
Orban, B. (1947). *Am. J. Orthodont.* **33**, 637–657.
Orban, B. and Weinmann, J. P. (1942). *J. Periodont.* **13**, 31–45.
Reynolds, E. S. (1963). *J. Cell Biol.* **17**, 208–212.
Schroeder, H. E. (1973). *Helv. odont. Acta* **17**, 6–18.
Schroeder, H. E. (1977). In *Borderland between Caries and Periodontal Disease* (T. Lehner, ed.), pp. 43–78, Academic Press, London.
Schroeder, H. E. and Attström, R. (1979). *Scand. J. dent. Res.* **87**, 279–287.
Skillen, W. G. (1930). *J. Am. dent. Assoc.* **17**, 1088–1110.
Slots, J. (1979). *J. clin. Periodont.* **6**, 351–382.
Slots, J. and Gibbons, R. J. (1978). *Infect. Immun.* **19**, 254–264.
Smith, A. L. (1976). *Microbiology and Pathology*, 11th edn, Mosby, St. Louis, pp. 31–33.
Socransky, S. S. (1977). *J. Periodont.* **48**, 497–504.
Waerhaug, J. (1952). *Ondont. Tidskr.* **60**, Suppl. 1.
Waerhaug, J. (1976). *J. Periodont.* **47**, 636–642.
Waerhaug, J. (1978a). *J. Periodont.* **49**, 1–8.
Waerhaug, J. (1978b). *J. Periodont.* **49**, 119–134.
Waerhaug, J. (1979). *J. Periodont.* **50**, 355–365.
WHO (1978). *Epidemiology, Etiology and Prevention of Periodontal Diseases*, Technical Report Series no. 621, WHO, Geneva.
Wilkinson, F. C. (1935). *Dent. Rec.* **55**, 145–147.

8. Stimulation of Gingival Lymphocytes by Antigens from Oral Bacteria

L. IVANYI

Introduction

It has been reported previously that peripheral blood lymphocytes from patients with gingival or periodontal disease respond by enhanced *in vitro* proliferation to antigens from oral bacteria and dental plaque, as compared with subjects with clinically healthy gingiva (Ivanyi and Lehner, 1970, 1971; Horton *et al.*, 1972; Baker *et al.*, 1976; Patters *et al.*, 1976). Furthermore, no significant stimulation by *Veillonella* and plaque antigens is observed in lymphocyte cultures from patients with severe periodontitis (Ivanyi *et al.*, 1973; Baker *et al.*, 1978), although this finding is challenged by other authors (Patters *et al.*, 1976). However, the question of the reactivity of the lymphocytes localized within the gingival tissue has not been explored previously.

The aims of this study were to find out if lymphocytes isolated from the gingiva of patients undergoing periodontal surgery would respond *in vitro* to oral bacterial antigens. Furthermore, the pattern of response of gingival and peripheral blood lymphocytes was compared in individual patients.

Materials and Methods

Patients

Forty-two patients with periodontal disease were investigated. Each patient underwent a course of therapy to remove plaque and to reduce gingival inflammation before periodontal surgery. Russell's periodontal index (PI) was used to determine the degree of severity of periodontal disease, since this index has been used in our previous studies and we wished to compare these investigations. Pocket depth and bone loss were also measured. Two groups of patients were evaluated. Group 1 consisted of 23 patients (12 males and 11 females) ranging in age from 23 to 56 years with moderate periodontitis (MP; PI <4.0, pocket depth up to 5 mm; bone resorption up to half of the root). Group 2 consisted of 19 patients (9 males and 10 females) ranging in age from 26 to 58 years with severe periodontitis (SP; PI >4.0, pocket depth over 5 mm, bone resorption over half of the root). Many of these patients required a combination of periodontal surgery and extractions because of extensive bone loss.

Gingival tissue was excised from both facial and oral aspects of at least six teeth in each patient undergoing periodontal surgery. Twelve biopsies came from the upper right, 10 from the upper left, 10 from the lower left and 10 from the lower right quadrants before the surgery was carried out. On this occasion each patient had a blood specimen taken.

Stimulants

Veillonella alcalescens (V) and a human strain of *Actinomyces viscosus* (A) were cultured and disintegrated by ultrasonication as described previously (Ivanyi and Lehner, 1970) and used at the optimal concentration of 20 µg of protein per millilitre of culture for V and 10 µg of protein per millilitre of culture for A (Ivanyi and Lehner, 1978). Phytohaemagglutinin (PHA) (Wellcome Reagents, Beckenham, U.K.) was used at a dilution of 1:100 per millilitre of culture.

Lymphoid Cell Suspensions and DNA Synthesis

Gingival tissue was minced with scalpel and scissors in medium TC 199 enriched with added L-glutamine (2 mmol/ml), penicillin (100 IU/ml) and streptomycin (100 µg/ml), and passed through a stainless steel sieve (100 mesh) to retain debris and epithelial cells. To avoid bacterial contamination, all suspensions were also passed through a gradient of fetal calf serum (1200 r.p.m. for 10 min), washed three times and then counted. More than 90% of lymphocytes were viable, as assessed by the trypan blue exclusion test. Duplicate cultures were set up at a concentration of 4×10^5 lymphocytes per millilitre of culture in the presence of erythrocytes. The cultures were supplemented with 20% autologous serum.

Peripheral blood lymphocytes were isolated from heparinized blood using Ficoll-Triosil, washed three times and their concentration was adjusted to 4×10^5 per millilitre of culture, supplemented with 20% autologous serum.

The cultures were maintained for 5 days and then harvested and assessed as described previously (Ivanyi and Lehner, 1970). The results were expressed as counts per minute (c.p.m.) per 4×10^5 viable lymphocytes and as stimulation indices (SI), which is the ratio between [^{14}C]thymidine uptake in antigen- and saline-stimulated cultures. Analysis of unstimulated cultures showed that a ratio of 2 (for gingival and blood lymphocytes) included three standard deviations above the mean and represented a significant degree of stimulation ($P = 0.01$).

Evaluation of Factors which Might Affect Gingival Lymphocyte Cultures

We first considered whether intravascular lymphocytes represented a significant contamination of gingival lymphocyte cultures. The degree of contamination by intravascular lymphocytes was calculated from the formulae

$$\frac{\text{Number of erythrocytes}}{1700} = \text{Number of blood lymphocytes}$$

and

$$\frac{\text{Number of blood lymphocytes}}{\text{Total number of lymphocytes}} \times 100 = \text{Contamination (\%)}.$$

These formulae were based on the lymphocyte/erythrocyte ratio of one lymphocyte to 1700 erythrocytes in 1 mm^3 of peripheral blood and make the assumption that intravascular lymphocytes and erythrocytes will be in the same ratio.

The results of 13 experiments which yielded gingival cell suspensions containing between 0.8 and 4.6×10^6 lymphocytes and between 0.6 and 2.2×10^7 erythrocytes showed only 0.3% contamination on average with capillary lymphocytes (Table I). Those suspensions which contained less than a total of 2.6×10^6 lymphocytes were discarded.

TABLE I
Percentage Contamination of Gingival Lymphocytes by Capillary Lymphocytes

Patient number	Total yield		Contamination with capillary lymphocytes (%)
	Lymphocytes ($\times 10^6$)	Erythrocytes ($\times 10^7$)	
1	3.5	2.0	0.3
2	2.6	2.1	0.4
3	4.6	1.8	0.2
4	4.2	2.1	0.2
5	2.8	1.2	0.2
6	2.7	1.3	0.1
7	3.0	1.0	0.2
8	3.3	1.2	0.4
9	3.9	1.6	0.2
10	3.3	2.2	0.4
11	1.2	0.6	0.2
12	0.8	0.8	0.5
13	1.9	0.6	0.1
Mean ± S.E.	2.9 ± 0.30	1.4 ± 0.16	0.3 ± 0.03

TABLE II
The Effect of Addition of Erythrocytes on Blood Lymphocyte Stimulation Induced by Veillonella in 5 Patients

Cell suspension		Veillonella	Saline
Lymphocytes	Erythrocytes	(mean c.p.m. ± s.e.)	(mean c.p.m. ± s.e.)
4×10^5	2×10^6	511 ± 148.1	211 ± 26.7
4×10^5	None	461 ± 111.9	197 ± 18.6

c.p.m., counts per minute.

As the suspensions contained approximately a fivefold excess of red cells, we assessed the possible effect of erythrocytes on lymphocyte cultures (Table II). Peripheral blood lymphocytes were cultured either in the absence or presence of erythrocytes, at the same ratio as in the gingival cultures. The results indicated that addition of erythrocytes had no effect on lymphocyte stimulation induced by *Veillonella* (mean c.p.m. of 511 ± 148 and 461 ± 111) or on control cultures with saline (mean c.p.m. of 211 ± 26 and 197 ± 18).

As the gingival tissue was obtained under local anaesthesia, with about 4 ml of xylocaine per quadrant being injected into the buccal sulcus and palatal mucosa for maxillary gingiva and an inferior dental block for the mandibular gingiva, we investigated the effect of local anaesthetic on *in vitro* lymphocyte stimulation (Table III). Peripheral blood lymphocytes were preincubated for 1 h in medium TC 199 alone, or in medium with xylocaine at a dilution of 1:10 or 1:50. The cells were then washed twice and cultures were set up with various stimulants. Preincubation of cells with xylocaine as compared with those

TABLE III
The Effect of Local Anaesthetic on Blood Lymphocyte Stimulation Induced by Various Stimulants

	Stimulants (c.p.m.)			
Xylocaine	PHA*	Veillonella	Actinomyces	Saline
0	34 225	1197	996	240
1:10	39 182	1151	961	232
1:50	36 251	1173	1017	218

* Mean values from two experiments.
c.p.m., counts per minute.

without xylocaine (Table III) had no effect on the extent of lymphocyte stimulation induced by PHA (mean c.p.m. of 34 225, 39 182, 36 251), *Veillonella* (mean c.p.m. of 1197, 1151, 1173) or *Actinomyces* (mean c.p.m. of 996, 961, 1017).

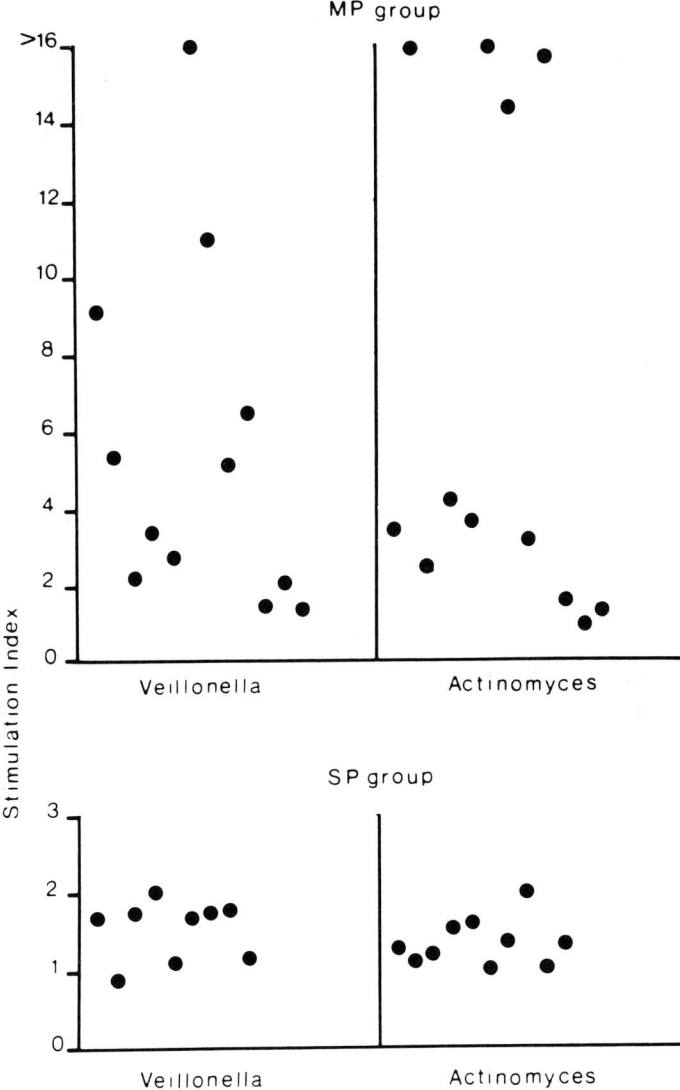

Fig. 1 Stimulation of gingival lymphocytes in two groups of patients. MP group, patients with moderate periodontitis; SP group, patients with severe periodontitis.

Results

In vitro Stimulation of Gingival Lymphocytes in Two Groups of Patients

Gingival lymphocytes from 12 patients with moderate periodontitis (MP group) and from 10 patients with severe periodontitis (SP group) were cultured in the presence of *Veillonella* and *Actinomyces* (Fig. 1). In the MP group gingival lymphocytes from eight patients responded by enhanced DNA synthesis to *Veillonella* (mean SI of 6.6 ± 2.32) and the lymphocytes from seven patients responded to *Actinomyces* (mean SI of 8.8 ± 2.83). However, the values of stimulation indices with both antigens varied considerably, from 0.8 up to 20. In the SP group, gingival lymphocytes from nine patients were not stimulated to a significant degree by *Veillonella* (mean SI of 1.5 ± 0.12) or *Actinomyces* (mean SI of 1.3 ± 0.11). This lack of stimulation was observed in cultures over a range of antigen concentrations (results not presented).

The *in vitro* response of gingival lymphocytes to the T-cell mitogen PHA in the two groups of patients are shown in Table IV. No difference in the degree of stimulation by PHA was observed between the two groups; between 12 000 and 38 000 c.p.m. in the MP group and between 14 000 and 36 000 c.p.m. in the SP group. The results indicate that the lack of *in vitro* lymphocyte response in the SP group was specific for antigens from oral bacteria.

TABLE IV
Stimulation of Gingival Lymphocytes by Phytohaemagglutinin

Patient number	Group	PHA (c.p.m.)	*Veillonella* (c.p.m.)	Saline (c.p.m.)
1	MP	28 128	5097	169
2	MP	15 231	514	122
3	MP	38 343	2230	73
4	MP	17 584	1932	191
5	MP	12 150	491	94
6	SP	14 321	204	123
7	SP	15 830	283	119
8	SP	36 242	273	225
9	SP	16 830	161	119
10	SP	15 973	171	96

MP, moderate periodontitis; SP, severe periodontitis; c.p.m., counts per minute.

Comparison of *in vitro* Responses of Gingival and Blood Lymphocytes

Gingival and blood lymphocytes from 11 patients from the MP group and from nine patients from the SP group were cultured in the presence of

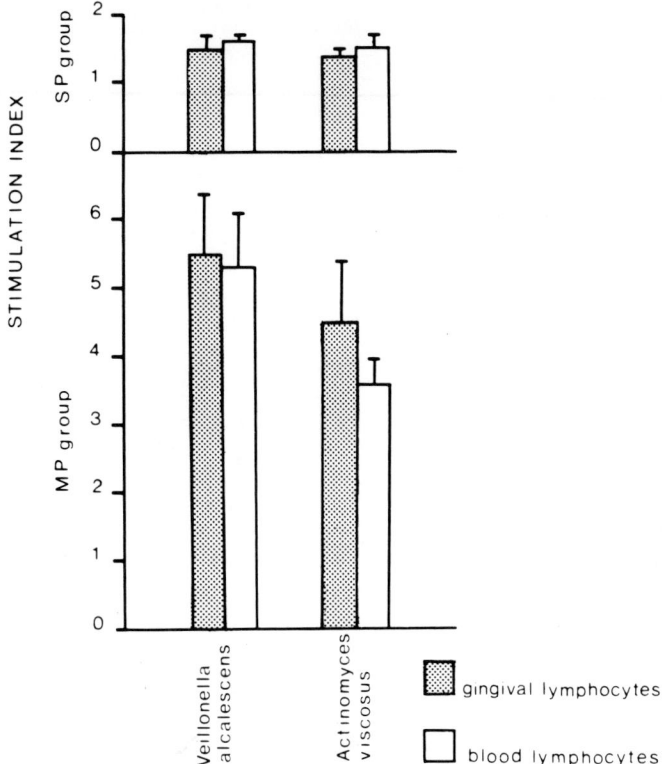

Fig. 2 The *in vitro* response of gingival and blood lymphocytes in patients with periodontal disease. MP group, patients with moderate periodontitis; SP group, patients with severe periodontitis.

Veillonella and *Actinomyces* (Fig. 2). In the MP group, both gingival and blood lymphocytes responded by enhanced DNA synthesis to *Veillonella* (mean SI of 5.5 ± 0.95 and 5.3 ± 0.83) and to *Actinomyces* (mean SI of 4.5 ± 0.92 and 3.6 ± 0.46). In the SP group no significant degree of stimulation was observed in the presence of *Veillonella* (mean SI of 1.5 ± 0.12 and 1.6 ± 0.12) and *Actinomyces* (mean SI of 1.4 ± 0.12 and 1.5 ± 0.17).

The degree of stimulation of gingival and blood lymphocytes was compared in individual patients by Spearman's rank correlation method (Fig. 3). In the MP group a significant positive correlation was found between gingival and blood stimulation indices in cultures with *Veillonella* ($r = 0.68$, $P < 0.02$) and *Actinomyces* ($r = 0.78$, $P < 0.01$). In the SP group the values of stimulation indices were too low to establish any correlation.

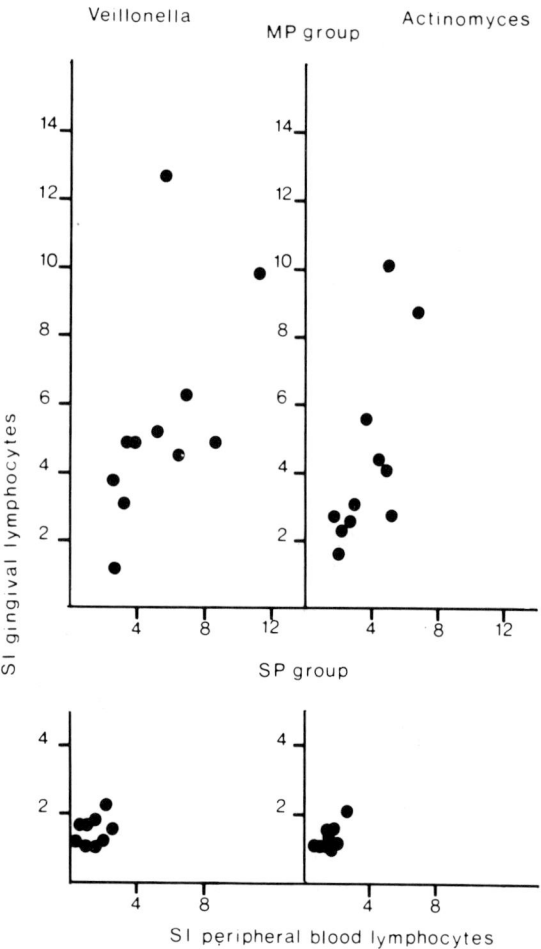

Fig. 3 Correlation between stimulation of gingival and blood lymphocytes in patients with periodontal disease. MP group, patients with moderate periodontitis; SP group, patients with severe perodontitis; SI, stimulation index.

Discussion

In all previous studies of *in vitro* cellular immunity in patients with periodontal disease only peripheral blood lymphocytes have been used. However, the immune reactions to oral bacterial and plaque antigens probably occur within the gingival tissue. Therefore, the first step in this investigation was to isolate lymphocytes from the gingival tissue in order to use them in *in vitro* culture. Gingival lymphocyte suspensions were prepared by a mechanical method, avoiding the use of proteolytic enzymes which may affect the cell surface receptors (Fakhri and Tan, 1975; Viac et al., 1977). Examination of gingival fragments remaining after mechanical treatment revealed the presence of some retained cells. The identification of lymphocyte types within these fragments by immunofluorescent and histochemical techniques suggested that gross lymphocyte selectivity had not occurred during isolation (Topic and L. Ivanyi, in preparation). It was not possible to separate successfully gingival lymphocytes from the erythrocytes on a Ficoll–Triosil gradient. However, the presence of an excess of erythrocytes in the cultures had no effect on the extent of lymphocyte stimulation induced by various stimulants.

The results show that gingival lymphocytes from a large proportion of patients with moderate periodontitis have the functional capacity to respond by *in vitro* proliferation to sonicates from oral bacteria, *V. alcalescens* and *A. viscosus*. Furthermore, the degree of stimulation correlated with that of peripheral blood lymphocytes in individual patients. In contrast, gingival lymphocytes from patients with severe periodontitis failed to respond to oral bacterial antigens. The lack of response seemed to be specific, as these cells responded to the T-cell mitogen PHA. Similar results showing a lack of response of lymphocytes from patients with severe periodontitis to plaque antigens have been reported by other investigators (Baker et al., 1978). These authors have also shown that after therapy (either full extractions or combination of extractions with periodontal surgery) lymphocytes from the same subjects responded significantly to plaque antigens.

The interpretation of these findings would be as follows: Prolonged sensitization with oral bacterial antigens results in systemic immunity. T-lymphocytes become sensitized in lymph nodes and probably also in the spleen, which is followed by their recirculation, as detected by their presence in peripheral blood. The finding of sensitized T-cells within the gingival tissue indicates that they return to the site of antigenic challenge where they may carry out their functional activities. There is some evidence that cellular immunity may play a protective role in the hamster periodontium (Barefoot and Silverman, 1977).

Summary

Lymphocytes isolated from the gingival tissue from patients with moderate periodontitis responded by *in vitro* proliferation to sonicates from oral bacteria, *Veillonella alcalescens* and *Actinomyces viscosus*. In contrast, gingival lymphocytes from patients with severe periodontitis failed to respond to oral bacterial antigens. This lack of response seemed to be specific, as these cells responded to the T-cell mitogen phytohaemagglutinin. The degree of stimulation of gingival lymphocytes correlated with that of peripheral blood lymphocytes in individual patients.

Acknowledgement

I wish to thank Dr J. M. A. Wilton for the supply of *Veillonella* and *Actinomyces* antigens. This investigation was carried out under a Medical Research Council grant.

References

Baker, J. J., Chan, S. P., Socransky, S. S., Oppenheim, J. J. and Mergenhagen, S. E. (1976). *Infect. Immun.* **13**, 1363–1368.
Baker, J. J., Wright, W. E., Chan, S. P. and Oppenheim, J. J. (1978). *Clin. exp. Immunol.* **34**, 199–205.
Barefoot, D. H. and Silverman, M. S. (1977). *J. Periodont.* **48**, 699–704.
Fakhri, O. and Tan, R. S. H. (1975). *Cell. Immunol.* **15**, 452–457.
Horton, J. E., Leiken, S. and Oppenheim, J. J. (1972). *J. Periodont.* **43**, 522–527.
Ivanyi, L. and Lehner, T. (1970). *Archs oral Biol.* **15**, 1089–1096.
Ivanyi, L. and Lehner, T. (1971). *Archs oral Biol.* **16**, 1117–1121.
Ivanyi, L. and Lehner, T. (1978). *Clin. exp. Immunol.* **30**, 252–258.
Ivanyi, L., Challacombe, S. J. and Lehner, T. (1973). *Clin. exp. Immunol.* **14**, 491–500.
Patters, M. R., Genco, R. J., Reed, M. J. and Mashimo, P. A. (1976). *Infect. Immun.* **14**, 1213–1220.
Viac, J., Bustmante, R. and Thivolet, J. (1977). *Br J. Dermat.* **97**, 1–10.

9. Cellular Autoimmunity in Periodontal Disease

E. BOLANOS, D. GNANASEKHAR, G. SINGH,
H. CHURCH and A. E. DOLBY

Autoimmunity: General Concepts

Autoimmunity, the existence of a humoral or cellular immune response to self components, is known to occur in several diseases. The autoimmune response may be organ-specific, as for example in autoimmune thyroiditis where antibody to thyroglobulin is increased, or non-organ-specific, as in systemic lupus erythematosus where antibody to nucleoprotein is detectable.

The awareness of the existence of autoimmune disease is such that immunological theory has had to account for its presence in any overall explanation of the immune response. The original concept of the elimination of self-reactive clones of lymphocytes in fetal life (Burnet, 1957) has had to be modified in the light of the knowledge that there are antibodies to host components, even if in small amounts, in normal animals (Primi et al., 1978). These naturally occurring antibodies are thought to be held at low level or suppressed by specific thymus-derived suppressor cells (Cunningham, 1976; Werkele, 1977), since thymic abnormalities play an important role in the expression of autoimmunity. An immune response to non-self antigens may activate lymphocytes that bear anti-self receptors and had been formerly suppressed. This may occur when the non-self antigens are similar to, but not identical with, self antigens, such as occurs for example in rheumatic heart disease where Group 2a streptoccocal antigens cross-react to varying degrees with antigen of heart muscle (Kaplan and Suchy, 1964).

Some autoimmune responses are undoubtedly pathogenic. Antibody to glomerular basement membrane in acute glomerulo-nephritis is, again, an example of an antibody to a cross-reacting antigen (Lehner et al., 1967). Not only is the active filtration effect of the glomerular basement membrane impaired, but polymorphonuclear leukocytes are attracted to the site of deposition of the anitgen–antibody complexes, with secondary damage occurring due to lysosomal enzyme release (Cochrane, 1969).

All the foregoing comments relate to autoimmunity based upon an abnormal humoral immune response. Cellular autoimmunity implies the reaction of thymus-derived cells with endogenous antigen. Although cellular autoimmunity has been detected in certain diseases, for example enhanced cellular immunity to collagen in rheumatoid arthritis (Trentham et al., 1977), the major evidence for the existence of the phenomenon has come from experiments in animals. The diseases are characterized histologically by an invasive destructive lesion of the organ affected, in which small lymphocytes appear to be closely associated with the damage (Waksman, 1962).

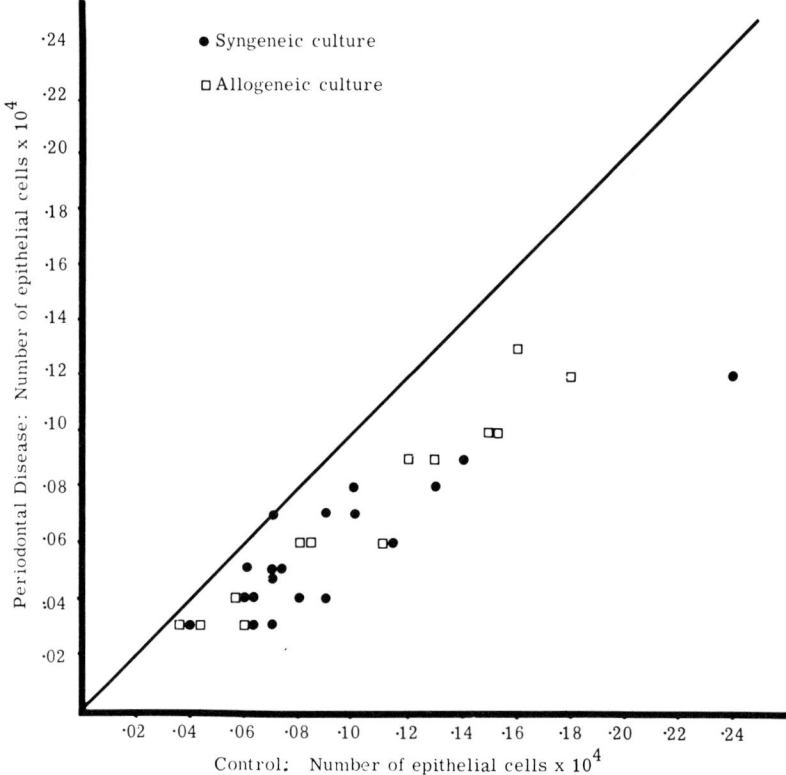

Fig. 1 Relationship of survival of the epithelial cells in the paired cultures from gingiva (0.25% trypsin for 2 h at 37°C) and washed three times (TC 199). Lymphocytes were separated from peripheral blood of patients and control subjects (Coulson and Chalmers, 1964); 10% were non-specific esterase positive. Cultures were incubated in 96-well microculture trays in triplicate for 18 h in a humidified CO_2/air mixture at 37 °C. The number of epithelial cells added to each well was from 1000 to 6000 (mean 2100 ± S.D. 1100); lymphocytes were added in a ratio of 20/1. Additional wells contained epithelial cells with the volume of medium added with the lymphocytes to the mixed cultures. After 18 h samples were counted in a Fuchs Rosenthal counting chamber and viability recorded (0.1% trypan blue exclusion). Each □ or ● represents a paired periodontal disease/control subject experiment with the mean (of three cultures) number of viable epithelial cells compared directly.

Autoimmunity in Periodontal Disease: Lymphocytotoxicity for Oral Epithelial Cells

The possibility that a cellular autoimmune phenomenon may exist in periodontal disease was first raised by the findings of Movius et al., (1975) that there was an impaired survival of gingival epithelial cells when these were cultured with peripheral blood lymphocytes of patients with periodontal disease, compared with their survival when cultured with lymphocytes from healthy, control subjects.

In an extension (Bolanos et al.,1979) of the experiments conducted by Movius et al. (1975), oral epithelial cells obtained from patients suffering from periodontal disease were incubated with lymphocytes from the same subjects ("syngeneic cultures"), from other subjects with periodontal disease ("allogeneic cultures"), or from subjects who were free of periodontal disease (periodontal index, PI <0.5) (Russell, 1956). Thus, in the syngeneic experiments control lymphocytes were not necessarily histocompatible with the epithelial target cells and in the allogenetic experiments neither the patients' lymphocytes nor the control lymphocytes were necessarily histocompatible with the epithelial target cells. Survival of the epithelial cells was generally better with the addition of control, rather than periodontal disease lymphocytes (Fig. 1). The cytotoxicity,

$$\text{Cytotoxicity } (\%) = \left(1 - \frac{\text{Epithelial cells} + \text{Lymphocytes}}{\text{Epithelial cells alone}}\right) \times 100,$$

of the lymphocytes from 32 patients has been related to the severity of periodontal disease (Fig. 2). The cytotoxicity tended to increase linearly with the severity of the disease in the range of periodontal disease considered ($r=0.564$, d.f. $=30$, $p < 0.01$).

Nature of the Cytotoxicity: Comparison with Antibody-dependent Cell-mediated Cytotoxicity

Several possible lymphocytotoxic mechanisms may be responsible for this phenomenon. Although the lymphocytotoxicity of periodontal disease is detectable within 18 h of culture and occurs in a serum-free medium (Movius et al., 1975), sufficient cell surface antibody could be released in the medium to invoke the cytotoxic mechanism known as antibody-dependent cell-mediated cytotoxicity or ADCC (MacLennan, 1969), since the amount of antibody required is very small. The effector cells are known as K or killer cells and although they have a lymphocyte-like morphology they also have cell surface markers which distinguish them from both T and B lymphocytes. The Fc

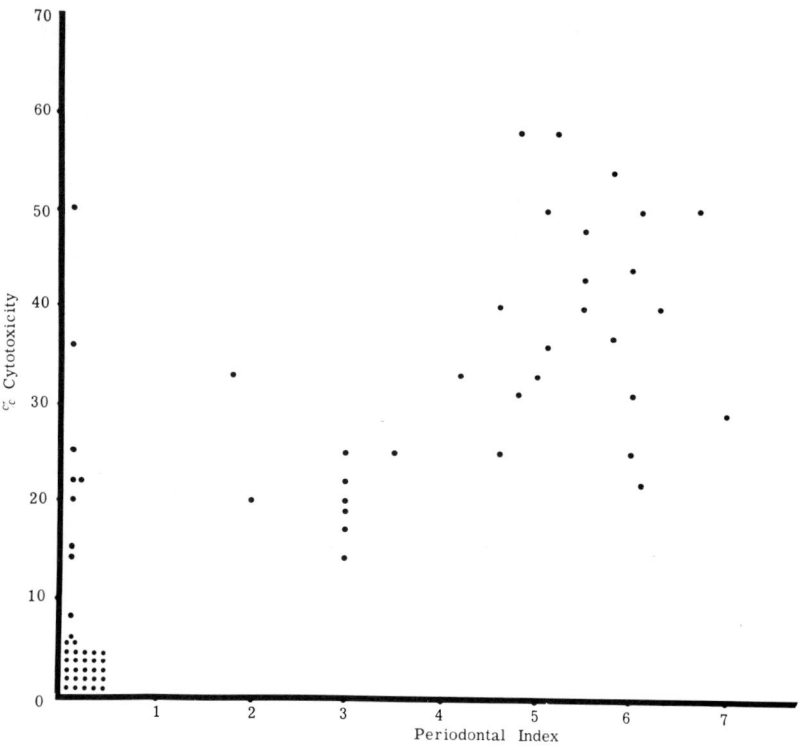

Fig. 2 Relationship of cytotoxicity of lymphocytes for oral epithelial cells to the degree of periodontal disease:

$$\text{Cytotoxicity (\%)} = \left(1 - \frac{\text{Epithelial cells} + \text{Lymphocytes}}{\text{Epithelial cells alone}}\right) \times 100.$$

receptors of these cells permit them to bind to the Fc portion of complexed antibody on the surface of the target cell. The cells are not phagocytic when adhering to the IgG antibody-coated target cell; they kill the cell by an extracellular mechanism. The Fc portion of the antibody molecule is apparently essential since binding of Fab fragments alone will not lead to ADCC (MacLennan, 1972; Perlman *et al.*, 1972). To examine the possibility that the mechanism observed by Movius *et al.* (1975) was in fact ADCC an artificial model was established *in vitro* (Bolanos *et al.*, 1979). Anti-epithelial cell serum was obtained by immunizing New Zealand White rabbits with human oral epithelial cells. Gingival epithelial cells separated from gingivectomy specimens were washed three times in tissue culture medium TC 199 and incubated for 30 min at 37 C with a 1/100 dilution of the antiserum in

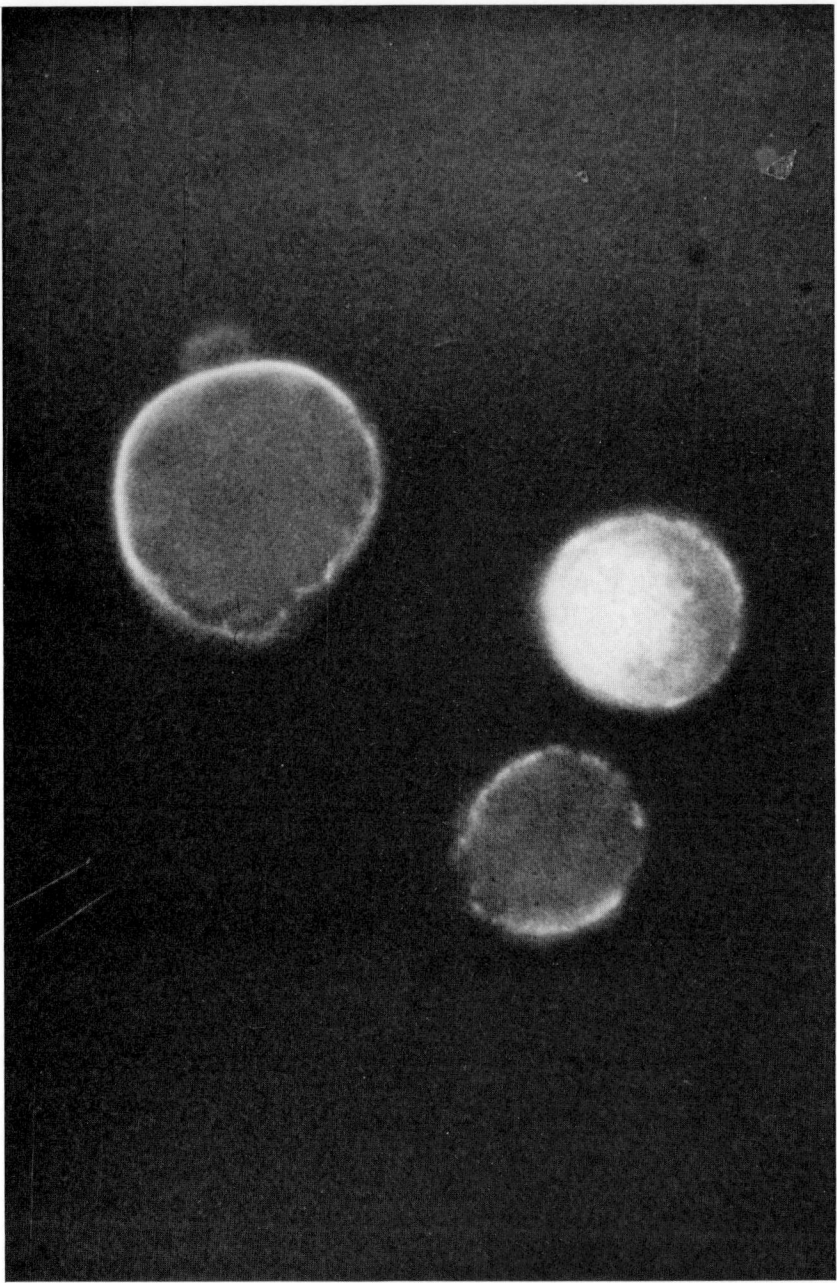

Fig. 3 Anti-oral epithelial cell serum was produced by injecting New Zealand White rabbits with freshly derived (0.25% trypsin for 2 h at 37 °C) gingival epithelial cells (3.0×10^6 cells total) in Freunds's complete adjuvant at multiple intradermal sites on two occasions 10 days apart. After a further 10 days the animals were bled and the sera separated and decomplemented by heating at 56 °C for 30 min. Cells were incubated in antiserum (1/100 dilution in phosphate-buffered saline for 30 min at 37 °C) and reincubated in a 1/10 dilution of commercial fluorescent goat anti-rabbit immunoglobulin. Viewed with ultraviolet light, BG 12 and OG515 filters. Magnification ×400.

phosphate-buffered saline (Fig. 3). Parallel suspensions of epithelial cells were incubated with an equvalent dilution of normal rabbit serum or phosphate-buffered saline alone. After incubation the treated cells were washed three times in TC 199 and added to the lymphocyte cultures. In those cultures where epithelial cells had been pre-incubated in anti-epithelial cell serum prior to the addition of lymphocytes from control subjects, there was a significant reduction in the viability of the epithelial cells, compared with those pre-incubated with normal rabbit serum.

Cell preparations made from these cultures and compared with those obtained from cultures containing epithelial cells and lymphocytes from patients with periodontal diseases revealed two features that appeared to distinguish the two sets of cultures. In the ADCC cultures a large number of lymphocytes were adherent to the epithelial cells (Fig. 4), whereas "ballooning" of the epithelial cells was more common in the lymphocytototoxicity of periodontal disease (Fig. 5). Although the findings would suggest that ADCC is not involved in the periodontal disease lymphocytotoxicity, the experiments are by no means conclusive and do not exclude ADCC as a contributory mechanism. Thus, the lymphocyte attachment to epithelial cells in such disproportionate amounts in the two mechanisms of cytotoxicity may be a reflection of the titre of the anti-epithelial cell antiserum chosen, rather than represent a distinction between the two cytotoxic mechanisms. However, the "ballooning" phenomenon seen in the cultures associated with lymphocytes from patients with periodontal disease is not a feature of antibody-dependent cell-mediated cytotoxicity, either in the simulated form recorded here or in other reports (Rosenau and Tsoukas, 1976) and may be a distinguishing feature of *in vitro* periodontal lymphocytotoxicity.

The Role of T-cell-mediated Cytotoxicity

An additional mechanism which may be responsible for the lymphocytotoxicity of periodontal disease is direct T-cell-mediated cytotoxicity. In this, contact is essential between lymphocytes and the target cell (Gately *et al.*, 1976), antibody is not required and there is apparently no release of toxic soluble mediator (Granger and Williams, 1968; Rosenau and Tsoukas, 1976). *In vitro* studies of cell-mediated cytotoxicity by T-lymphpcytes have established that immune T-lymphocytes exhibit specific cytotoxic activity against target cells carrying the corresponding immunizing antigens (Cerrottini and Brunner, 1974; Lonai *et al.*, 1971). T-lymphocyte-mediated cytotoxicity is inhibited by colchicine (Henney *et al.*, 1974) and vinblastine (Shacks and Granger, 1971; Rosenau and Tsoukas, 1976). The two inhibitors, colchicine and vinblastine, may also serve to distinguish the T-

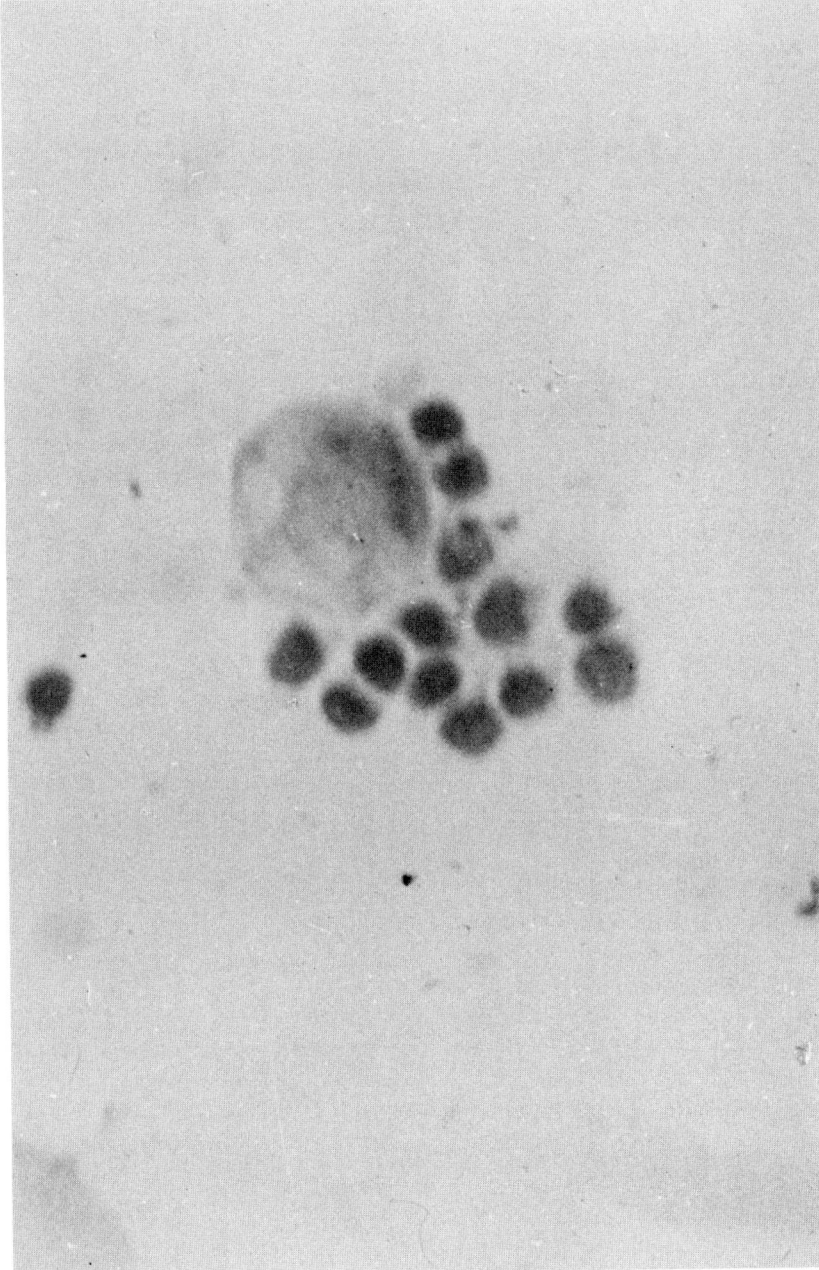

Fig. 4 "Clustering" of lymphocytes to oral epithelial cell observed in epithelial cell/lymphocyte cultures. Termination of culture, 18 h. Leishman stain. Magnification ×400.

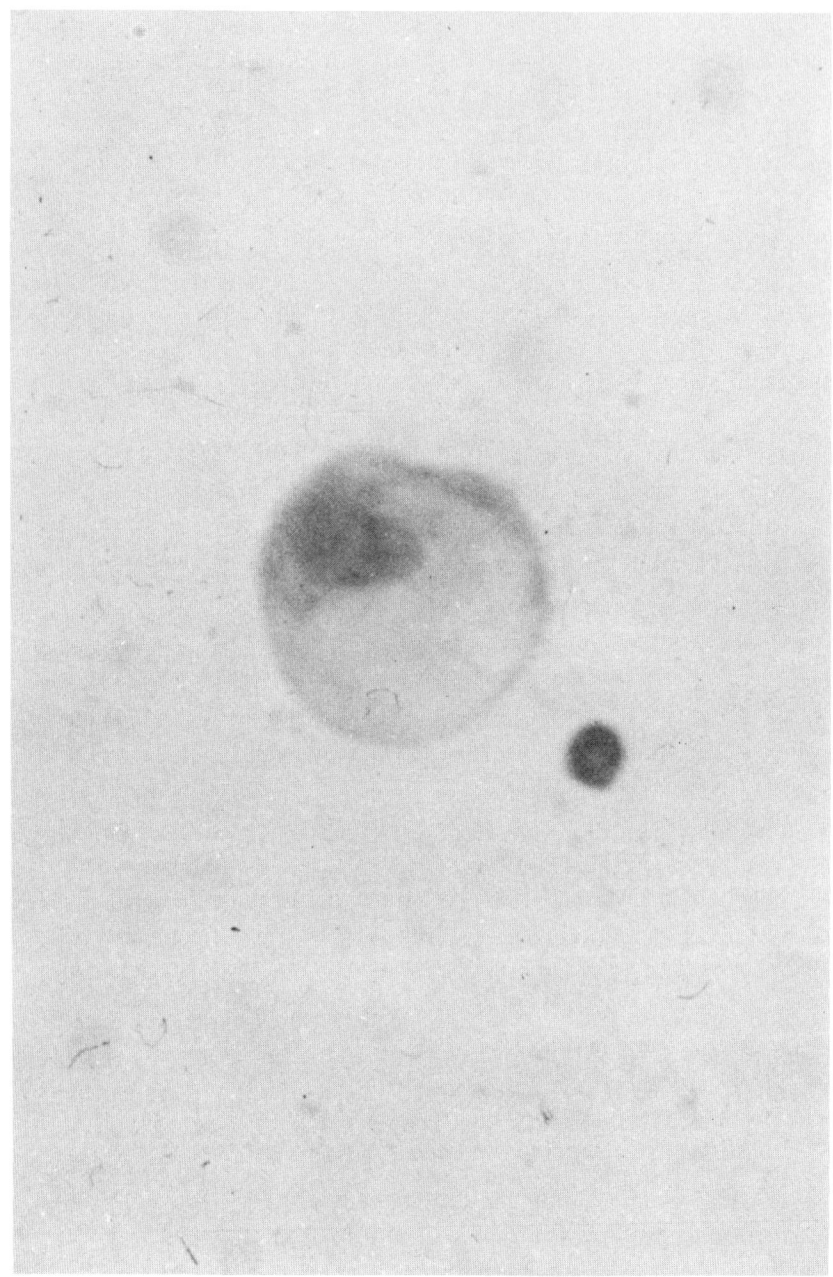

Fig. 5 "Ballooning" of epithelial cells observed in epithelial cell/lymphocyte cultures. Termination of culture, 18 h. Leishman stain. Magnification ×400.

mediated cytotoxicity from the lymphocytotoxicity dependent upon the production of lymphotoxin, a soluble toxic mediator released by antigen- and mitogen-activated lymphocytes (Granger and Williams, 1968). Thus, for example, cytochalasin B inhibits the production of lymphotoxin (Yoshida et al., 1972), whereas cholchicine or vinblastine do not (Shacks and Granger, 1971; Henney et al., 1974; Rosenau and Tsoukas, 1976).

In cultures in which peripheral blood lymphocytes from patients with periodontal disease and control subjects were pre-incubated in vinblastine or cholchicine (Bolanos et al., 1979) pre-treatment of the lymphocytes with vinblastine and colchicine significantly ($p > 0.02$ and $p > 0.01$, respectively) improved the level of survival of the epithelial cells, compared with the untreated lymphocyte/epithelial cell cultures (Fig. 6) and this would offer

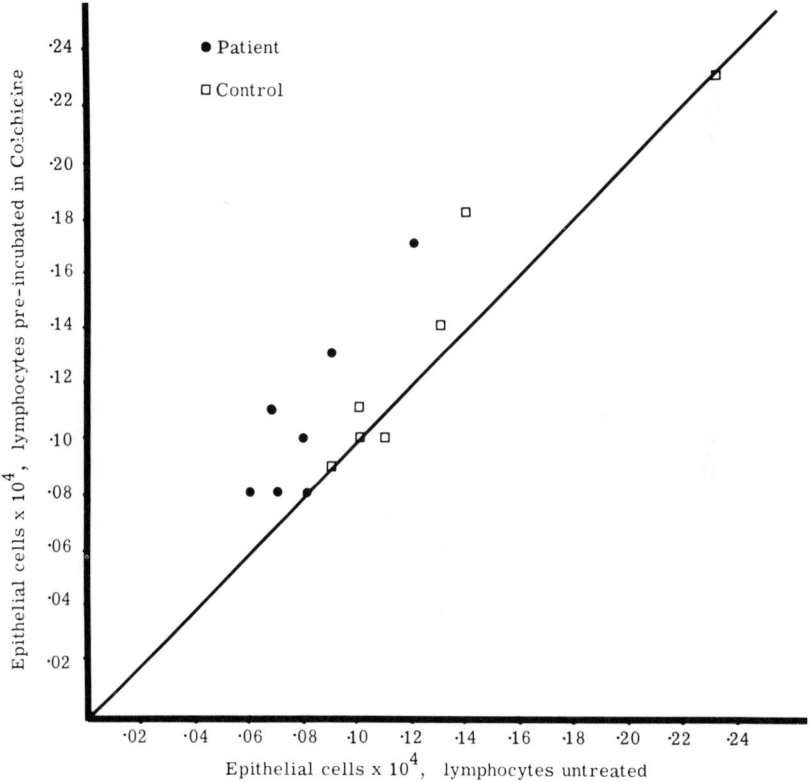

Fig. 6 Relationship of the the survival of the epithelial cells in the paired cultures following pre-incubation in vinblastine or colchicine (3×10^{-4} M). Lymphocytes were centrifuged (60g), supernatant removed and re-incubated with 0.5 ml of 3×10^{-4} M concentration of the drug. The lymphocytes were then washed three times in TC199 and resuspended in TC199. In control cultures the lymphocytes were treated with saline.

support for the mechanism being due to T-lymphocyte-mediated cytotoxicity.

Thymus-derived lymphocytes may be separated from other peripheral blood lymphocytes by making use of the knowledge that they form rosettes with sheep red cells. This method was employed to culture epithelial cells with lymphocytes from patients with periodontal disease which had been separated into two populations, thymus-derived and others. The two populations of lymphocytes from patients with periodontal disease were added to epithelial cells in culture in three separate experiments. The removal of the T-cells (i.e. SRBC rosette-forming lymphocytes) markedly impaired the cytotoxicity; equally, the difference between the survival with SRBC "positive" lymphocytes from the patient and a control culture was markedly increased (Table 1).

The Role of Trypsin in the Cytotoxicity

The possible implication of the T-lymphocyte in the mechanism focuses attention on the surface of the epithelial cell, since it is of such importance in T-mediated cytolysis (Gately et al., 1976). In all the experiments describing this phenomenon (Movius et al., 1975; Bolanos et al., 1979) the gingival epithelial cells had been derived from gingiva by trypsinization (0.25% trypsin for 2 h at 37°C). The possibility arises that the phenomenon is dependent upon the unmasking of antigens of the epithelial cell which were previously hidden. In parallel culture experiments, the lymphocyte cytotoxicity of periodontal disease was studied by making use of trypsin-derived cells and oral epithelial cells which had been derived without the use of trypsinization (Gnanasekhar et al., 1980). Gingival fragments left in culture medium only for 84 h release a considerable number of epithelial cells into the surrounding medium and the viability of these epithelial cells can be improved by centrifugation through serum.

There were several complicating factors in the design of these experiments. In the first place the different methods of derivation of the gingival epithelial cells, trypsinized and autolytically released, meant that the cells used as targets were derived from different patients. In the first series of six experiments (Fig. 7, procedure 1) the peripheral blood lymphocytes from periodontal disease patients to be used in the autolysis/trypsinization comparison were derived from different patients, although an attempt was made to match these patients for the degree of periodontal disease. In a second series of six experiments (Fig. 7, procedure 2) the comparability was improved by obtaining the peripheral blood lymphocytes from one patient and one control subject in each experiment. However, the gingival epithelial cells autolytically released or trypsinized were again obtained from separate patients who were matched, as closely as possible, for the degree of periodontal disease. In a third series of

TABLE I

Total Viable Epithelial Cells at the Termination of the Culture with Lymphocytes from Patients and Control Subjects (Periodontal Index <0.5).

Case no.	Original epithelial count	Total viable epithelial cells $\times 10^4$/well $\pm$ s.d.				Epithelial cells alone
		With patients' lymphocytes		With control lymphocytes		
		Pellet	Interface	Pellet	Interface	
1	0.20	0.05 ± 0.004	0.11 ± 0.009	0.10 ± 0.01	0.14 ± 0.013	0.12 ± 0.010
2	0.31	0.15 ± 0.007	0.20 ± 0.011	0.20 ± 0.009	0.22 ± 0.016	0.17 ± 0.011
3	0.24	0.08 ± 0.006	0.13 ± 0.009	0.11 ± 0.008	0.14 ± 0.01	0.13 ± 0.008

Peripheral blood lymphocytes (Triosil-Ficoll separation in MEM-HEPES) were added to 1% sheep red blood cells (SRBC) in fetal calf serum. After preincubation at 4°C for 1 h lymphocytes were layered on Triosil-Ficoll, centrifuged at 60 g for 10 min and at 400 g for 25 min. The interface was removed and washed three times with MEM-HEPES, the pellet washed once with phosphate-buffered saline and SRBC lysed with distilled water. The lymphocytes remaining in the interface were predominantly SRBC rosette depleted and the lymphocytes forming the pellet were predominantly SRBC rosette enriched.

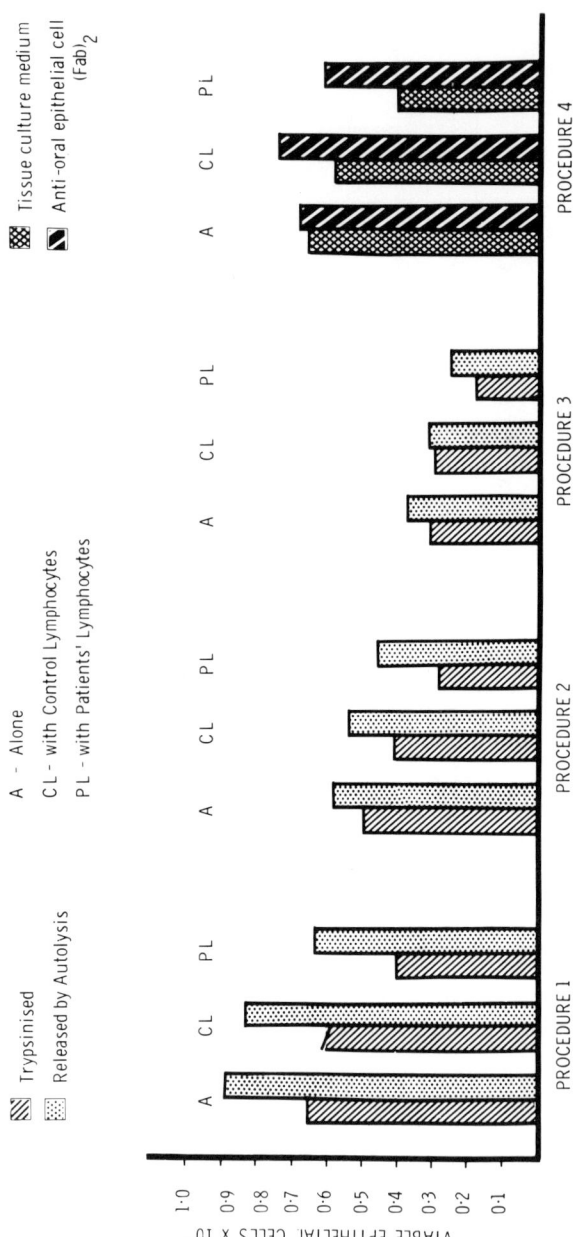

Fig. 7 Viability of epithelial cells on their own, and when cultured with control lymphocytes and with patients' lymphocytes under the specified conditions.

experiments (Fig. 7, procedure 3), one half of a suspension of oral epithelial cells released by autolysis from the gingiva of one patient was incubated in 0.0005% trypsin for 2 h and the cells washed twice in TC 199. The two suspensions of cells, enzyme-treated and untreated, were further divided and incubated with lymphocytes from one patient and from one control subject as previously described. Three experiments, involving three patients and three control subjects, were carried out using this procedure. The level of trypsin in these three experiments was the highest compatible with the survival of epithelial cells suitable for use as targets. The cultural conditions and cytotoxic assay were as described previously. In all the experiments the survival of the epithelial cells was greater with the addition of control lymphocytes than with the addition of lymphocytes from patients with periodontal disease (Fig. 7). Higher mean values of survival were obtained with autolytically released cells than with trypsin-released or trypsin-treated cells. The cytotoxic effect of lymphocytes from patients with periodontal disease is apparent both in trypsinized and autolysed cultures; however, trypsinization appears to enhance a cytotoxic effect in the presence of patients' lymphocytes (Table II).

Several possible explanations exist for this apparent effect of trypsin. Tryspin inhibits protein synthesis in rabbit alveolar macrophages (Ulrich, 1976). This may be the case with the trypsinized oral epithelial cells used in this investigation, wherein the epithelial cells, due to trypsin-induced changes in their metabolism, may be in a state in which they cannot withstand the additional metabolic insult which may arise from the lymphocytes. Loss of trypsin-sensitive surface glycoproteins may expose or unmask receptors or antigens which are normally hidden. These sites may equate with antigens of dental plaque or disintegrating epithelial cells which may have given rise to immunological stimulation during the course of periodontal disease. If this had occurred to the oral epithelial cells in this series of experiments, they would have presumably become more suitable targets for the sensitized lymphocytes. Trypsin has also been shown to potentiate the response of hamster lymphoid cells to lipopolysaccharide (Hart and Streilein, 1977) and to exert a mitogenic effect on human peripheral blood lymphocytes (Kaplan and Bona, 1974). It is conceivable that the increased lymphocytotoxicity for trypsinized oral epithelial cells observed could have resulted from the stimulation of the peripheral blood lymphocytes by the trypsin in the culture medium, either released from the trypsinized oral epithelial cells or present as residual trypsin. This would indeed seem possible as three washes of the trypsinized epithelial cells would give an estimated effective dilution of approximately 0.005% trypsin, which is very near to that dilution of trypsin (0.1–0.3 µg/ml) observed by Kaplan and Bona (1974) to stimulate human peripheral blood lymphocytes. If such a stimulation of the lymphocytes by the

TABLE II

The Survival of Oral Epithelial Cells when Cultured with Lymphocytes from Patients with Periodontal Disease and Control Subjects: the Effect of Trypsin Treatment and Pre-incubation in Anti-oral Epithelial Cell $F(ab')_2$ IgG of the Oral Epithelial Cells Used as the Target

Experiment	Derivation of OEC*	No. of patients	Original epithelial cell count	Row	Viable epithelial cells × 10³ after 18 h culture		
					Alone	With control lymphocytes	With patients' lymphocytes
Autolysed/trypsinized OEC dissimilar patients	Trypsinized	6	1.0×10^3	1	0.66 ± 0.16	0.60 ± 0.15	0.40 ± 0.04
					——— <0.05 ———	——— <0.005 ———	
	Autolysed	6		2	0.89 ± 0.18	0.84 ± 0.30	0.64 ± 0.12
					——— NS ———	——— <0.025 ———	
Autolysed/Trypsinized OEC same patients	Trypsinized	6	1.0×10^3	3	0.50 ± 0.17	0.40 ± 0.12	0.28 ± 0.04
						——— <0.01 ———	——— <0.01 ———
	Autolysed	6		4	0.59 ± 0.21	0.54 ± 0.16	0.46 ± 0.07
					——— NS ———	——— <0.01 ———	
Autolysed and 0.0005% trypsinized/autolysed only OEC	Autolysed and 0.0005% trypsinized	3	0.6×10^3	5	0.31 ± 0.05	0.30 ± 0.08	0.18 ± 0.03
					——— NS ———	——— NS ———	
	Autolysed	3		6	0.37 ± 0.08	0.31 ± 0.04	0.25 ± 0.02
					——— NS ———	——— <0.025 ———	
Anti-OEC $(Fab')_2$ treated OEC untreated OEC	Trypsinized OEC pre-incubated in TC 199†	6	1.0×10^3	7	0.65 ± 0.45	0.59 ± 0.36	0.40 ± 0.13
					——— NS ———	——— <0.005 ———	
	Trypsinized OEC pre-incubated in anti-OEC $(Fab')_2$	6		8	0.68 ± 0.43	0.73 ± 0.45	0.61 ± 0.18
					——— NS ———	——— <0.005 ———	

* OEC, oral epithelial cells.
† TC 199, tissue culture medium 199.

Each value represents the mean ± S.D. of six experiments (three in experiment 3) involving different patients and control subjects. Although the absolute differences in the first two comparisons (CL vs. PL) in rows 1 and 2 are the same (0.60 − 0.40 = 0.20; 0.84 − 0.14 = 0.20), in relative magnitudes the cytotoxic effect within the trypsinized cultures (−0.4/0.6 = 0.33) is greater than in the autolysed cultures (1 − 0.64/0.84 = 0.23). A similarly enhanced cytotoxic effect is observed with trypsinization in the other comparisons.

p values represent paired t-test for survival values with lymphocytes and alone. NS, not significant.

residual or released trypsin were in fact the explanation for the phenomenon, then it can be seen that the lymphocytes of patients with periodontal disease are more susceptible to this stimulatory effect of trypsin than are the lymphocytes from control subjects.

Specificity: The Role of the Epithelial Cell Surface

The specificity of T-cell-mediated lymphocytotoxicity is a well-established fact (Cerottini and Brunner, 1974; Rosenau and Tsoukas, 1976; Dennert, 1976). The specific nature of the *in vitro* lymphocytotoxicity in periodontal disease was examined in an initial experiment (Gnanasekher *et al.*, 1980) by incubating lymphocytes from subjects with and without periodontal disease with HEp-2 cells (human carcinoma of larynx; Toolan, 1954). This cell line was chosen because it is derived from tissue found in close proximity to the oral cavity. However, the original stratified squamous epithelium of the mucous membrane of the larynx would almost certainly have undergone changes in terms of the surface of the individual cells. The changes that are likely to have occurred are the appearance of tumour-specific transplantation antigens, appearance of carcinoembryonic antigens and loss of tissue-specific antigens (Rapin and Burger, 1974). It was observed that the survival of the HEp-2 cells with the lymphocytes was lower than when they were cultured alone. However, there was no difference in this apparent cytotoxicity of the lymphocytes when subjects with and without periodontal disease were compared in a series of four experiments. The reduction in the level of survival of the HEp-2 cells may be due to the tissue culture exhaustion or toxicity of metabolic products of the added lymphocytes. Conversely, the phenomenon may represent spontaneous cytotoxicity. Spontaneous cytotoxicity, the effector cells often being termed natural killer (NK) cells, occurs predominantly where the target cells are one of continuous cell lines (Kiessling *et al.*, 1975) and would be expected in this experimental situation involving HEp-2 cells. Thus it is conceivable that a proportion of the cytotoxicity observed in the cultures involving oral epithelial cells and patients' lymphocytes may also represent spontaneous cytotoxicity, although the nature of the target cell, an end cell culture, may preclude this. The findings would also suggest that there may be some degree of specificity with regard to the lymphocytotoxicity for oral epithelial cells in periodontal disease.

In the experiments described earlier (Bolanos *et al.*, 1979), use was made of an antiserum to the oral epithelial cells to simulate antibody-dependent cell-mediated cytotoxicity or ADCC. If the Fc fragment of the IgG portion of this antiserum is removed, the phenomenon would no longer occur and one would have available an antibody which would bind to the surface of the oral epithelial cell and which could be used to study the role of the target cell surface in the cytotoxicity of periodontal disease (Gnanasekhar *et al.*, 1980).

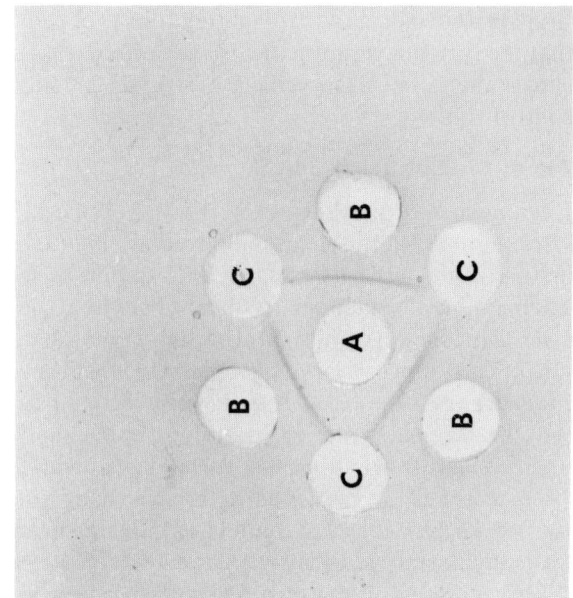
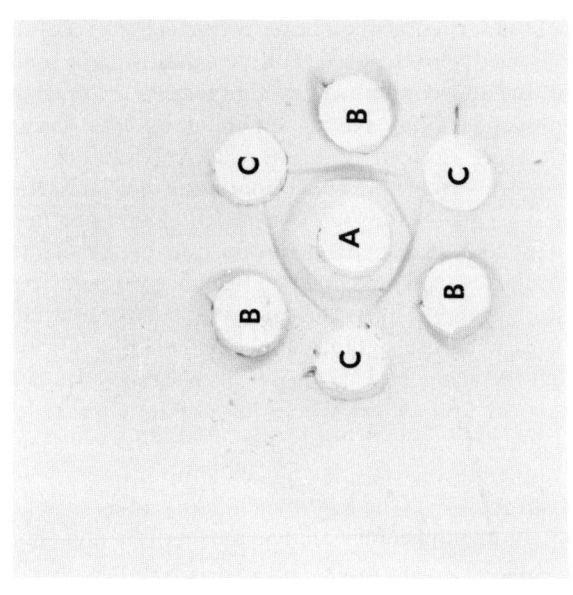

Fig. 8 (a) Gel diffusion method used to confirm digestion of the Fc portion of the rabbit anti-epithelial cell IgG by pepsin treatment. A, swine anti-rabbit IgG; B, rabbit anti-epithelial cell IgG; C, pepsin-treated rabbit anti-epithelial cell IgG. (b) Gel diffusion method used to detect the presence of Fc fragment of IgG in the pepsin-treated rabbit anti-epithelial cell IgG. A, swine anti-rabbit Fc; B, rabbit anti-epithelial cell IgG; C, pepsin-treated rabbit anti-epithelial cell IgG.

Following separation of the IgG fraction from the anti-epithelial cell serum, the Fc fragment was removed by pepsin digestion and confirmed by immunodiffusion (Fig. 8). In a series of six experiments epithelial cells to be used as targets were pre-treated either with medium or with $F(ab)^2$ fragments of anti-epithelial cell serum prior to incubation with lymphocytes from patients with periodontal disease or control subjects. The cytotoxicity of lymphocytes from patients with periodontal disease was significantly higher ($p > 0.005$) for oral epithelial cells not treated with anti-epithelial cell IgG $F(ab')_2$ when compared with the cytotoxicity for oral epithelial cells pre-treated with anti-epithelial cell IgG $F(ab')_2$ (Table II and Fig. 7). Thus, masking of the surface of the oral epithelial cell appeared to impair the cytotoxic effect, suggesting that the cell surface was of considerable importance in the phenomenon. The IgG $F(ab')_2$ used in the investigation was absorbed with red blood cells (RBC), white blood cells (WBC), and platelets from the patients from whom oral epithelial cells were obtained. This was undertaken in an effort to remove antibodies directed against histocompatibility antigens (Davies and Staines, 1976) present on the surface of the oral epithelial cells. Blood group antigen A, present also on the surface of oral epithelial cells (Dabelsteen and Fejerskov, 1974) would also have been absorbed. Absorption of these antigens from the antiserum was confirmed by the observation that after the final absorption, the RBC, WBC and platelets did not show binding of fluorescent anti-rabbit IgG. Thus, the blood group antigen A and HLA antigens would not appear to be of importance in the lymphocytotoxicity of periodontal disease. This is in agreement with the initial (Movius *et al.*, 1975) and later (Bolanos *et al.*, 1979) investigations in which there was no apparent difference in the cytotoxicity observed in syngeneic and allogeneic cultures of epithelial cells and lymphocytes from patients with periodontal disease.

T-cell-mediated cytotoxicity is thought to be most effective when the major histocompatibility complex (MHC) of antigens, such as the HLA of man, are available to the effector cell (Doherty *et al.*, 1976). Two methods are proposed for this mechanism: the first (a) that the MHC site is itself modified, so leading to activation of the effector cell; alternatively (b) that a minimum of two sites is required for activation, one of which is the MHC of the cell. If T-cell-mediated cytotoxicity is of importance in the lymphocytotoxicity of periodontal disease, then it would seem not to be due to the first proposed mechanism, that is the modification of the MHC site itself, since this was apparently uncovered in this last series of experiments.

Relationship to Dental Bacterial Plaque Antigen

One possible source of antigen responsible for this apparent T-cell stimulation could be dental bacterial plaque (DBP). Extracts of DBP have been shown to lead to the induction of non-specific cytotoxicity in peripheral blood lymphocytes in patients with periodontal disease (Ivanyi et al., 1972; Horton et al., 1973). It has been shown that it is possible to "arrest" the stimulation of T-lymphocytes with antigen by the addition of the chemical 5-bromodeoxyuridine (5-BUdR) to the lymphocyte/antigen culture (Zoschke and Bach, 1971). This material is apparently taken up by the lymphocytes responding to antigen, and the inclusion of the thymidine analogue into the cellular DNA induces alterations at the transcriptional level (Fitzmaurice and Barker, 1974; Flickinger, 1975). Such cells are killed if exposed to light in the visible or near visible region of the spectrum (Zoschke and Bach, 1971). Pre-incubation in DBP extract followed by the addition of BUdR and exposure to light significantly reduced the cytotoxic effect exhibited by the lymphocytes from patients with periodontal disease (Fig. 9).

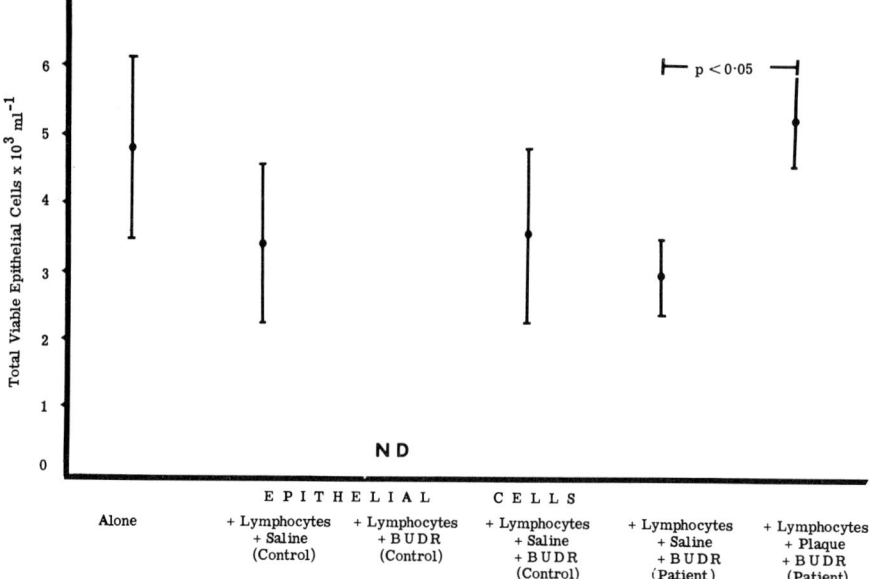

Fig. 9 Effect upon the *in vitro* lymphocytotoxicity of pre-culture of lymphocytes with dental bacterial plaque (DBP) extract and treatment with 5-BUdR. DBP extract was prepared by ultrasonication (8 μ, 8 min) of aliquots of pooled, cooled plaque. The supernatant (20 000 g) was dialysed overnight against distilled water and was added to lymphocyte cultures from patients with periodontal disease. Parallel cultures contained saline. At 72 h 5-BUdR (10^{-5} M) was added; 24 h later cultures with DBP extract and saline were exposed to fluorescent light (90 min). Cells were then washed three times in TC 199, adjusted to 10^6 viable lymphocytes per millilitre, added to triplicate cultures of oral epithelial cells derived from the donor of the lymphocytes the same day (lymphocyte/epithelial cell ratio 20/1). Total viable epithelial cell count was determined 18 h later. The *in vitro* cytotoxic effect of lymphocytes from patients with periodontal disease is still apparent, but does not reach significance within the three experiments.

Several possible explanations exist for this apparent reduction in lymphocytotoxicity. DBP antigen may reside upon the oral epithelial cells used as the target in the experiments described above and may have been acquired *in vivo* or *in vitro*. However, it should be remembered that trypsin has been used and that with it the cytotoxicity is enhanced (Ghanasekhar *et al.*, 1980). In addition, the more superficial cells of the epithelium, such as the squames, which are derived during the cell separation process and could presumably carry the greatest bacterial antigen load, are not included in the total count and viability (Bolanos *et al.*, 1980; Gnanasekhar *et al.*, 1980). An additional possibility is that the antigen is cross-reactive with DBP antigen, that is, that there is a structural similarity between the glycoprotein/lipoprotein of the oral epithelial cell and bacterial antigen. The third explanation of the result is that extracts of the DBP included epithelial cell antigen. This is a real possibility since examination of dental plaque shows that there is a population of approximately 20 000 epithelial cells per gram w/w of dental plaque (A. Ahmed and G. Singh, unpublished results). In addition there are presumably fragments of epithelial cells and epithelial cell antigen in solution.

If it is the case that there is a T-cell response to epithelial cell antigen in periodontal disease which leads to the cytotoxic phenomenon, then this may also be detected by other methods which assay T-cell responses. One of these is T-cell blastogenesis, and this possibility was studied using epithelial cells derived from gingivectomy specimens, that is from patients suffering from periodontal disease, and from gingiva removed at the time of tooth extraction in patients who did not suffer from periodontal disease. The peripheral blood lymphocytes and the autologous cells were cultured together for 5 days, tritiated thymidine was added and the uptake of thymidine was assayed by precipitation of the nucleoprotein, addition to scintillant fluid and counting in a beta counter. All of these cultures represent the co-culture of histocompatible cells. It was therefore surprising to see relatively high stimulation indices (ratio of counts per minute with epithelial cells to counts per minute with saline) obtained with the cultures of oral epithelial cells and lymphocytes from patients with periodontal disease. Insignificant stimulation indices were recorded with the control subjects (Fig. 10).

Lymphoblastic responses to allogeneic cells are thought to arise from stimulation by HLA-DR antigens of the major histocompatibility complex-coded classical transplantation antigens which are present on cells of the immune system, (Shreffler and Davis, 1975) or Langerhans cells of the epidermis (Rowden *et al.*, 1977) and on sperm (Hammerling *et al.*, 1975). More recently they have been detected in several epithelial tissues (Wiman *et al.*, 1978), or at least antigens which react with an antiserum specific for HLA-DR antigens, the human counterparts of the murine Ia antigens.

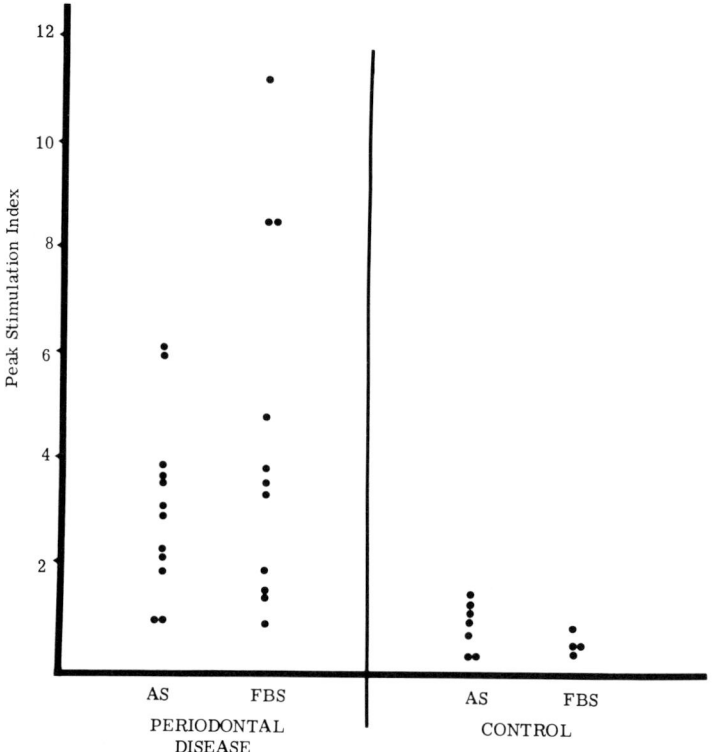

Fig. 10 Peak lymphoblastic responses to autologous epithelial cells in patients with periodontal disease and control subjects. Epithelial cells derived from gingiva by trypsinization (0.25% at 37 C for 2 h, washed and added to microcultures of lymphocytes for 120 h (lymphocyte/epithelial cell ratio approximately 20:1). Tritiated thymidine (0.1 μCi) was added for 12 h, nucleoprotein precipitated and added to scintillant for assay of β emission. Values are means of triplicate cultures. Stimulation index.

$$\text{Stimulation index} = \frac{\text{c.p.m. with epithelial cells}}{\text{c.p.m. with saline}}.$$

Unusually high lymphoblastogenic responses to autologous cells have been recorded with mouse neonate thymus/adult spleen cells (Howe *et al.*, 1970; Boehmer, 1974; Boehmer and Byrd, 1972), rat thymus/spleen cells (Llacer and Uyeki, 1969) and rabbit white blood cells, spleen cells/gut-associated lymphoid cells (Milthorp and Richter, 1979). These enhanced responses suggest that the responder cells may detect the "foreignness" of the autologous stimulator cells (Milthorp and Richter, 1979).

The investigations recorded above lead to the supposition that an autoimmune response has been promoted in patients with periodontal disease. In addition, in so far as the cytotoxicity experiments are a manifestation of cell-mediated immunity, the autoimmunity appears to increase with the increasing severity of the disease. This apparent loss of tolerance for self-antigens may arise in a variety of ways. First, as had been suggested above, the experiments may represent the interaction of sensitized lymphocytes with bacterial antigen carried by the target or stimulator epithelial cells. Alternatively, there may be immunological cross-reactivity between antigens of the oral epithelial cells and bacterial antigen to which patients with periodontal disease have been previously sensitized. This cross-reactivity may also lead to a loss of tolerance to self-antigens by the activation of lymphocytes that bear receptors and have been formerly suppressed.

T-lymphocytes, capable of recognizing self-antigens, can apparently be easily induced in experimental situations and the mechanisms behind the inhibition of expression of these self-reactive T-cells are still unknown (Primi *et al.*, 1978). B-cell loss of tolerance, that is the existence of self-reactive B-lymphocytes, is known to occur more readily in the presence of materials termed polyclonal B-cell activators (PBA) (Primi *et al.*, 1977). A large number of infective microorganisms possess intrinsic PBA activating capacity (Biberfield and Gronowicz, 1976; Greenwood and Rosalind, 1975; Sultzer and Nilsson, 1972). They are also common in dental plaque and one, lipopolysaccharide, can enhance or suppress antigen-induced T-cell proliferation *in vitro* (Ivanyi, 1976). Lipopolysaccharide has also been shown to influence transplantation reactions (Thomason and Jutila, 1974; Rose *et al.*, 1976). Thus, the presence of these bacterial materials in dental plaque may encourage a loss of tolerance to self-antigens. Lastly, lysosomal enzyme release is apparently a common phenomenon in chronic periodontal disease, a process which may lead to the uncovering of new antigenic determinants in the cells and tissues of the periodontium.

The experimentally induced loss of tolerance described above by, for example, the presence of PBAs or *in vitro* culture (Cohen and Wekerle, 1976; Wekerle, 1977) leads to the production of modest amounts of auto-antibody which are apparently of little pathogenic significance. It remains to be seen whether the phenomenon first described by Movius *et al.* (1975) plays a role in the destructive process of periodontal disease and is representitive of a local disturbance in immune homeostasis which contributes to the progression of the disease.

Summary

Several features of chronic periodontal disease may promote the development of a cellular autoimmune response within the gingiva. The *in vitro* killing of oral epithelial cells by peripheral blood cells from patients with periodontal disease may represent such a cellular autoimmune response to antigens which are either intrinsic to the epithelial cell surface or have been acquired from the local environment. This *in vitro* cytotoxicity correlated ($r = 0.07$) with the degree of periodontal disease in a group of 32 patients (periodontal index, 0.4–7.4) and was reduced by removal of thymus-derived lymphocytes from the "killer" population or by the treatment of this population with colchicine or vinblastine (3×10^{-4} M). Oral epithelial cells derived without the use of trypsin were also susceptible to the *in vitro* killing, although enzyme treatment increased the cytotoxic effect. Pre-incubation of the "killer" population with dental plaque ultrasonicate and 5-deoxybromomuridine, to eliminate lymphocytes responding to antigen in the dental plaque, resulted in a population with reduced cytotoxic activity for trypsinized oral epithelial cells. Enhanced lymphoblastic responses were observed when peripheral blood lymphocytes from patients with periodontal disease were cultured with autologous oral epithelial cells. Thus the antigen, which is presumably associated with the cytotoxicity, may have originated from dental plaque or might be an epithelial cell antigen which is cross-reacting with dental plaque antigen.

Acknowledgements

This work was supported in part by the Medical Research Council. We are also grateful to Jean Thomas and Susan Walker for undertaking the BUdR study and to Dr T. Khosla for statistical advice. E. Bolanos was on a visiting research studentship from the University of Costa Rica during the course of this investigation.

References

Biberfeld, G. and Gronowicz, E. (1976). *Nature, Lond.* **261**, 238.
Boemer, H. V. and Byrd, W. J. (1972). *Nature new Biol.* **235**, 50.
Boemer, H. V. (1974). In *Proceedings of the Eighth Leukocyte Culture Conference*. (K. Lindahl-Kiessling and D. Osoba, eds), p. 289, Academic Press, New York.
Bolanos, E., Church, H. and Dolby, A. E. (1979). *J. dent. Res.* **58**, Special Issue C, 1227, abstract 25.
Burnet, F. M. (1957). *Aust. J. Sci.* **20**, 67.
Cerottini, J. C. and Brunner, K. T. (1974). *Adv. Immunol.* **18**, 67.
Cochrane, C. G. (1969). *Transplant. Proc.* **1**, 949–955.
Cohen, R. I. and Werkele, H. (1976). *Science, N.Y.* **194**, 1324.
Coulson, A. S. and Chalmers, D. G. (1964). *Lancet* 29 Feb., 468.
Cunningham, A. J. (1976). *Transplant. Rev.* **31**, 22–43.
Dabelsteen, B. and Fejerskov, O. (1974). *Scand. J. dent. Res.* **82**, 206.
Davies, D. A. L. and Staines, N. A. (1976). *Transplant. Rev.* **30**, 19.
Dennert, G. (1976). *Transplant. Rev.* **29**, 59.
Doherty, P., Blander, R. V. and Zinkernagel, R. H. (1976). *Transplant. Rev.* **29**, 89.
Fitzmaurice, L. C. and Baker, R. F. (1974). *J. cell. comp. Physiol.* **83**, 295.
Flickinger, R. A. (1975). *Cell Differentiation* **4**, 295.
Gately, M. K., Mayer, M. and Henney, C. (1976). *Cell. Immunol.* **27**, 82.
Gnanasekhar, D., Singh, G. and Dolby, A. E. (1980). *J. dent. Res.* in press.

Granger, G. A., and Williams, T. W. (1968). *Nature, Lond.* **218,** 1253.
Greenwood, B. M. and Rosalind, M. V. (1975). *Nature, Lond.* **257,** 592.
Hammerling, G. J., Mauve, G., Goldberg, E. and McDevitt, H. O. (1975). *Immunogenetics* **5,** 428.
Hart, D. A. and Streilein, J. S. (1977). *Expl Cell Res.* **107,** 434.
Henney, C. S., Gaffney, J. and Bloom, B. R. (1974). *J. exp. Med.* **140,** 837.
Horton, J. E., Oppenheim, J. J. and Mergenhagen, S. E. (1973). *Clin. exp. Immunol.* **13,** 383–393.
Howe, M. L., Goldstein, A. L. and Batisto, J. R. (1970). *Proc. natn. Acad. Sci. U.S.A.* **67,** 673.
Ivanyi, L. (1976). *Clin. exp. Immunol.* **23,** 385–388.
Ivanyi, L., Wilton, J. M. A. and Lehner, T. (1972). *Immunology* **22,** 141–145.
Kaplan, J. G. and Bona, G. (1974). *Expl Cell Res.* **88,** 388.
Kaplan, M. H. and Suchy, M. L. (1964). *J. exp. Med.* **119,** 643.
Kiessling, R., Klein, E., Pross, H. and Wigzell, H. (1975). *Eur. J. Immunol.* **5,** 117.
Lehner, R. A., Glassock, R. J. and Dixon, F. J. (1967). *J. exp. Med.* **126,** 989–1004.
Llacer, V. and Uyeki, E. M. (1969). *Int. Archs Allergy* **35,** 88.
Lonai, P., Clark, W. R. and Feldman, M. (1971). *Nature new Biol.* **229,** 566.
MacLennan, I. C. M. (1969). *Ann. rheum. Dis.* **28,** 328.
MacLennan, I. C. M. (1972). *Transplant. Rev.* **13,** 67.
Milthorp, P. and Richter, M. (1979). *Immunology* **37,** 375.
Movius, D. L., Rogers, R. S. and Reeve, C. M. (1975). *J. Periodont.* **46,** 271–276.
Perlmann, P., Perlmann, H. and Wigzell, H. (1972). *Transplant. Rev.* **13,** 91.
Primi, D., Hammarström, L., Smith, C. I. E. and Moller, G. (1977). *J. exp. Med.* **145,** 21.
Primi, D. Smith, C. I. E. and Hammarström, L. (1978). *Scand. J. Immunol.* **7,** 121–126.
Rapin, A. M. C. and Burger, M. M. (1974). *Adv. Cancer Res.* **20,** 1.
Rose, W. C., Rodey, G. E., Rimm, A. A., Truitt, R. L. and Bortin, M. M. (1976). *Expl Hemat.* **4,** 90.
Rosenau, W. and Tsoukas, C. D. (1976). *Am. J. Path.* **84,** 580.
Rowden, G., Lewis, M. G. and Sullivan, A. K. (1977). *Nature, Lond.* **268,** 247.
Russell, A. L. (1956). *J. dent. Res.* **35,** 350–358.
Shacks, S. J. and Granger, G. A. (1971). *J. reticuloendothelial Soc.* **10,** 28.
Shreffler, D. C. and Davis, C. S. (1975). *Adv. Immunol.* **20,** 125.
Sultzer, B. M. and Nilsson, B. S. (1972). *Nature, Lond.* **240,** 198.
Thomason, P. E. and Jutila, J. W. (1974). *J. reticuloendothelial Soc.* **16,** 327.
Toolan, H. W. (1954). *Cancer Res.* **14,** 660.
Trentham, D. E., Townes, J. and Kang, H. (1977). *J. exp. Med.* **146,** 857–867.
Ulrich, F. (1976). *Expl Cell Res.* **101,** 267.
Waksman, B. H. (1962). In *Proceedings of the Second International Symposium on Immunopathology* (P. Grabar and P. Miescher, eds), p. 146, Karger, Basel.
Werkerle, H. (1977). *Nature, Lond.* **267,** 357.
Wiman, K., Curman, B., Forsum, U., Klareskog, L., Malmnas Tjernlund, U., Rask, L., Tradgardh, L. and Peterson, P. A. (1978). *Nature, Lond.* **276,** 711.
Yoshida, M., Waksman, B. H. and Malawista, S. E. (1972). *Science, N.Y.* **176,** 1147.
Zoschke, D. C. and Bach, F. H. (1971). *J. immunol. Methods* **55,** 56.

10. Bacteria and Oral Fluid Components: Report of the Oral Condition in Hypogammaglobulinaemic Patients

DOUGLAS BRATTHALL and JANNE BJÖRKANDER

Introduction

Bacteria in the oral cavity are subjected to a variety of host protective systems in saliva or in crevicular fluid (for reviews see Bowen, 1974; Cimasoni *et al.*, 1977). Among the non-specific factors, lysozyme, lactoferrin and lactoperoxidase have been specially noted. Specific factors include antibodies and possibly the salivary agglutinins. Interest was raised in protective mechanisms specific for certain types of bacteria with the demonstration of the transmissible caries-inducing *Streptococcus mutans* by Keyes in 1960. Since then, many investigations have been performed aimed at preventing this specific target microorganism from colonizing the teeth by stimulation of some oral fluid components. However, it is striking how many of our current ideas are being recycled from the time when the lactobacillus was thought to be the principal cariogenic organism (see Jay *et al.*, 1933).

As an illustration of the recent interest in local immunity and in the immunological approach to the prevention of dental caries, many reports at several symposia can be mentioned: "International Symposium on the Immunoglobulin A System", Birmingham, Alabama, 1973; "Immunological Aspects of Dental Caries", New York City, 1975; "International Symposium on the Secretory Immune System and Caries Immunity", Birmingham, Alabama, 1977; "Saliva and Dental Caries", Stony Brook, New York, 1978. The proceedings from these meetings cover the subject in great detail. Also, at the "Borderland between Caries and Periodontal Disease" meeting in 1977, extensive reviews were presented by Lehner (1977) and by Brandtzaeg and Tolo (1977). In this brief review we wish to confine ourselves to some aspects of oral defence mechanisms. We also wish to present clinical data from a study of hypogammaglobulinaemic patients; this study may give some clues concerning the importance of antibodies and agglutinins in oral fluid.

Bacteria and Immunoglobulins

Antibodies reach the oral cavity through major and minor salivary glands and through crevicular fluid. Whilst secretory IgA (sIgA) is dominant among the Ig classes in salivary secretions, IgG as well as IgA and IgM are present in crevicular fluid (Brandtzaeg, 1965). In a recent review, Bowen and Guggenheim (1978) pointed out that several independent groups have successfully immunized various animals against dental caries. However, they also mentioned that satisfactory interpretations of these findings are still lacking. Inhibition of adherence of specific pathogenic bacteria by sIgA may represent one major way, but several findings also argue for the protective effects of IgG via other mechanisms (Lehner et al., 1978). The possible effects of this antibody class have been discussed by Challacombe et al. (1978). Among various possibilities they mention inhibition of glucosyltransferase (GTS) activity, inhibition of adherence, complement-dependent antibacterial reactions and enhancement of phagocytosis. Thus, bacteria in the oral cavity may react with local antibodies, although it should be observed that bacteria not common in the populations under investigation may also react with salivary antibodies (Arnold et al., 1976; Bratthall et al., 1978). Several bacterial antigens can be responsible for such reactions and these are not necessarily strain specific. For example Bratthall et al. (1979) have shown that lipotheichoic acid (LTA), which is cross-reactive among several strains, reacts with salivary IgA antibodies. Thus, it is not necessary that a bacterial strain which reacts with salivary immunoglobulins must have been the one responsible for the original antibody formation.

Bacteria and Salivary Agglutinins

Another salivary substance, or group of substances, with the capacity to agglutinate oral bacteria has been known for at least 10 years. These are described as high molecular weight glycoproteins, aggregating factors or agglutinins, but our knowledge about their actual composition is much less compared to what is known about immunoglobulins. Some data are available (Hay et al., 1971; Ericsson et al., 1976; Kaskhet and Guilmette, 1978; Levine et al., 1978; Mirth et al., 1979a,b) and it seems clear that they can be separated from the salivary immunoglobulins by column chromatography (Kaskhet and Guilmette, 1978). However, as observed by Ericson et al. (1979a) the streptococcal agglutinating activity of whole parotid saliva can be completely abolished after the addition of anti-IgA serum. This observation suggests that antibodies and agglutinins may be associated with each other in saliva. Agglutinins have been reported to interfere with dental plaque formation (Magnusson and Ericson, 1976) and to prevent adhesion of bacteria to epithelial cells *in vitro* (Williams and Gibbons, 1975). There seem to be some contradictory results as to how the agglutinating capacity varies between different subjects. Bratthall and Carlén (1978) found a striking similarity between parotid saliva from three different subjects. Submandibular saliva, however, differed between the subjects for a few bacterial strains. Other papers seem to indicate more variations from subject to subject with parotid saliva as well.

Bacteria and Other Salivary Components

Saliva and crevicular fluid certainly contain other substances than antibodies with an ability to react with bacteria. In a recent study, Ericson et al. (1979b) tested 31 oral streptococci for the possible binding of haptoglobin, haemoglobin, fibrinogen and aggregated β_2-microglobulin. They also investigated the possibility of bacterial binding to the Fc part of human immunoglobulins G, G1, G2, G3, G4, A1, A2, M1 and M2. The study showed that only β_2-microglobulin was bound by several types of streptococci. Also, IgA1 showed positive binding to one strain. Furthermore, Myhre and Kronvall (1980) showed that albumin may be adsorbed to certain streptococci. These results indicate that not only antibodies and agglutinins may affect bacteria in the oral cavity but also other host factors. In addition, foods contain components which may also bind to the bacteria. For example, Bratthall (1978) has shown that carrots (*Daucus carrota*) can bind certain types of streptococci and an extract from carrots may agglutinate *Strep. mutans*.

These data suggest that many types of reactions exist between bacteria and oral fluid components and that these probably may interact, preventing reactions of other substances or perhaps enhancing them. Therefore, it must be rather difficult to define the exact role of a single substance, such as antibodies, with respect to caries or periodontitis in man. Variations in oral hygiene, dietary regimens or fluorides might mask even major effects. In a discussion Good (1978) pointed out the difficulties in interpreting studies of this sort. He stressed that useful data could be obtained by studying a small number of unique populations, for example patients with immunodeficiencies. Indeed, it has been suggested that individuals suffering from immunoglobulin deficiencies are more susceptible to dental caries than normal individuals (Robertson and Cooper, 1974; Cole *et al.*, 1977; Arnold *et al.*, 1979). To extend further our knowledge about these types of defects, we have studied the oral condition in a group of adults with hypogammaglobulinaemia and we have investigated their salivary agglutinins.

A Study of Hypogammaglobulinaemic Patients

Subjects

Eleven hypogammaglobulinaemic patients had oral examinations. The patients had been referred to Sahlgren's Hospital, Göteborg, for a detailed

TABLE I
Some Medical Data of Hypogammaglobulinaemic Patients Included in the Study

Age/Sex	Clinical manifestations	Height (cm)	Weight (kg)	Duration of symptoms (years)
25 m	Chronic bronchitis Chronic blepharitis Corneal cicatrization	172	40	25
29 m	Chronic bronchitis Pulmonary emphysema Bronchiectasis	175	59	26
29 f	Chronic bronchitis Pulmonary emphysema Entero-colitis (non-specific)	155	53	22
31 f	Bronchiectasia Emphysema Chronic sinusitis	158	41	31
35 f	Diabetes mellitus Chronic sinusitis Entero-colitis Arthralgia	167	47	30
37 f	Entero-colitis	165	51	11
40 m	Chronic bronchitis Bronchiectasis Chronic sinusitis Gastro-duodenitis	170	62	34
51 f	Urticaria Entero-colitis Arthralgia	155	54	23
57 f	Bronchiectasis Entero-colitis Arthralgia	161	57	33
66 m	Chronic bronchitis Chronic sinusitis	178	94	34
66 f	Chronic bronchitis Bronchiectasis Pernicious anaemia Osteoarthritis	154	55	32

clinical and immunological investigation. Some data from the medical examination are listed in Table I and the serum immunoglobulins are shown in Table II. The patients were given codes of numbers indicating their age and m (male) or f (female) for their sex. Thus, "66 f" is a 66-year-old woman. Every second or third week the patients received injections of 20–30 ml gammaglobulins. The examinations listed below were performed at least 2 weeks after the last injection. Data from a Swedish epidemiological study including 1000 subjects were used for comparison (Axelsson et al., 1976). Saliva controls were obtained from six healthy subjects of 25–40 years of age.

TABLE II
Immunoglobulin G, A, M and E Concentrations in Serum of the Hypogammaglobulinaemic Patients

Subjects	IgG (g/l)	IgA (g/l)	IgM (g/l)	IgE (µg/l)
25 m	2.4	0	0	<5
29 m	3.3	0	0	<5
29 f	3.2	0	0.4	<5
31 f	Trace	0·	0	<5
35 f	3.6	0.1	0.2	11
37 f	0.7	0	0.8	<5
40 m	3.5	0	0.1	<5
51 f	6.6	0	1.0	<5
57 f	3.0	0	0	<5
66 m	3.6	0.7	0.5	<5
66 f	1.6	0	0	<5
Range	6.6–trace	0.7–0.1	1.0–0	11–<5
Normal values range	17–7	3.5–0.5	1.8–0.5	

Oral Examination

The oral examination included registration of a number of teeth (third molar excluded), bitewing radiographs, caries experience (decayed or filled surfaces), percentage of tooth surfaces with visible plaque (Silness and Löe, 1964; score 2 and 3), gingivitis (Löe and Silness, 1963; score 2 and 3) and pocket formation (probing depth), i.e. a gingival crevice of 4 mm or more. All measurements were performed on the four surfaces of each tooth.

Saliva and Microbial Analyses

Three saliva samples were collected. First an unstimulated whole saliva sample was obtained. About 0.3–0.5 ml was collected and used for the determination of IgG, IgA or IgM by the technique of Mancini et al. (1965), using Behringwerke antisera. Another paraffin-stimulated whole saliva sample was collected. It was used to determine the secretion rate, buffer capacity and pH (Ericsson, 1959). One millilitre of this sample was used for enumeration of *Strep. mutans* and lactobacilli, using standard methods (see Klock and Krasse, 1977). The third saliva sample consisted of parotid saliva. Eleven millilitres of saliva stimulated with citric acid was collected with Curby cups over a period of about 30 min. The parotid saliva was tested for the presence of IgA antibodies reacting with *Strep. mutans* strain KPSK2 (serotype c) and B13 (d) and *Strep. sanguis* strain ATCC 10556 and DB 401. The modified ELISA technique was used (Bratthall *et al.*, 1978). Parotid saliva was also used for aggregation experiments with *Strep. mutans* KPSK2 and *Strep. sanguis* DB 401. The technique described by Ericson *et al.* (1975) was adopted. Furthermore, aggregation inhibition experiments were performed as described by Ericson *et al* (1979*a*). The anti-immunoglobulin antisera were obtained from Behringwerke.

Results

Three patients (40 m, 57 f, 66 f) were completely edentulous. Subject 40 m had lost his teeth at about the age of 26. Subject 57 f had lost her maxillary teeth at the age of 17 and the mandibular teeth about 10 years later. Subject 66 f had all her teeth extracted at about the age of 30. One patient, 66 m, had only two teeth left. He had lost most of his teeth when he was about 25 years old. Subjects 40 m and 66 m seemed to be certain that the reason for the extractions was that the teeth had become loose rather rapidly. The other two patients were not certain but believed that both caries and periodontitis had been present.

Seven patients had most of their teeth left. However, 29 f had only 20 teeth, about six teeth less than the age-matched controls.

These data are summarized in Table III.

Number of decayed and filled teeth
With only one exception (37 f), all patients had more surfaces attacked by caries than their controls (see Table III).

Plaque, gingivitis and pocket formation
All patients had more surfaces covered by plaque and more surfaces had gingivitis, except for patient 37 f. Pocket formation was specially evident in patients 29 f and 35 f.

Secretion rate, pH and buffer capacity
A normal secretion rate with paraffin stimulation is 1–3 ml/min (Ericsson and Hardwick, 1978). Six patients fell in this group. Three patients had higher rates and two lower. Saliva pHs were generally close to normal (7.0–7.5), whilst five patients had a rather low buffer capacity (normal end pH 5.75–6.50).

TABLE III

Data from the Oral Examinations of Hypogammaglobulinaemic Patients in Comparison with Control Groups

Subjects	Number of teeth		Number of decayed or filled surfaces	Percentage of tooth surfaces with		
	Male	Female		Plaque	Gingivitis	Pocket formation
Controls, 20 years	27.5	26.9	35.1	29.1	34.5	1.2
Patient 25 m	25		65	51	55	7
Patient 29 m	27		73	70	56	4
Patient 29 f		20	62	90	93	33
Controls, 30 years	25.8	25.8	48.4	30.3	23.9	3.1
Patient 31 f		28	53	81	56	3
Patient 35 f		26	88	63	61	14
Patient 37 f		28	14	10	1	0
Controls, 40 years	23.1	23.5	52.6	40.4	32.7	7.5
Patient 40 m	0					
Controls, 50 years	19.5	20.5	50.5	44.3	38.5	8.5
Patient 51 f		27	86	59	31	3
Patient 57 f		0				
Controls, 60 years	14.5	14.9	49.0	49.7	43.5	10.8
Patient 66 m	2		(10)*	(75)*	(75)*	
Patient 66 f		0				
Controls, 70 years	8.9	8.1	41.0	66.2	60.2	14.4

* Based on two teeth only.

TABLE IV
Examination of the Secretion Rate, pH, Buffer Capacity and Bacterial Contents in Saliva

Subjects	Stimulated, whole saliva			Number of colony forming units per millilitre of saliva		Comments
	Secretion rate (ml/min)	pH	Buffer capacity	Strep. mutans	Lactobacilli	
25 m	2.30	7.61	7.67			
29 m	1.33	7.28	4.28	170 000	750 000	
29 f	1.32	6.83	3.38	1 370 000	450 000	
31 f	3.55	7.34	3.50	1 330 000	7 800	
35 f	0.85	7.24	6.29	80 000	184 000	
37 f	1.55	7.73	7.85	119 000	3 500	Good oral health
40 m	5.25	7.49	7.60	9 800	600	No teeth
51 f	1.67	7.23	4.43			
57 f	2.30	7.66	6.70	<100	137 000	No teeth
66 m	4.25	7.47	7.92	1 250 000	32 000	Only two teeth
66 f	0.88	6.90	4.16	<100	30 000	No teeth

TABLE V
Parotid IgA Antibody Levels of Hypogammaglobulinaemic Patients and Control Subjects (C1–C6) as Determined by the ELISA Technique

Subject	Strep. mutans KPSK2	Strep. mutans B13	Strep. sanguis ATCC 10556	Strep. sanguis DB401	Saliva control
25 m	0.12	0.09	0.06	0.06	0.03
25 m*	0.09	0.07	0.06	0.03	0.04
29 m	0.07	0.03	0.05	0.04	0.01
29 f	0.08	0.04	0.05	0.04	0.02
31 f	0.10	0.07	0.07	0.05	0.02
35 f	0.09	0.05	0.04	0.03	0.01
37 f	0.08	0.06	0.07	0.04	0.02
37 f*	0.08	0.08	0.06	0.05	0.02
40 f	0.10	0.05	0.05	0.04	0.02
51 f	0.10	0.05	0.07	0.03	0.02
57 f	0.12	0.05	0.07	0.06	0.01
66 m	0.16	0.18	0.21	0.24	0.09
66 f	0.06	0.04	0.05	003	0.02
C 1	0.91	0.75	0.86	0.80	0.07
C 2	1.29	1.57	2.23	2.41	0.08
C 3	1.62	1.61	1.35	1.46	0.11
C 4	1.23	1.75	2.85	3.18	0.11
C 5	2.15	2.83	3.28	3.12	0.09
C 6	1.63	1.60	1.61	1.45	—
Bacteria control	0.12	0.08	0.09	0.06	—

ELISA values are based on spectrophotometer readings at 405 nm and the mean of four determinations are given. 'Saliva control' indicates tubes without bacteria. 'Bacteria control' is the total procedure without saliva added. For further details see Bratthall et al. (1978).

* Saliva collected 1 day after the patient had received an injection of 20–30 ml γ-globulin. In all other cases, salivas were collected at least 14 days after the last injection of γ-globulin.

Strep. mutans *and lactobacilli*

Based on clinical experience, we use > 1 million *Strep. mutans* per millilitre of saliva as indicating a high bacterial count. Three of the dentulous patients had a high count. For lactobacilli, 100 000–1 million per millilitre of saliva is considered to be a high count. One subject reached 750 000 (29 m) and another 450 000 (29 f). The patient with good oral health (37 f) had only 3500 lactobacilli per mililitre of saliva.

Immunoglobulins in saliva
In unstimulated whole saliva only one patient, 37 f, showed trace amounts of IgA. In subjects 35 f and 51 f, some IgG could be detected (0.09 and 0.01 g/l, respectively). No other patient showed IgG, IgA or IgM either in unstimulated whole saliva or in stimulated parotid saliva.

Another sample of saliva was collected from two patients (25 m, 37 f) just 1 day after they had received γ-globulin injections (20–30 ml). No immunoglobulins could be detected in these saliva samples.

Parotid IgA antibodies reacting with specific strains of *Strep. mutans* and *Strep. sanguis* were tested with the ELISA technique (Table V). The ELISA readings for the hypogammaglobulinaemic patients were close to the buffer controls. Parotid saliva from control subjects showed considerably higher values.

Bacterial aggregation induced by parotid saliva
Aggregation curves for *Strep. mutans* KPSK 2 are shown in Fig. 1. The pattern obtained with saliva from patient 25 m is very similar to that of the control subject.

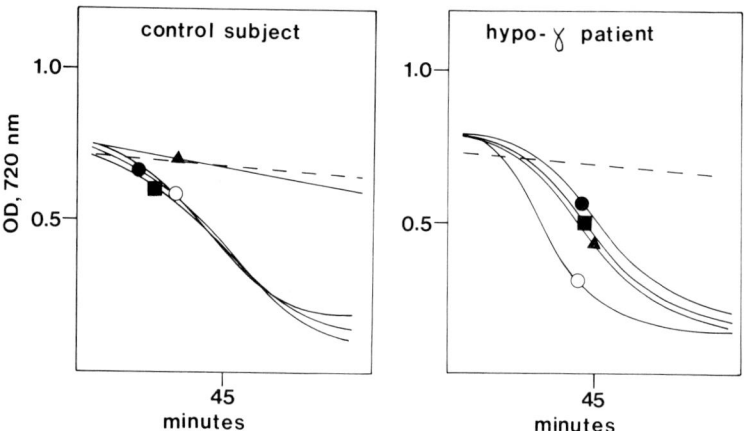

Fig. 1 Aggregation of *Strep. mutans*, strain KPSK 2 (serotype c) by saliva of a control subject and a hypogammaglobulinaemic patient (25-year-old male). ○——○, parotid saliva and bacteria; ●——●, parotid saliva, anti-IgG and bacteria; ■——■, parotid saliva, anti-IgM and bacteria; ▲——▲, parotid saliva, anti-IgA and bacteria; ---, bacteria only (control).

The reaction mixtures consisted of 0.5 ml parotid saliva, 0.1 ml 0.01 M potassium phosphate buffer, pH 7.0 containing 0.15 M NaCl (PBS) and 1.2 ml bacterial suspension in PBS; O.D. 1.5 at 700 nm. In the inhibition experiments 0.1 ml PBS was replaced by 0.1 ml anti-IgG, IgA or IgM antisera (Behringweke), diluted 1:2 in PBS. In these studies, saliva and anti-Ig were mixed 90 min prior to the addition of bacteria. For further details, see Ericson *et al.* (1979a).

10. Oral Condition in Hypogammaglobulinaemic Patients 169

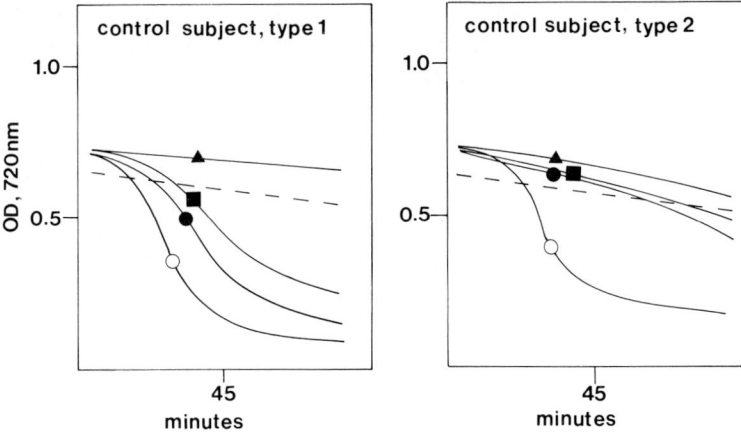

Fig. 2 Aggregation of *Strep. sanguis* strain DB401 induced by parotid saliva of healthy, control subjects. Reaction mixtures consisted of saliva, PBS and bacteria (O———O), or saliva, bacteria and anti-IgG (●———●), anti-IgM (■———■) or anti-IgA (▲———▲). – – – denotes bacteria without saliva (control). See Fig. 1 for details.

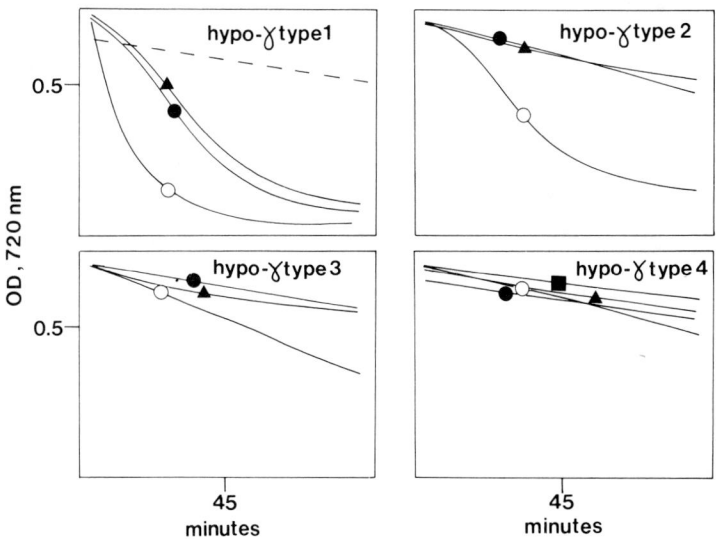

Fig. 3 Aggregation of *Strep. sanguis* strain DB401 induced by parotid saliva of hypogammaglobulinaemic patients. Reaction mixtures consisted of saliva, PBS and bacteria (O———O), or saliva, bacteria and anti-IgG (●———●), anti-IgM (■———■) or anti-IgA (▲———▲). – – – denotes bacteria without saliva (control). See Fig. 1 for details. Data are given for the following subjects: 40 m (type 1); 51 f (type 2); 31 f (type 3); 37 f (type 4).

Adding anti-IgA but not IgM or IgG sera inhibited the aggregation of bacteria by saliva from the control subjects. For the hypogammaglobulinaemic patient, however, anti-IgA had no effect. The individual curves shown are representative for all patients, controls as well as the hypogammaglobulinaemic patients, respectively.

Aggregation curves for *Strep. sanguis* are shown in Figs 2 and 3. Saliva from all control subjects aggregated *Strep. sanguis* DB 401. When anti-immunoglobulin antisera were added two types of reactions occurred. For five subjects, only anti-IgA inhibited the reaction; for one subject, anti-IgA, IgM and IgG prevented the reaction (Fig. 2).

The hypogammaglobulinaemic patients showed four types of reactions (Fig. 3): (i) aggregation with no inhibition by anti-IgG, IgA and IgM; (ii) aggregation with inhibition of anti-immunoglobulin antisera; (iii) aggregation to a limited extent with inhibition of anti-immunoglobulin antisera and (iv) no aggregation.

Discussion

Although many laboratory studies have indicated important roles for various salivary components reacting with bacteria, there have been rather few observations concerning their clinical significance. The difficulties in such studies have already been pointed out. All our hypogammaglobulinaemic patients had very low levels of immunoglobulins in their sera and little if any immunoglobulins in their saliva. All patients, with one exception, showed more plaque, more gingivitis and more decayed and filled tooth surfaces compared to age-matched controls. However, these indices are not necessarily strong indicators of specific immunoglobulin effects. As the patients have long medical records, oral hygiene may have been neglected. Medications may have increased caries activity, as sucrose is a common ingredient in many medicines and the salivary flow may also have been affected. However, the rapid loss of teeth between the ages of 20 and 30 years seems to be an unusual observation. Indeed, after this study had been completed 10 additional hypogammaglobulinaemic patients were checked for dental disease. Two of these patients had lost all their teeth between 25 and 30 years of age and one patient had had all his maxillary teeth extracted. This means that seven out of 21 patients showed severe loss of teeth at an early age. Although this study does not present direct evidence that a lack of immunoglobulins is the causative factor, it points to these patients as a risk group. It also suggests that, although many of the inflammatory and destructive effects of periodontitis presumably result from hypersensitivity responses, the protective functions of the immune system should not be overlooked.

Saliva from the hypogammaglobulinaemic patients and control subjects induced aggregation of *Strep. mutans* in a similar way. However, anti-IgA had no effect if added to saliva from patients with hypogammaglobulinaemia. If salivary IgA under normal conditions interacts with agglutinins (Ericson *et al.*, 1979a; Mirth *et al.*, 1979a), the agglutination capacity would be changed by adding anti-IgA. Consequently, the reactions of the hypogammaglobulinaemic patients would be unaffected. Unlike with *Strep. mutans*, the reactions with the *Strep. sanguis* strain were complicated. Probably the salivary receptors for *Strep. sanguis* are different from those on *Strep. mutans*. Thus, if the salivary aggregating factors play an important part in the defence mechanism, these patients may have the factors for certain species of streptococci and not for others.

Summary

Bacteria in the oral cavity are exposed to a variety of host protective mechanisms in the saliva or in the crevicular fluid. Among the non-specific factors, lysozyme, lactoferrin and lactoperoxidase have been specially emphasized. Antibodies and possibly the salivary agglutinins are considered to be more specific. In view of the successful results of several animal immunization experiments against caries, considerable interest has been focused on the role of secretory antibodies. Although there are some data about the effects of antibodies and agglutinins, some confusion exists concerning their role in the regulation of the oral bacterial flora in man. Saliva and crevicular fluid also contain other substances with a potential ability to react with bacteria e.g. β_2-microglobulin. In addition, substances from food may bind to bacteria.

The development of both caries and periodontal disease is dependent on several factors, such as the amount of plaque, types of bacteria, diet, etc. It is therefore difficult to describe the exact role of mucosal immunity in these diseases. However, studies of immunodeficient patients might at least give some indication of the role of immunity in dental disease. A group of 11 hypogammaglobulinaemic patients with low IgG, IgA or IgM in serum were examined for the number of teeth, caries experience (DMFS), gingival and periodontal status and plaque scores. Salivary samples were analysed for immunoglobulins, secretion rate, pH, buffer capacity, IgA antibodies reacting with *Strep. mutans* and *Strep. sanguis* and for agglutinins against these bacteria. The numbers of lactobacilli and *Strep. mutans* in saliva were also determined. Data from a Swedish epidemiological study comprising 1000 subjects were used as controls.

The results showed that the hypogammaglobulinaemic patients (in all cases but one) had higher DMFS compared to age-matched controls, as well as more dental plaque and pocket formation. No salivary antibodies were found but all salivas agglutinated *Strep. mutans* normally. All patients harboured

Strep. mutans and lactobacilli. The most striking observation was, however, that four of the patients gave a history of rapid loss of teeth between the ages of 20 and 30 years. Another group of 10 hypogammaglobulinaemic patients were studied and two of these also had lost their teeth between 25 and 30 years of age and one had had all his maxillary teeth extracted. Thus, seven out of 21 patients showed severe loss of teeth at an early age. It is suggested that these data illustrate a possible role of antibodies in the protection of teeth against caries and periodontal disease.

Acknowledgements

This study was supported by the Swedish Medical Research Council, Project No. 4548. We wish to acknowledge the expert technical assistance of Miss Anette Carlén, Department of Cariology, Faculty of Odontology, University of Göteborg, Göteborg, Sweden.

References

Arnold, R. R., Mestecky, J. and McGhee, J. R. (1976). *Infect. Immun.* **14**, 355–362.
Arnold, R. R., Pruitt, K. M., Cole, M. F., Adamson, J. M. and McGhee, R. R. (1979). In *Saliva and Dental Caries* (I. Kleinberg, S. A. Ellison and I. D. Mandel, eds), pp. 449–462, Special Supplement to *Microbiology Abstracts*
Axelsson, P., Göland, U., Hugoson, A., Koch, G., Paulander, G., Pettersson, S., Rasmusson, C-G., Schmidt, G. and Thilander, H. (1975). *Tandläkartidn* **11**, 656–667.
Bowen, W. H. (1974). *J. oral Path.* **3**, 266–278.
Bowen, W. H. and Guggenheim, B. (1978). *Acta odont. scand.* **36**, 185–198.
Brandtzaeg, P. (1965). *Archs oral biol.* **10**, 795–803.
Brandtzaeg, P. and Tolo, K. (1977). In *Borderland between Caries and Periodontal Disease* (T. Lehner, ed), pp. 145–183, Academic Press, London and Grune and Stratton, New York.
Bratthall, D. (1978). In *Secretory Immunity and Infection* (J. R. McGhee and J. Mestecky, eds), pp. 327–333, Plenum Press, New York and London.
Bratthall, D. and Carlén, A. (1978). *Scand. J. dent. Res.* **86**, 430–443.
Bratthall, D., Gahnberg, L. and Krasse, B. (1978). *Archs oral Biol.* **23**, 843–849.
Bratthall, D., Carlén, A., Knox, K. W. and Wicken, A. J. (1979). *Acta path. microbiol. scand.* **87**, 251–255.
Challacombe, S. J., Russell, M. W. and Hawkes, J. (1978). *Clin. exp. Immunol.* **34**, 417–422.
Cimasoni, G., Ishikawa, I. and Jaccard, F. (1977). In *Borderland between Caries and Periodontal Disease* (T. Lehner, ed), pp. 13–41. Academic Press, London and Grune and Stratton, New York.
Cole, M. F., Arnold, R. R., Rhodes, M. J. and McGhee, J. R. (1977). *J. dent. Res.* **56**, 198–204.
Ericsson, Y. (1959). *Acta odont. scand.* **17**, 131–165.
Ericsson, Y. and Hardwick, L. (1978). *Caries Res.* **12**, 94–102.

Ericson, Th., Pruitt, K. and Wedel, H. (1975). *J. oral Path.* **4**, 307–323.
Ericson, Th., Carlén, A. and Dagerskog, L. (1976). In *Microbial Aspects of Dental Caries* (M. M. Stiles, W. J. Loesche and T. C. O'Brien, eds), Information Retrieval Inc., Washington, D. C.
Ericson, Th., Bratthall, D. and Rundegren, J. (1979a). In *Saliva and Dental Caries* (I. Kleinberg, S. A. Ellison and I. D. Mandel, eds), pp. 243–254, Special Supplement to *Microbiology Abstracts*.
Ericson, D., Bratthall, D., Björk, L., Myhre, E. and Kronvall, G. (1979b). *Infect. Immun.* **25**, 279–283.
Good, R. A. (1978). In *Secretory Immunity and Infection* (J. R. McGhee, J. Mestecky and J. L. Babb, eds), pp. 395, Plenum Press, New York and London.
Hay, E. J., Gibbons, R. J. and Spinell, D. M. (1971). *Caries Res.* **5**, 111–123.
Jay, P., Crowley, M., Hadley, F. F. and Bunting, R. W. (1933). *J. Am. dent. Assoc.* **20**, 2130–2148.
Kashket, S. and Guilmette, K. M. (1978). *Caries Res.* **12**, 170–172.
Keyes, P. H. (1960). *Archs oral Biol.* **1**, 304–320.
Klock, B. and Krasse, B. (1977). *Scand. J. dent. Res.* **85**, 56–63.
Lehner, T. (1977). In *Borderland between Caries and Periodontal Disease* (T. Lehner, ed.), pp. 129–144, Academic Press, London and Grune and Stratton, New York.
Lehner, T., Murray, J. J., Winter, G. and Caldwell, J. 1978). *Archs oral Biol.* **23**, 1061–1067.
Levine, M. J., Hertzberg, M. C., Levine, M. S., Ellison, S. A., Stinson, M. W., Li, H. C. and Dyke, T. (1978). *Infect. Immun.* **19**, 107–115.
Löe, H. and Silness, J. (1963). *Acta odont. scand.* **21**, 533–551.
Mancini, G., Carbonara, A. and Heremans, J. (1965). *Immunochemistry* **2**, 235–254.
Magnusson, I. and Ericson, Th (1976). *Caries Res.* **10**, 273–286.
Mirth, D. B., Miller, C. J., Kingman, A. and Bowen, W. H. (1979a). In *Saliva and Dental Caries* (I. Kleinberg, S. A. Ellison and I. D. Mandel, eds), pp. 255–266, Special Supplement to *Microbiology Abstracts*
Mirth, D. B., Miller, C. J., Kingman, A. and Bowen, W. H. (1979b). *Caries Res.* **13**, 121–131.
Myhre, E. B. and Kronvall, G. (1980). *Infect. Immun.* **27**, 6–14.
Robertson, P. B. and Cooper, M. D. (1974). In *The Immunoglobulin A System* (J. Mestecky and A. R. Lawton, eds), pp. 497–503, Plenum Press, New York and London.
Silness, J. and Löe, H. (1964). *Acta odont. scand.* **22**, 121–135.
Williams, R. and Gibbons, R. (1975). *Infect. Immun.* **11**, 711–718.

11. Effects of Immunization on Periodontal Disease and Caries in Gnotobiotic Rats Associated with *Actinomyces viscosus*

B. GUGGENHEIM

Actinomyces viscosus: Cariogenic and Periodontopathic Bacterium

Rodent model systems initiated the present trend in oral microbiology of correlating distinct disease entities with specific microorganisms. In 1960, Fitzgerald and Keyes demonstrated the aetiological role of strains of *Streptococcus mutans* in experimental caries. At that time the original observations of J. K. Clarke (1924) on the cariogenicity of this species in man had been forgotten. However, these findings were confirmed by Krasse *et al.* (1968) and de Stoppelaar *et al.* (1969). The situation was similar with periodontal disease. Experimental periodontitis was induced by a Gram-positive, filamentous bacterium, now classified as *Actinomyces viscosus* (George *et al.*, 1969), in hamsters by Jordan and Keyes (1965) and in gnotobiotic rats by Jordan *et al.* (1965). The role of *A. viscosus* in the aetiology of human periodontal diseases is less convincingly documented. Proportions of *A. viscosus* and *A. israelii* were found to be positively correlated with the gingival inflammatory index score (Loesche and Syed, 1978). More indirect evidence for the participation of *A. viscosus* in the aetiology of the disease was gained through immunological studies. Peripheral blood lymphocytes from gingivitis and periodontitis patients showed an increased blastogenesis in the presence of crude *A. viscosus* antigens (Ivanyi *et al.*, 1972; Lang and Smith, 1977). Nevertheless, the microflora associated with human periodontal disease seems to be much more complex and not related to a single genus of bacteria. This area has been recently reviewed (Slots, 1979). It is premature to speculate whether the different forms of human periodontal disease are the result of (a) the host response to a particular bacterial species, (b) the host response to certain ecological communities, (c) a mixture of both, (d) a response to a particular species living within a nutritionally interrelated community.

It was our aim some years ago to study the effect of bacterial interactions on caries and periodontal disease in the gnotobiotic rat. *A. viscosus* Ny 1 and *Streptococcus mutans* OMZ 26 (serotype d) were mono- and di-associated in germ-free RIC-rats. At an average age of 21 days, two animals from each of four litters were transferred to three isolators. On days 31 and 32, the animals in the first treatment were mono-associated with *A. viscosus* Ny 1, the rats in the second treatment with *Strep. mutans* OMZ 26, while those in the third group were di-associated with both organisms. The animals received the γ-irradiated (2.5 Mrd) cariogenic vitaminized diet 580 (Gustafson, 1963) and autoclaved water *ad libitum*. All rats were killed on day 73 (42 experimental days). Plaque was scored according to Regolati and Hotz (1972); bone loss in mandibles was measured using the modified methods described by Keyes and Gold (1955) and Costich (1955). Dental caries in mandibular molars was assessed as described by Keyes (1958) and König (1966). General procedures used in our gnotobiotic animals have been published (Guggenheim and Schroeder, 1974). Details of this particular experiment formed part of a thesis (Wuhrmann, 1977).

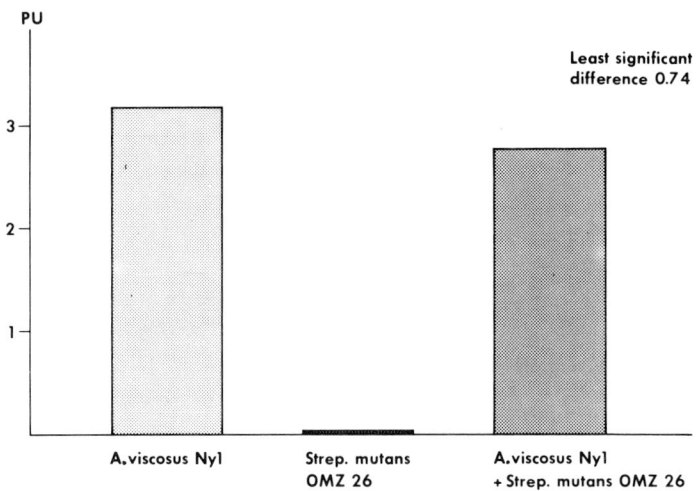

Fig. 1 Smooth surface plaque units (PU) of gnotobiotic rats mono- or di-associated with *A. viscosus* Ny 1 and *Strep. mutans* OMZ 26 for 42 days; 4 units at risk.

As shown in Fig. 1, the rats mono-associated with *Strep. mutans* developed practically no smooth surface plaque, while *A. viscosus* Ny 1 mono-or di-associated with *Strep. mutans* OMZ 26 covered almost all surfaces with a voluminous layer. *A. viscosus* in mono-association was responsible for a moderate incidence of smooth surface caries, while this particular strain of *Strep. mutans* alone or di-associated with *A. viscosus* caused only a negligible number of lesions (Fig. 2). A reverse pattern was found with regard to fissure

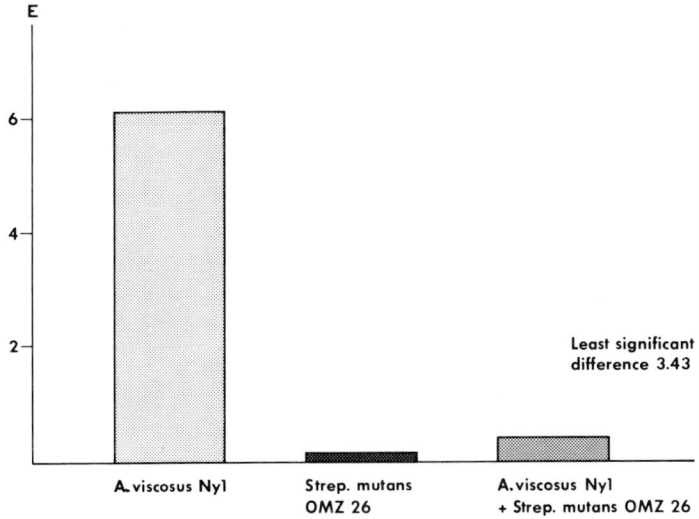

Fig. 2 Smooth surface caries score (E) of gnotobiotic rats mono-or di-associated with *A. viscosus* Ny 1 and *Strep. mutans* OMZ 26 for 42 days; 24 units at risk.

caries (Fig. 3). *A. viscosus* Ny 1 failed to produce fissure caries in mono-association. *Strep. mutans* OMZ 26 was only weakly cariogenic, but in di-association these strains showed an increased cariogenic activity. The nature of these interactions remain to be resolved. The evaluation of periodontal

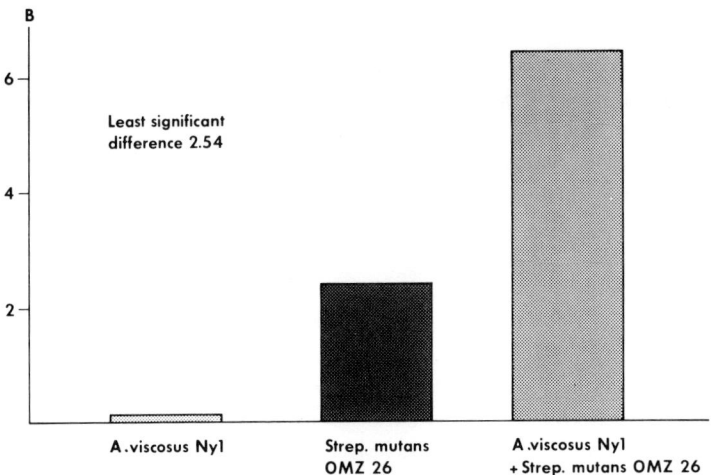

Fig. 3 Advanced dentinal fissure lesions (B) of gnotobiotic rats mono- or di-associated with *A. viscosus* Ny 1 and *Strep. mutans* OMZ 26 for 42 days; 12 units at risk.

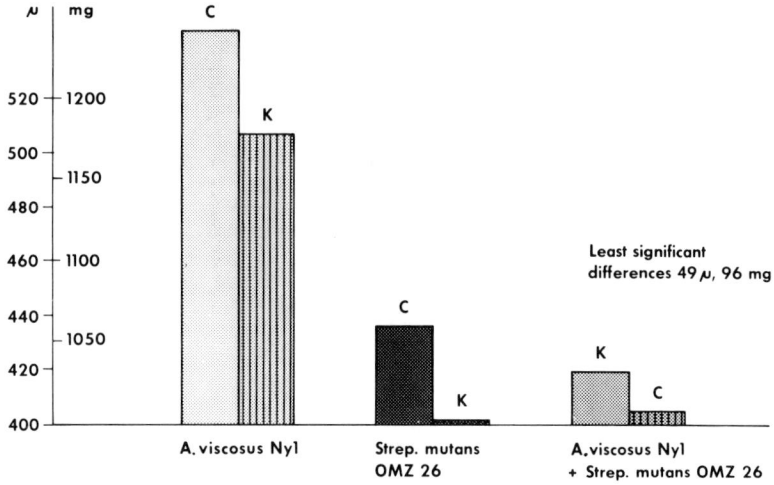

Fig. 4 Mandibular alveolar bone loss of gnotobiotic rats mono- or di-associated with *A. viscosus* Ny 1 and *Strep. mutans* OMZ 26 for 42 days. Evaluation according to Costich (1955) (C) and according to Keyes and Gold (1955) (K).

bone loss (Fig. 4) showed that animals mono-associated with *A. viscosus* Ny 1 had experienced significantly more bone loss compared to the other two treatments. The combined flora had no osteolytic effect, although the amount of plaque was not significantly different in mono- from di-associated rats (Figs 1, 4).

The following conclusions were drawn from this experiment. *A. viscosus* Ny 1 caused smooth surface caries and periodontitis when mono-associated in RIC-rats. In animals di-associated with *Strep. mutans* and *A. viscosus* antagonistic and synergistic interactions were found. In the di-associated animals smooth surface caries and bone loss were significantly reduced, while fissure caries was significantly enhanced as compared with rats mono-associated with *A. viscosus*.

It follows from this and other experiments in conventional or gnotobiotic rodents (König and Guggenheim, 1968; Regolati *et al.*, 1972; Mikx *et al.*, 1975, 1976a,b) that the cariogenic potential of a given bacterium may be largely modified by the accompanying microflora. The weak cariogenicity of *Strep. mutans* OMZ 26 in this experiment is not surprising because it has repeatedly been observed that rats above the age of 30 days showed a rapidly decreasing caries susceptibility. This has been interpreted as "enamel maturation" (reviewed by König, 1966) and by a decreased oral colonization of *Strep. mutans* during ageing in rats (van Houte *et al.*, 1977). A possible change in the immune response has not been studied systematically. Nevertheless, it should be borne in mind that testing for pathogenicity of oral bacteria in animals, and especially in gnotobiotic animals, serves a limited purpose (Socransky, 1979) and to extrapolate those findings to man is unwarranted.

Difficulties in the Assessment of Cellular Immunity in Gnotobiotic Rats

Morphometric analysis of the infiltrated connective tissue of rats mono-associated with *A. viscosus* (Guggenheim and Schroeder, 1974) revealed a similar sequence of events to that observed in human periodontal lesions (reviewed by Page and Schroeder, 1976).

As judged by the cellular composition of the infiltrate after an acute inflammatory phase, a classical delayed hypersensitivity reaction developed which then changed into a dense and later a plasma cell infiltration. To substantiate the role of cell-mediated immune reactions, rat lymphocyte cultures did not seem to confront us with major problems in view of the work accomplished with human peripheral lymphoid cells (Ivanyi *et al.*, 1972; Mackler *et al.*, 1974; Baker *et al.*, 1976). Although the immunological history of syngeneic mono-associated rats is known and experimental factors are easy to control, the development of periodontitis in gnotobiotic animals has never been associated with delayed hypersensitivity.

The collection of peripheral blood as source of rat lymphocytes was not feasible because of the insufficient yield of cells. Lymphocytes were therefore separated mainly from spleens. While establishing optimum cultural conditions for these cells from unsensitized germ-free animals, it was observed that *A. viscosus* antigens induced a strong lympho-proliferative response. Under these circumstances it seemed impossible to monitor changes of cell-mediated immunity in rats mono-associated with *A. viscosus*.

B-cell Mitogenicity of *A. viscosus* Antigens

It was evident that the lympho-proliferative response of cells from germ-free animals could be explained by a mitogenic property of the antigen preparation used. This was demonstrated independently by Burckhardt *et al.* (1977) and Engel *et al.* (1977). It was shown that crude antigen preparations—and in our study also a purified extracellular heteroglycan—stimulated spleen cells from germ-free rats and conventional mice and those from athymic nude mice. Such spleen cells developed direct plaque-forming cells against densely coupled TNP-sheep red blood cells. The mitogenic properties of the antigen preparations could be diminished considerably by mild alkaline hydrolysis, treatment with bacterial protease or treatment with metaperiodate.

The B-cell mitogenicity of *Actinomyces* fractions, and most probably also human plaque, does not seem to have interfered with human lymphocyte cultures (Ivanyi et al., 1972; Lang and Smith, 1977; Baker et al., 1976). This may be explained by different modes of antigen preparation or differences in the culture conditions. It is, however, not due to a differential reactivity of lymphocytes from rodents and man, because purified fractions of *A. viscosus* are strongly mitogenic for human B-cells (J. J. Burckhardt, unpublished data).

Under these conditions an *in vitro* test system reflecting the cell-mediated immune status of rats mono-associated with *A. viscosus* could only be established by eliminating the "background" response to the B-cell mitogens. Two solutions to this problem seemed possible, the elimination of B-cells on a preparative scale or, alternatively, the preparation of mitogen-free antigens. The second possibility was dismissed. Initially it seemed important to work with a crude antigen mixture, because it is not known whether certain antigens are critical for triggering the chronic inflammatory response. The loss of such antigens during purification could have obscured the picture. On the other hand, purification of the mitogens of *A. viscosus* is of interest and is being pursued.

Purification of Rat T-lymphocytes

T-lymphocytes present in rat spleen cell suspensions were separated by filtration through Degalan beads coated with anti-rat IgG serum (Wigzell, 1976). This column filtration method is highly efficient in removing B-lymphocytes, by reacting with cells containing surface IgG, while B-cells expressing other Ig class specificities are retained by anti-light chain antibodies or via Fc receptors. The reactivity of T-lymphocytes from spleens of RIC Sprague–Dawley rats, primed several months earlier with cells of *A. viscosus*, was carefully analysed (Burckhardt, 1978, 1979). T-cells from primed donors showed a strong proliferative, response on antigenic challenge *in vitro*, whereas T-cells of non-immunized conventional or germ-free controls showed only a slight response to a crude *A. viscosus* antigen preparation and were not activated by the purified extracellular heteroglycan prepared from this organism. T-cells from primed animals, as assayed by the uptake of [^{3}H]-thymidine, gave a maximum response after 4 days of culture, at a concentration of 10 μg per culture, with either of the above-mentioned antigens. The T-cell mitogen phytohaemagglutinin (PHA) induced a maximum proliferation of lymphocytes, irrespective of whether T-cells originated from primed or unprimed, conventional or germ-free animals. In addition, it could be demonstrated by culturing T-lymphocytes with protein-coated silica (a macrophage toxin) for 24 h or 4 days that the response to PHA or concanavalin A (Con A) was not macrophage dependent. In contrast, T-cells from primed rats were dependent on the help of macrophage precursors for the manifestation of an *in vitro* anamnestic response to *A. viscosus* antigens.

The removal of cells which responded non-specifically to B-cell mitogens allowed us to monitor changes in cell-mediated immunity of rats during the development of periodontitis.

Immune Status and Alveolar Bone Loss

Development of Immunological Sensitization and Alveolar Bone Loss in Rats Mono-associated with *A. viscosus* Ny 1

The development of cell-mediated immunity, antibody response and alveolar bone loss was investigated in rats mono-associated with *A. viscosus* Ny 1. Forty-three germ-free inbred RIC Sprague–Dawley rats from four litters were weaned and transferred to two plastic isolators at 22 days of age. Diet 2000 S, sterilized by γ-radiation and autoclaved tap water were available *ad libitum*. The rats in one isolator were orally mono-associated on day 27 and 28. The rats in the second isolator remained germ-free. At 26, 46, 60 and 88 days of age animals from each isolator were removed and weighed. Individual blood samples were collected after decapitation. Heat-inactivated serum samples were used to determine antibody titres against *A. viscosus* in a microagglutination test. The rats were spleenectomized and pooled spleen cells suspensions were prepared from each group of animals. T-cells were separated as discussed above. T-cell cultures were established in Eagle's high amino acid medium, supplemented with 1% syngeneic serum (Burckhardt, 1978). Experimental details and complete results are published elsewhere (Burckhardt *et al.*, 1980).

The measurement of horizontal alveolar bone loss, as performed previously, was based on a modified method of Costich (1955) and proved to be inadequate. The prominent craterform, intra-alveolar molar bone pockets, which were regularly observed, were hidden by the more elevated facial and oral alveolar bone crest and could therefore not be measured.

Accurate measurement of vertical bone loss was achieved by hemisectioning jaw quadrants mesiodistally, from the first to the third molar. The resulting lingual and palatal parts were radiographed under standardized conditions. Vertical distances between cemento-enamel junction and the deepest point of bone resorption were measured at defined sites on positive prints which had been enlarged on a fixed scale. Three or five positions per quadrant were measured, depending on whether the third molar was included or not. The resulting six or 10 values per maxilla or mandible were expressed as the average distance per animal. Statistical differences were calculated by using Student's *t*-test and one degree of freedom per animal. Further details on the methodology will be described elsewhere (Gaegauf *et al.*, 1980).

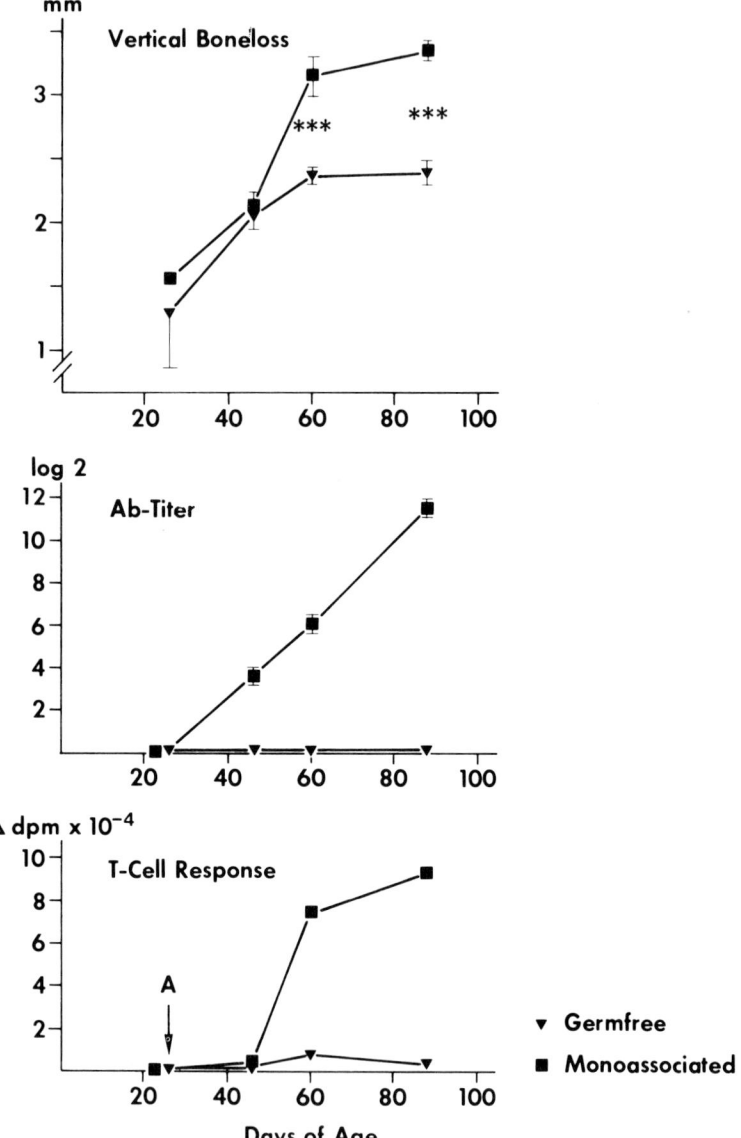

Fig. 5 Mean vertical bone loss ± s.d. of first and second maxillary molars, mean antibody titre ± s.d., and *in vitro* T-cell response of germ-free and gnotobiotic rats mono-associated with *A. viscosus*. Standard deviations are not shown if smaller than the symbols. The T-cell response was determined by the uptake of [^{3}H]thymidine in 96 h cultures, in the presence or absence of a crude antigen preparation of *A. viscosus* (BCS). The data are expressed as Δd.p.m. and refer to the mean of the peak response to BCS ($n = 3$) minus the mean of the control value in the absence of an antigen ($n = 12$); *** $P_F < 0.001$.

A summary of the results is presented in Fig. 5. As expected, the germ-free animals lacked a proliferative response of T-cells in the presence of a mixture of soluble antigens (BCS) prepared from *A. viscosus* by mechanically disrupting the bacterial cells. In contrast, T-cells from mono-associated rats showed an increased uptake of [^{3}H]thymidine as early as 19 days after infection and a strong anamnestic response at 60 and 88 days of age. Antibody titres of the germ-free animals remained negative while the antibody titre of the mono-associated rats increased linearly after infection, up to $\log_2 12$ at the end of the experiment. The average vertical distance of the mandibular molars increased in the germ-free controls up to day 60. This has also been observed by Amstad-Jossi and Schroeder (1978) and was explained by a continuous eruption of the rat molars during growth which is not matched by a concomitant rate of bone apposition at the alveolar crest. In comparison to the controls, the infected animals lost significantly more bone between days 46 and 60 and to a lesser extent between days 60 and 80. It is evident that the course of bone loss parallels closely the development of the T-cell response. To a lesser degree, however, bone loss could also be related to the progressively increasing antibody response. In spite of these related events, the rate of bone loss after 60 days declined, while the T-cell response to *A. viscosus* antigens increased further. This could be due to the appearance of suppressor cells known to be activated in delayed-type hypersensitivity (Turk et al., 1976). Such suppressor T-cells possess Fc receptors (Hertel-Wulff and Rubin, 1976) and would have been eliminated by our T-cell preparation method. Hence, their action would have been missed in our *in vitro* T-lymphocyte cultures. Although interpreted differently, *in vitro* suppression of human lymphocytes from patients with severe periodontitis has been observed by Ivanyi and Lehner (1971) and with rat cells from gnotobiotic rats infected with *Eikonella corrodens* by Johnson et al. (1978).

Alveolar Bone Loss in Immunized Rats Mono-associated with *A. viscosus* Ny 1

In an earlier study (Guggenheim and Schroeder, 1974) it was observed that subcutaneous immunization of rats with *A. viscosus* before mono-association delayed periodontal inflammation and alveolar bone loss, while intravenous immunization had the reverse effect. At that time we were not able to monitor the development of cell-mediated immunity or hypersensitivity in these animals. It was therefore rather tempting to follow both, the formation of alveolar bone loss and the T-cell response in immunized, mono-associated rats. Anything from protection to enhancement of the disease could be expected.

Germ-free rats from six litters were weaned and transferred to screen bottom, stainless-steel cages in three plastic isolators at an average age of 19 days. On day 20, rats of groups 1 and 3 were immunized with *A. viscosus* Ny 1

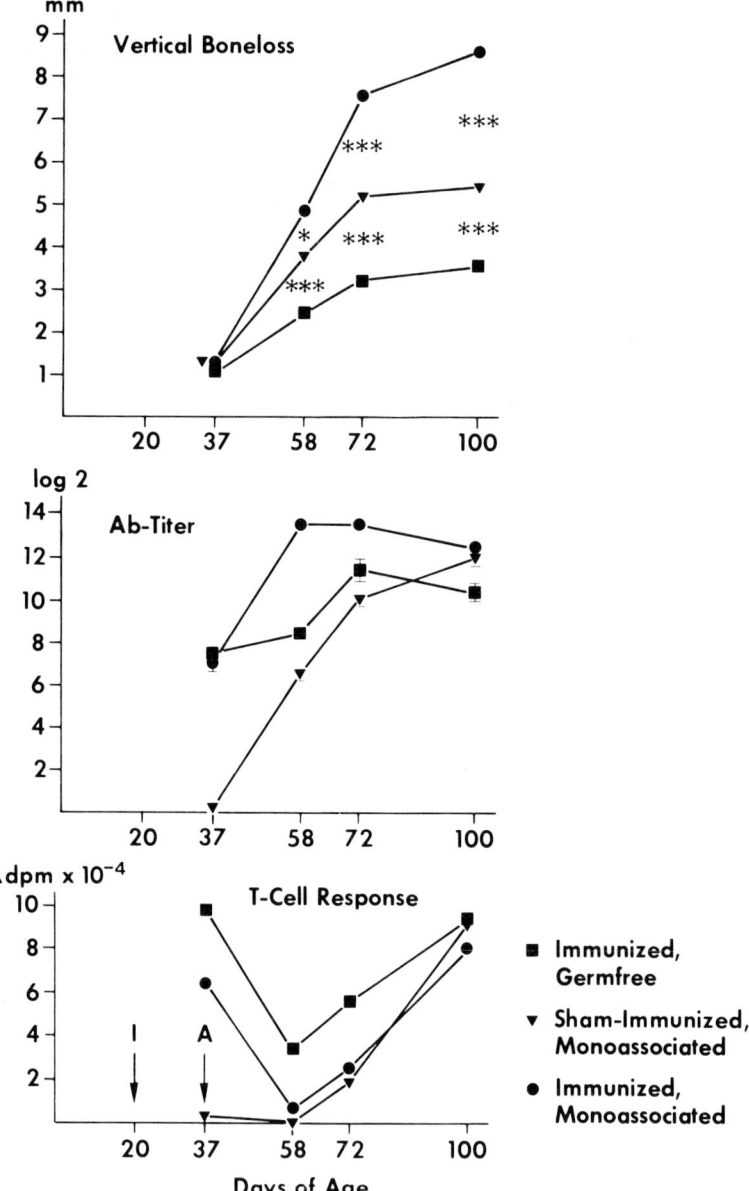

Fig. 6 Mean vertical bone loss ± S.D. first to third maxillary molars, mean antibody titre ± S.D. and *in vitro* T-cell response of immunized germ-free (group 1), sham-immunized mono-associated (group 2), and immunized mono-associated rats (group 3). The T-cell response was determined as shown in Fig. 5. Standard deviations are not shown if smaller than the symbols: $^*P_1 < 0.05$, $P_F < 0.001$.

grown in a defined medium (Bowden et al., 1976). A sample of 0.1 ml, containing 2 mg of lyophilized bacteria in equal parts of water and incomplete Freund's adjuvant (Difco), was injected subcutaneously at several ventro-lateral sites and into the hind footpads of each animal. Rats of group 2 were sham-immunized without the bacterial cells. On days 38 and 39, rats of groups 2 and 3 were mono-associated with *A. viscosus* Ny 1, while the animals of group 1 remained germ-free. At 37, 58, 72 and 100 days of age, animals from each group were removed and killed. All other experimental indices and methods of evaluation were as given earlier.

A summary of the results are given in Fig. 7. It is evident that the immunized rats showed a clear anamnestic *in vitro* lympho-proliferative response at an age of 37 days, while cells of the sham-immunized group were not stimulated. The reason for the difference of the proliferative response between the immunized animals of group 1 and 3 is not known. Between day 37 and 72 a reduction in the proliferative response of the T-cells of the immunized groups was observed. The T-cells derived from the sham-immunized, mono-associated rats were still unresponsive. However, from day 72 to the end of the experiment, T-cells from all three groups showed an increasing response, and at the age of 100 days there was virtually no difference in the magnitude of proliferation of T-cells from the three groups. Because the germ-free immunized group lacked a secondary *in vivo* challenge by *Actinomyces* cells, the conversion of the T-cell reactivity after day 58 is interesting and could indicate a cyclic regulation of the cell-mediated response. The continuous antigenic challenge by *A. viscosus* plaque in mono-associated rats induced a general depression of the T-cell response at an age of 58 days, as is evident from stimulation by the T-cell mitogens PHA and Con A which were also strongly reduced (data not shown). However, this depression was only of short duration, after day 58 the reactivity of the T-cells derived from the immunized mono-associated group 3 was fully regained. In addition the sham-immunized rats developed a strong T-cell response against BCS antigens due to the continuous antigenic stimulation by *Actinomyces* cells colonizing the teeth in the form of massive dental plaques. As already mentioned, the observed suppression is unlikely to be due to the presence of a suppressor T-cell population in our cultures, because such Fc receptor positive cells would have been retained during the separation of T-lymphocytes.

The antibody response of the rats in these experiments is more comprehensible. The immunized groups developed appreciable antibody titres on day 37, while the animals in the sham-immunized group 2 showed no antibody response. The titres in the mono-associated immunized group 3 increased further until day 58, due to the continuous antigenic challenge, and remained virtually at the same level until the end of the experiment. A further increase in titre was also observed in the immunized germ-free group 1. An almost linear increase of the antibody titre after day 37 was noticed in the sham-immunized, mono-associated group 2. At the end of the experiment, the antibody titres of all treatments were very close.

Clear-cut differences in vertical maxillary bone loss between the three groups were observed at the ages of 58 and 20 days after mono-association, until the end of the experiment. As could be expected, the germ-free animals experienced no bone loss above the physiological level, despite a strong humoral and cellular response against *A. viscosus* antigens.

The immunized mono-associated rats lost significantly more alveolar bone than the sham-immunized infected animals. The vertical bone loss of the latter group was again significantly higher than that in the immunized germ-free control. If one compares the development of bone loss and the *in vitro* T-cell response to BCS antigens it is obvious that there is no simple relation between these phenomena. Bone was lost early in the experiment, between days 37 and 58, in both mono-associated immunized and sham-immunized rats, during a period when the T-cell response in the immunized animals was declining and was not measurable in the sham-immunized group. On the other hand, there was an increase in bone loss and T-cell response in both these groups between days 58 and 72. In contrast, the rate of bone loss declined in both mono-associated groups, as the T-cell response rose to a maximum. It must be stressed, however, that immunization or better hypersensitization and mono-association had a most dramatic effect on the amount of alveolar bone loss. It is therefore concluded that the purified T-cell population, lacking suppressor T-cells, may not reflect accurately the immune status of the rats. It seems highly probable that cell-mediated hypersensitivity is one of the mechanisms participating in periodontal disease, but periods of exacerbation and quiescence depend on delicate interactions of lymphoid cells and effector cells. On the basis of these results one would be inclined to dismiss the participation of antibodies as far as bone loss is concerned. Although it would be easy to construct a statistically significant correlation between titres and bone loss in some periods of the experiment, the fact that the rate of bone loss was declining when the antibody titres were at their maximum (group 3) or still increasing (group 2) points to an epiphenomenon.

If any role *is* to be attributed to antibodies, the decline of the rate of bone loss could be speculated to be the result of a protective effect of antibodies. It is conceivable that antigens are complexed with antibodies, present in the interstitial fluid of the connective tissue, and these might prevent activation of T-lymphocytes in inflammatory infiltrates. Protection of alveolar bone loss following immunization has been reported by Guggenheim and Schroeder (1974), Rylander *et al.* (1976) and Crawford *et al.* (1978). The last-mentioned group reported a definite trend towards a reduction in bone loss in gnotobiotic rats mono-associated with *A. naeslundii* or *Strep. mutans* due to a secretory IgA response which reduced the degree of colonization of these organisms in dental plaque. Delayed hypersensitivity against *A. viscosus*, estimated by skin-testing, was accompanied by an increase in vertical bone loss (Crawford et al., 1978). In our experiment (Guggenheim and Schroeder, 1974) protection was most probably mediated by tolerance. The subcutaneously immunized group in that experiment received a dose of 9.6 mg lyophilized *A. viscosus* cells in complete Freund's adjuvant which was administered in four injections. This experiment was repeated (data not shown) and it could be demonstrated that a complete B- and T-cell tolerance was induced which was, however, gradually broken. Induction of a specific tolerance seems, at least in gnotobiotic animals, to be a practical way to confer partial protection against periodontal disease.

Effects of Immunization and Immunosuppression on Smooth Surface Caries in Gnotobiotic Rats Mono-associated with *A. viscosus* Ny 1

The experiments so far discussed were pursued in order to study periodontal disease; caries was only of peripheral interest. However, when examining defleshed jaws, particularly in two experiments, it struck us that some of the mandibular molars showed extensive smooth surface caries while others had no or a few lesions only. Smooth surface caries was therefore evaluated in these experiments, using methods described earlier.

The first experiment was designed to investigate whether T-cell suppression with cyclosporin A (CS-A) had an effect on the establishment and progression of periodontal disease in rats mono-associated with *A. viscosus* Ny 1. The experimental protocol, methods and results concerning dental caries have been previously published (Guggenheim et al., 1978), whilst the effect of CS-A on periodontal disease are presented elsewhere (Guggenheim et al., 1980).

In brief, the experiment was carried out with two treatments (16 rats each) in two isolators. In one of the isolators, CS-A was added to the high sucrose diet 2000, aiming at a dosage of 15 mg per day and per kilogram body weight. In a second isolator (control), the same diet was fed without CS-A. At days 24, 38, 52 and 65, four animals from each group were removed from the isolators. Dental plaque, dental caries and alveolar bone loss were evaluated. In addition, antibody titres and the T-cell suppressor effect of individual sera of all animals were determined. Despite distinct differences between the two groups in antibody titres, as well as an interference of the sera of the CS-A-treated animals with the Con A-dependent lymphocyte activation, bone loss was observed in both groups. It was concluded that periodontal disease seems to be the result of a multitude of pathological mechanisms and that it was not strictly correlated with T-cell-dependent hypersensitivity.

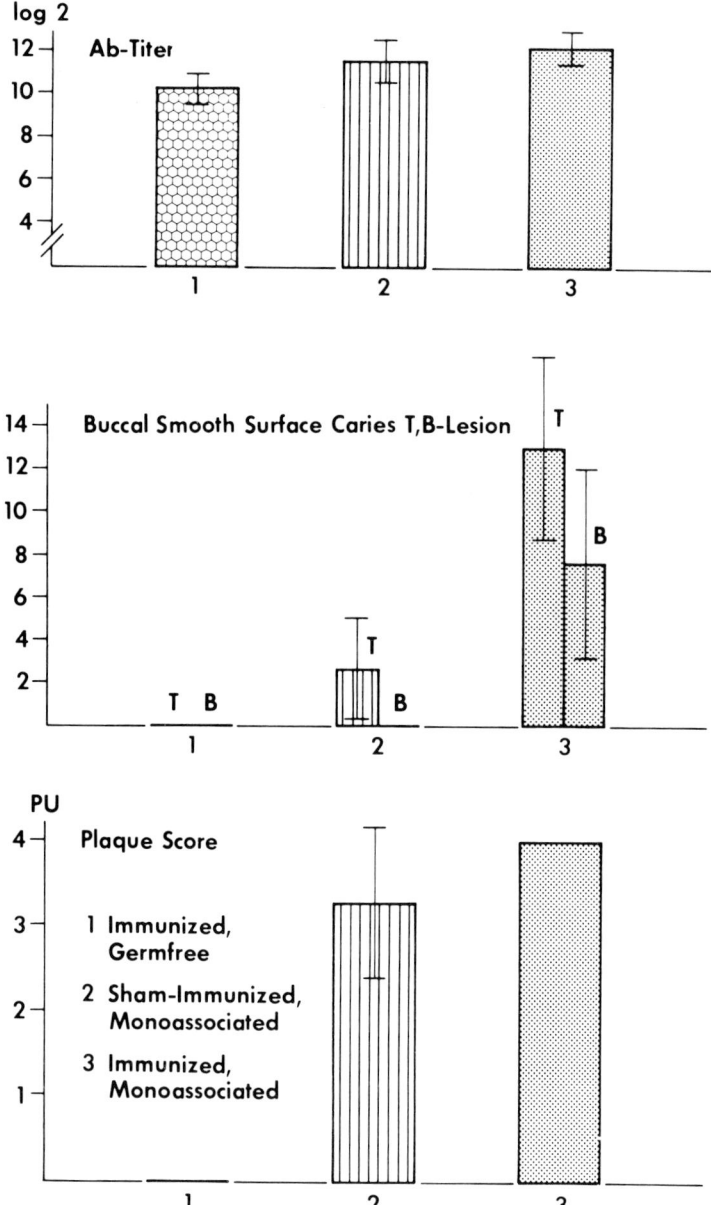

Fig. 7 Mean antibody titres ± s.d., buccal smooth surface caries lesions (T, B) and plaque score (PU) of immunized germ-free (groups 1), sham-immunized mono-associated (group 2) and immunized mono-associated rats (group 3).

The prevalence of buccal smooth surface caries in the control and the CS-A treatments differed greatly. Contrary to what was expected, almost a maximum prevalence in caries in the controls was reached after 38 days of the experiment. After 65 days an increase of the caries score in the CS-A group was also observed; however, evaluation not only of carious areas but also of the severity of the lesions revealed 6.75 + 1.0 dentinal lesions in the control, while the rats in the CS-A group had only a score of 1.0 $\pm$ 0.4 (n = 4). Although carefully investigated, this statistically significant difference ($P_F <$ 0.01) could not be attributed to a non-specific effect, i.e. differences in the feeding habits or a bacteriostatic or bacteriocidal property of the drug. To explain these results a rather challenging hypothesis was put forward. It was postulated that antibodies produced against T-helper-cell-dependent antigens which occurred only in the non-immune suppressed control animals had a caries promoting effect, while antibodies formed in response to the B-cell mitogens of *A. viscosus* were protective. A caries promoting effect of immunization against *Strep. mutans* has been previously reported (Guggenheim *et al.*, 1970; Tanzer *et al.*, 1973; Bowen *et al.*, 1975).

The second experiment in which an increased caries activity in immunized animals was observed has been outlined above and has been published recently (Burckhardt and Guggenheim, 1980). In this experiment both mono-associated groups, the sham-immunized and the immunized groups 2 and 3, showed nearly maximum caries incidence on the buccal surface of the mandibular molars at an age of 72 days or 34 days after mono-association. The sham-immunized group experienced no lingual smooth surface caries at that time. In contrast, the immunized group had 5.8 $\pm$ 6.0 (n = 5) lesions. At the end of the experiment, at 100 days of age (62 days after infection), the buccal smooth surface caries scores of both groups, evaluated by the Keyes's (1958) area score, were again very high, but not significantly different (19.3 $\pm$ 3.7 for group 2 vs. 22.7 $\pm$ 1.6 for group 3; n = 6). When the severity of these lesions was evaluated according to the method of König *et al.* (1958) the picture changed (Fig. 7). The sham-immunized group 2 had 2.7 $\pm$ 2.3 dentinal lesions (T) and no advanced dentinal lesions (B), whilst the score in the immunized group was 13.5 $\pm$ 4.3 (T) and 7.7 $\pm$ 4.4 (B) lesions. The mean antibody titre and plaque score of these two groups were not significantly different.

The reasons for these differences are not known. Again it seems not unlikely that differences in the specificity of antibodies and/or immunoglobulin classes (Lehner *et al.*, 1978) could have been responsible for this difference.

Summary

Rats mono-associated with *Actinomyces viscosus* develop periodontal disease. The cellular and humoral immune responses of these animals have been characterized during the development of this disease. Because *A. viscosus* contains components which have strong B-cell mitogenicity, it became necessary to prepare mitogen-free antigens or alternatively to prepare T-cell populations which are free of B-cells to monitor the cellular immune response.

An increased T-cell response was demonstrated in several animal experiments during the development of periodontal disease. However, the rats also developed high antibody titres. When other rats were sensitized with low doses of *A. viscosus* before oral infection, the inflammatory response was dramatically enhanced. However, high doses of antigens resulted in high zone tolerance which, although gradually broken, nevertheless retarded the disease. On the other hand, bone loss was not significantly affected by cyclosporin A, a compound which strongly interferes with T-cell activity. Furthermore, the importance of certain T-cell populations could be demonstrated *in vitro*, using a cytotoxicity model for fibroblasts; T-cells from sensitized animals killed fibroblast most efficiently.

In our studies, data on dental caries were only of peripheral interest. It could, however, be shown that animals sensitized with low doses of *A. viscosus* had significantly more smooth surface lesions than unsensitized controls. T-cell-suppressed animals had fewer lesions than unsuppressed controls, suggesting a protective effect of antibodies built up in response to polyclonal B-cell activators.

References

Amstad-Jossi, M. and Schroeder, H. E. (1978). *J. periodont. Res.* **13**, 76–90.
Baker, J. J., Chan, S. P., Socransky, S. S., Oppenheim, J. J. and Mergenhagen, S. E. (1976). *Infect. Immun.* **13**, 1363–1368.
Bowden, G. H., Hardie, J. M. and Fillery, E. D. (1976). *J. dent. Res.* **55**, A192–A204.
Bowden, W. H., Cohen, B. and Colman, G. (1975). *Br. dent. J.* **139**, 45–58.
Burckhardt, J. J. (1978). *Scand. J. Immunol.* **7**, 167–172.
Burckhardt, J. J. (1979). *Scand. J. Immunol.* **10**, 229–235.
Burckhardt, J. J. and Guggenheim, B. (1979). *Immunology* **26**, 753–757.
Burckhardt, J. J. and Guggenheim, B. (1980). *Caries Res.* **14**, 56–59.
Burckhardt, J. J., Guggenheim, B. and Hefti, A. (1977). *J. Immunol.* **118**, 1460–1465.
Burckhardt, J. J., Gaegauf, R. and Guggenheim, B. (1980). Submitted to *J. periodont. Res.*
Clarke, J. K. (1924). *Br. J. exp. Path.* **5**, 141–147.
Costich, E. R. (1955). *J. Periodont.* **26**, 301–305.
Crawford, J. M., Taubman, M. A. and Smith, D. J. (1978). *J. periodont. Res.* **13**, 445–459.
Engel, D., Clagett, J., Page, R. and Williams, B. (1977). *J. Immunol.* **118**, 1466–1471.
Fitzgerald, R. J. and Keyes, P. H. (1960). *Am. dent. Assoc.* **61**, 9–19.
Gaegauf, R., Burckhardt, J. J. and Guggenheim, B. (1980). Submitted to *J. periodont. Res.*
George, L. K., Pine, L. and Gerencser, M. A. (1969). *Int. J. syst. Bact.* **19**, 291–293.
Guggenheim, B. and Schroeder, H. E. (1974). *Infect. Immun.* **10**, 565–577.

Guggenheim, B., Hefti, A. and Burckhardt, J. J. (1978). In *Secretory Immunity and Infection* (J. R. McGhee, J. Mestecky and J. L. Babb, eds), pp. 293–301, Plenum Press, New York.
Guggenheim, B., Mühlemann, H. R., Regolati, B. and Schmid, R. (1970). In *Dental Plaque* (W. D. McHugh, ed.), pp. 287–296, E. & S. Livingstone Ltd, Edinburgh and London.
Guggenheim, B., Gaegauf, R., Hefti, A. and Burckhardt, J. J. (1980). Submitted to *J. periodont. Res.*
Gustafson, G. (1963). In *Germfree Life and Gnotobiology* (T. D. Luckey, ed.), p. 494, Academic Press, New York and London.
Hertel-Wulff, B. and Rubin, B. (1976). *Eur. J. Immunol.* **6**, 418–424.
van Houte, J., Upeslacis, V. N. and Edelstein, S. (1977). *Infect. Immun.* **16**, 203–212.
Ivanyi, L. and Lehner, T. (1971). *Int. Archs Allergy* **41**, 620–627.
Ivanyi, L., Wiltin, J. M. A. and Lehner, T. (1972). *Immunology* **22**, 141–145.
Johnson, D. A., Behling, U. H., Lai, C.-H., Listgarten, M., Socransky, S. and Nowotny, A. (1978). *Infect. Immun.* **19**, 246–253.
Jordan, H. V. and Keyes, P. H. (1965). *Am. J. Path.* **46**, 843–857.
Jordan, H. J., Fitzgerald, R. J. and Stanley, H. R. (1965). *Am. J. Path.* **47**, 1157–1167.
Keyes, P. H. (1958). *J. dent. Res.* **37**, 1088.
Keyes, P. H. and Gold, H. S. (1955). *Oral Surg.* **8**, 492–499.
König, G. K. (1966). *Möglichkeiten der Kariesprophylaxe beim Menschen und ihre Untersuchung im kurzfristigen Rattenexperiment*, Hans Huber Verlag, Bern and Stuttgart.
König, K. G. and Guggenheim, B. (1968). *Adv. oral Biol.* **3**, 217–252.
König, K. G., Marthaler, T. M. and Mühlemann, H. R. (1958). *Dt. Zahn-Mund-Kieferheilk.* **29**, 99–127.
Krasse, B., Jordan, H. V., Edwardsson, S., Svensson, I. and Trell, L. (1968). *Archs oral Biol.* **13**, 911–927.
Lang, N. P. and Smith, F. N. (1977). *J. periodont. Res.* **12**, 298–309.
Lehner, T., Russell, M. W., Wilton, J. M. A., Challacombe, S. J., Scully, C. M. and Hawkes, J. E. (1978). In *Secretory Immunity and Infection* (J. R. McGhee, J. Mestecky and J. L. Babb, eds), pp. 303–315, Plenum Press, New York.
Loesche, W. J. and Syed, S. A. (1978). *Infect. Immun.* **21**, 830–839.
Mackler, B. F., Altman, L. C., Wahl, S., Rosenstreich, D. L., Oppenheim, J. J. and Mergenhagen, S. E. (1974). *Infect. Immun.* **10**, 844–850.
Mikx, F. H. M., van der Hoeven, J. S., Plasschaert, A. J. M. and König, K. G. (1975). *Caries Res.* **9**, 1–20.
Mikx, F. H. M., van der Hoeven, J. S., Plasschaert, A. J. M. and Maltha, J. C. (1976a). *Caries Res.* **10**, 49–58.
Mikx, F. H. M., van der Hoeven, J. S., Plasschaert, A. J. M. and König, K. G. (1976b). *Caries Res.* **10**, 123–132.
Page, R. C. and Schroeder, H. E. (1976). *Lab. Invest.* **33**, 235–249.
Regolati, B. and Hotz, P. (1972). *Helv. odont. Acta* **16**, 13–18.
Regolati, B., Guggenheim, B. and Mühlemann, H. R. (1972). *Helv. odont. Acta* **16**, 84–88.
Rylander, H., Lindhe, J. and Ahlstedt, S. (1976). *J. periodont. Res.* **11**, 339–348.
Slots, J. (1979). *J. clin. Periodont.* **6**, 351–382.
Socransky, S. S. (1979). *J. clin. Peridont.* **6**, 16–21.
de Stoppelaar, J. D., van Houte, J. and Backer-Dirks, O. (1969). *Caries Res.* **3**, 190–199.

Tanzer, J. M., Hagenage, G. J. and Larson, R. H. (1973). *Archs oral Biol.* **18**, 1425–1439.
Turk, J. L., Polak, L. and Parker, D. (1976). *Br. med. Bull.* **32**, 165–170.
Wigzell, H. (1976). *Scand. J. Immunol.* **5**, Suppl. 5, 23.
Wuhrmann, H. C., (1977). *Quantititive und mikroskopische Beschreibung von parodontalen Veränderungen an keimfreien Ratten nach Inokulation zweier verschiedener Mikroorganismen,* Juris Druck + Verlag, Zurich.

12. The Role of Serum and Salivary Antibodies in Protection against Dental Caries

THOMAS LEHNER

Introduction

There are two principal immune mechanisms of protection against dental caries. The salivary secretory IgA antibodies affect the salivary domain, whereas the gingival crevicular fluid, containing IgG antibodies, complement and polymorphonuclear leukocytes, among other of the blood components, affect the gingival domain (Lehner *et al.*, 1976a). There is, however, no overwhelming evidence in favour of one or the other mechanism playing a predominant role in protection against caries and both mechanisms may operate under the particular experimental conditions.

Salivary IgA antibodies have been invoked as the protective agents in multiple subcutaneous immunization of rats near the salivary glands (Taubman and Smith, 1974). Furthermore, prolonged oral immunization of germ-free rats before and during dental implantation of *Streptococcus mutans* has led to a significant diminution in caries and this was attributed to an increase in salivary IgA antibodies (Michalek *et al.*, 1976). The role of secretory IgA in the mechanism of prevention of caries has been supported by transferring secretory antibodies in the milk of lactating germ-free rats to their litter which had minimal serum antibodies and showing that there was a significant reduction in caries (Michalek and McGhee, 1977). Although these experiments have been interpreted almost entirely in favour of secretory IgA antibodies, IgG antibodies in the serum, saliva or milk of the rats might have also played a part in these investigations.

The gingival crevicular fluid contains most of the immune components present in blood and these have direct access to the smooth and approximal surfaces of teeth and by mixing with saliva the resulting "oral fluid" may reach the occlusal surfaces. Subcutaneous and oral submucous immunization with *Strep. mutans* induces predominantly serum IgG, IgM and IgA antibodies and, to a much lesser extent, salivary IgA antibodies (Lehner *et al.*, 1975a, 1976b, 1977; Challacombe and Lehner, 1980). Protection against caries is related to serum IgG antibodies and there is no association with salivary IgA antibodies. Passive transfer of serum IgG, unlike IgA antibodies to *Strep. mutans*, has clearly shown that serum IgG antibodies can protect against dental caries, without a significant change in salivary IgA antibodies (Lehner et al., 1978a).

The object of this paper is to compare the systemic and salivary immune responses to active immunization by the oral and subcutaneous routes with *Strep. mutans* in Rhesus monkeys. The effect of oral followed by subcutaneous (s.c.) or the reverse sequence of immunization will be assessed in salivary and systemic immunity. The results of active immunization will be compared and assessed with those of passive transfer of IgG, IgA and IgM class of antibodies. The role of cell-mediated immunity will be also assessed in both active immunization and by means of transfer factor.

Animals and Methods

Thirty-eight young Rhesus monkeys weighing between 1.4 and 2.2 kg were caged and maintained on a human type of cariogenic diet, containing about 15% sucrose, as described previously (Lehner et al., 1975b). All monkeys had a fully erupted deciduous dentition and in some the first permanent molars were erupting. The duration of the experiment was up to 85 weeks.

Active Immunization and Animals

Twenty monkeys were randomly divided into five groups (Table 1).

TABLE I
Grouping and Schedules in Active Immunization of 20 Rhesus Monkeys

Group	No. of monkeys	Agent	Immunization		
			Route*	Times	Dose
1	6	Whole cells†	o.i.	130–170	5×10^{10} cells
2	2	Whole cells†	Gingival	44	10^{10} cells
3	4	Saline	s.c.	2	1 ml
4	3	Whole cells†	s.c.	1	5×10^{8} cells
5	5	Streptococcal antigen I/II	s.c.	2	5–10 mg

* o.i., oro-intestinal; s.c., subcutaneous.
† *Strep. mutans* (serotype c).

Group 1

Six monkeys were first immunized by administration of live *Strep. mutans* (serotype c) in the drinking water daily, for 18–24 weeks; this route of immunization will be referred to as the oro-intestinal route (o.i.). The streptococci were grown in Todd–Hewit broth without additional sucrose and these were administered to four monkeys, whilst two monkeys were given cells grown in the broth supplemented with 1% sucrose. The concentration of the streptococci was 10^8 cells per millilitre of water and about 500 ml of water was consumed by each monkey daily. Three of the monkeys were immunized (s.c.) on week 48 with 5×10^8 formalin-killed cells of *Strep. mutans* (serotype c) in Freund's incomplete adjuvant (FIA).

Group 2
Two monkeys were used for attempted topical gingival immunization. Live *Strep. mutans* (serotype c) was brushed adjacent to the gingival margin on four consecutive days, at 14 day intervals, 11 times using 10^{10} organisms mixed with Alhydrogel to a consistency of a paste. After week 48 the monkeys were immunized subcutaneously with 5×10^8 formalin-killed cells of *Strep. mutans* in FIA.

Group 3
Four monkeys were not immunized actively and were used as controls for the development of caries in the same experiments as those immunized by the oro-intestinal and gingival routes.

Group 4
Three monkeys were injected subcutaneously (s.c.) with 5×10^8 formalin-killed cells of *Strep. mutans* (serotype c) in FIA.

Group 5
Five monkeys had (s.c.) injections of 5–10 mg of streptococcal antigen I/II in FIA prepared as described previously (Russell and Lehner, 1978). A second injection of 5 mg of the corresponding antigen was administered on week 24. At week 70 of the experiment the monkeys were given live *Strep. mutans* (serotype c) in the drinking water, at a concentration of 10^8 cells/ml for 12 weeks. About 500 ml of water was consumed daily by each monkey.

Assessment of Caries

Caries was detected clinically and radiologically and the caries score indicates the mean of smooth surface and fissure cavities in the deciduous teeth and first permanent molars (Lehner *et al.*, 1977).

Assessment of Antibodies

Blood and whole saliva were collected as described previously (Lehner *et al.*, 1975*b*). Serum IgG, IgA and IgM antibody titres were determined by the indirect immunofluorescent method against air-dried smears of *Strep. mutans* (Lehner *et al.*, 1976*b*). Salivary agglutinating antibodies were determined by direct agglutination of the streptococcal cells (Challacombe, 1978). These were characterized for the IgA class specificity elsewhere (Challacombe and Lehner, 1980).

Skin Delayed Hypersensitivity (DH)

A sample of 0.05 ml of Mickle disintegrated cells of *Strep. mutans* (10^9 cells/ml) or physiological saline was injected intradermally into the shaved abdominal wall of the monkeys. Skin induration was measured with calipers at 6, 24 and 48 h after injection. The results were expressed as the mean specific increase in skin thickness due to *Strep. mutans*.

Culture of *Strep. mutans*

Plaque was collected with sterile probes from the cervical and approximal surfaces of the upper left deciduous molars and from the fissures of the adjacent first permanent molar. The samples were collected from the (o.i.) immunized and sham-immunized control monkeys, placed into transport medium and grown on TYC medium (Stopelaar et al., 1969). The colony-forming units (CFU) of *Strep. mutans* were determined as described previously (Caldwell et al., 1977).

Passive Immunization and Animals

Twenty-one young Rhesus monkeys, weighing 1.6–2.2 kg were used as recipients. They were given the human type of diet containing 15% sucrose, beginning on the day of passive transfer of plasma. Three monkeys were given intravenous infusions of 15 ml non-immune plasma and four monkeys received 15 ml of immune plasma, at intervals of 17–22 days. IgG, IgM and IgA were administered to seven monkeys (Table II) in the amounts calculated

TABLE II

Grouping and Schedules in Passive Immunization of 21 Rhesus Monkeys

Group	No. of monkeys	Immunization			
		Agent	Route*	Times	Dose
1	3	Non-immune plasma	i.v.	12	15 ml
2	4	Immune plasma	i.v.	12	15 ml
3	3	IgG	i.v.	12	177 (± 2.5) mg
4	2	IgM	i.v.	12	11.7 (± 1.1) mg
5	2	IgA	i.v.	12	28.4 (± 1.6) mg
6	3	Transfer factor	s.c.	3†	2.5×10^8‡
7	4	Saline	s.c.	2	1 ml

* s.c., subcutaneous; i.v., intravenous.
† Also plasma i.v. 12 times.
‡ Lymphocyte-derived transfer factor.

TABLE III

Immune Responses in Donor and Recipient Monkeys of Transfer Factor

Passive transfer			Donors						Recipients					
Transfer factor	Serum	Cellular immunity			Antibodies (mean log$_2$ ($\pm$ s.e.))			Cellular immunity			Antibodies (mean log$_2$ ($\pm$ s.e.))		
		LMI*	LyTr†	DH‡	IgG	IgM	IgA	LMI	LyTr	DH	IgG	IgM	IgA
Immune	Immune	66	6.5	0.9	8.9 ($\pm$0.2)	8.3 ($\pm$0.3)	4.8 ($\pm$0.4)	69	3.7	0.5	6.8 ($\pm$0.2)	5.2 (0.4)	4.2 ($\pm$0.3)
Immune	Control	66	6.5	0.9	0.9 ($\pm$0.3)	1.1 ($\pm$0.2)	1.1 ($\pm$0.2)	80	4.6	0.1	0.8 ($\pm$0.3)	0.3 ($\pm$0.3)	0.2 ($\pm$0.2)
Control	Immune	108	1.6	ND§	8.9 ($\pm$0.2)	5.3 ($\pm$0.3)	4.8 ($\pm$0.4)	78	ND	0	7.7 ($\pm$0.4)	4.1 ($\pm$0.5)	4.2 ($\pm$0.3)

* LMI, leukocyte migration inhibition.
† LyTr, lymphocyte transformation.
‡ DH, delayed hypersensitivity.
§ ND, not done.

to be present in 15 ml monkey plasma (Monte-Wicker et al., 1970). Four monkeys were sham-immunized with saline. The passive transfer of plasma or antibodies was carried out up to week 33. Transfer factor was injected (s.c.) in doses equivalent to 2.5×10^8 lymphocytes per animal at weeks 0, 8 and 21 and plasma was infused at intervals of 3 weeks, up to week 33. One monkey had immune plasma and non-immune transfer factor (TF), another had non-immune plasma and immune (TF), and the third had both immune plasma and immune (TF) (Table III).

Immune Plasma and Immunoglobulin

Immune or non-immune plasma and the separated IgG, IgA or IgM were prepared from 20 donor Rhesus monkeys weighing 4–7 kg (Lehner et al., 1978a). Fourteen donor monkeys were immunized with six s.c. injections of 5×10^8 heat-killed cells of Strep. mutans (serotype c), the first and last of these being given an equal volume (0.5 ml) of Freund's incomplete adjuvant. Six non-immunized donor monkeys had six injections of saline at the same time. The mean ($\pm$ S.E.) $\log_2$ serum fluorescent antibody titres (Lehner et al., 1978a) of the immunized donor monkeys were IgG 8.9 (± 0.2), IgM 5.3 (± 0.3), and IgA 4.8 (± 0.4). The corresponding titres in the sham-immunized donor monkeys were IgG 0.9 (± 0.3), IgM 1.1 (± 0.2) and IgA 1.1 (± 0.2). Each donor monkey had 40–60 ml of blood withdrawn about every 3 weeks. The blood was collected into sterile heparinized bottles and the plasma was separated from the cells by centrifugation.

Immunoglobulins were separated from 1.8 mol/l ammonium sulphate precipitate of pooled immune monkey serum by column chromatography (Lehner et al., 1978a). The IgG preparation contained 177 (± 2.5) mg IgG, <0.04 (± 0.04) mg IgM, and 2.75 (± 0.86) mg IgA. The IgM preparation contained 11.7 (± 1.1) mg IgM, <6 (± 1) mg IgG and 6.2 (± 1.7) mg IgA. The IgA preparation contained 28.4 (± 1.6) mg IgA, <1.6 (± 0.6) mg IgG and <0.3 (± 0.09) mg IgM.

Transfer Factor (TF)

Transfer factor was prepared (Lehner et al., 1978b) from one of the immunized monkeys which showed positive skin DH, lymphocyte transformation and leukocyte migration inhibition to Strep. mutans and from one of the control monkeys which failed to yield any of the three markers (Table III). TF was prepared from pooled lymphocytes from the spleen, and cervical, submandibular and mesenteric lymph nodes by five cycles of freezing and thawing. This was followed by digestion with ribonuclease and the material was dialysed and Millipore-filtered (Kirkpatrick et al., 1972). Both the dialysable and non-dialysable fractions were used (Baram and Condoulis, 1974).

Results

Active Immunization, Caries Score and CFU of *Strep. mutans*

Although the caries score was lower in monkeys immunized by the o.i. route than in controls, the difference was not significantly different for either smooth surface or fissure caries (Fig. 1). At the end of the experiment, at 64 weeks, the mean caries score ($\pm$ S.E.) in the o.i. immunized monkeys was 5.8 ($\pm$ 1.3), compared with 8.75 ($\pm$ 1.8) in the controls. The CFU of *Strep. mutans* showed little difference between the two groups of monkeys (Fig. 2). Somewhat surprisingly, topical gingival administration of *Strep. mutans* induced consistently higher caries scores than those found in controls. In contrast, monkeys immunized s.c. with whole cells of *Strep. mutans* showed a significant reduction in caries (2.7 $\pm$ 1.2) as compared with the controls ($t = 2.586$; $p < 0.05$). Caries in monkeys immunized with the streptococcal antigen are reported elsewhere (Lehner *et al.*, 1980).

Serum Antibodies

Subcutaneous injection of either cells (group 4) or the streptococcal antigens (group 5) in adjuvant elicited a prompt IgG antibody response (Fig. 3). However, only streptococcal cells elicited IgM antibodies (Fig. 4) and IgA

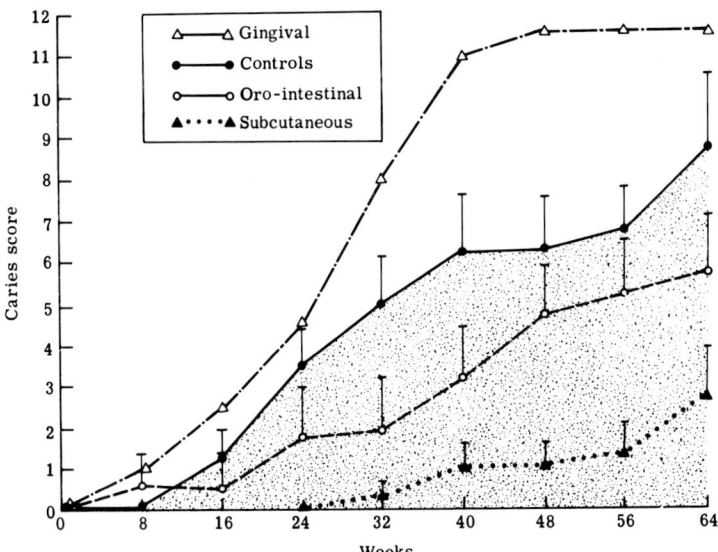

Fig. 1 Sequential development of dental caries in oro-intestinal, subcutaneous and gingival routes of immunization.

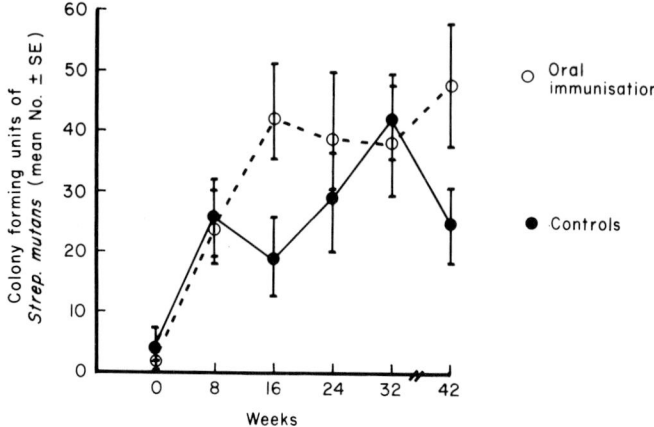

Fig. 2 *Strep. mutans* from smooth surfaces and fissures in orally immunized and control monkeys. Colony forming units (CFU) are expressed as a percentage of total CFU on TYC medium.

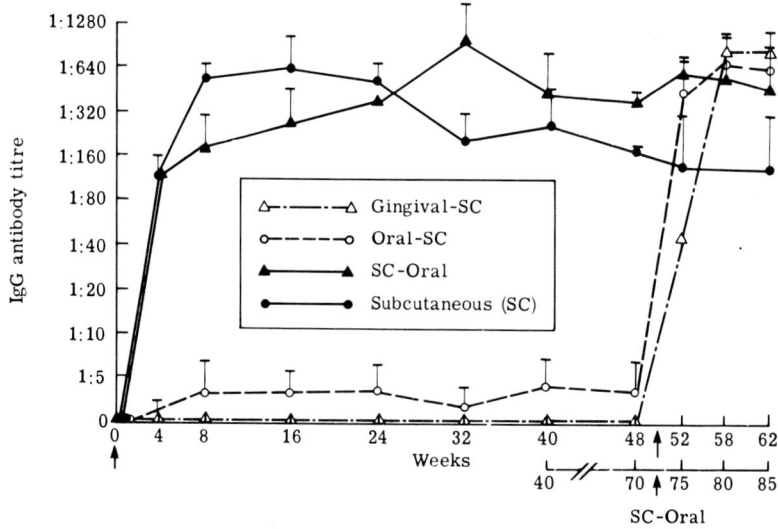

Fig. 3 IgG antibody titres in four groups of monkeys with sequential immunization by subcutaneous, oral or gingival routes. ▲——▲, Immunized with antigen I/II; other groups with whole cells of *Strep. mutans*.

12. Serum, Salivary Antibodies and Caries 201

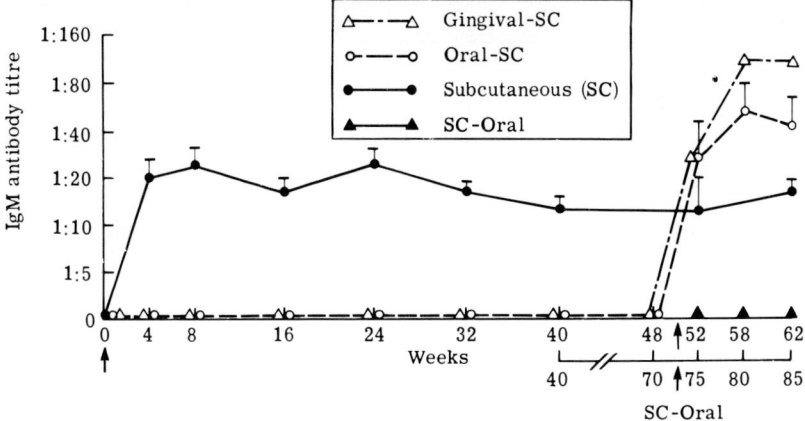

Fig. 4 IgM antibody titres in four groups of monkeys with sequential immunization by subcutaneous, oral or gingival routes. ▲——▲, Immunized with antigen I/II; other groups with whole cells of *Strep. mutans*.

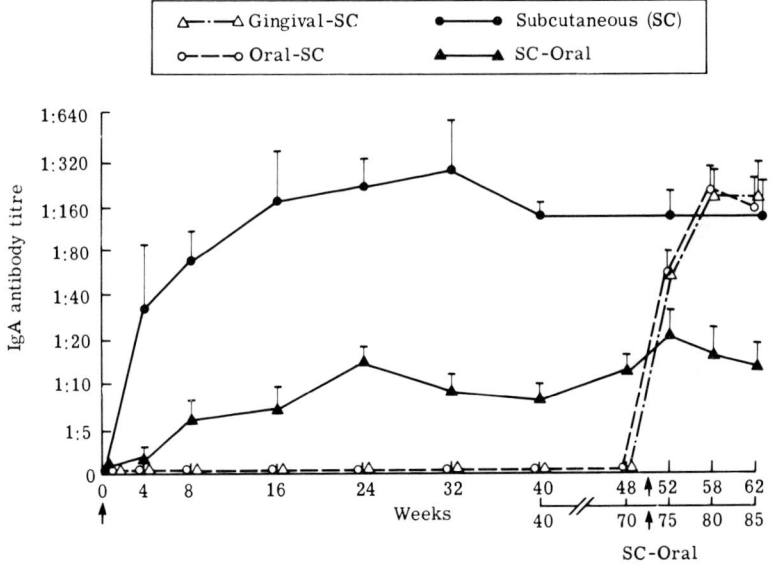

Fig. 5 IgA antibody titres in four groups of monkeys with sequential immunization by subcutaneous, oral or gingival routes. ▲——▲, Immunized with antigen I/II; other groups with whole cells of *Strep. mutans*.

antibody titres (Fig. 5) were significantly higher in the whole cell than the streptococcal antigen-immunized monkeys ($p < 0.01$ after week 4). Monkeys immunized by the o.i. or gingival route and the controls showed no serum IgG, IgA or IgM antibodies greater than 1:10 (Figs 3, 4, 5). However, after s.c. immunization with 5×10^8 killed cells of *Strep. mutans* in FIA at week 48, all monkeys in both groups (1 and 2) gave prompt IgG, IgA and IgM antibody titres, almost identical or slightly higher (especially IgM) than those resulting from immunization with cells at the start of the experiment (group 4). Feeding of cells of *Strep. mutans* to the s.c. immunized group of monkeys showed little change in the IgG or IgA antibody titres.

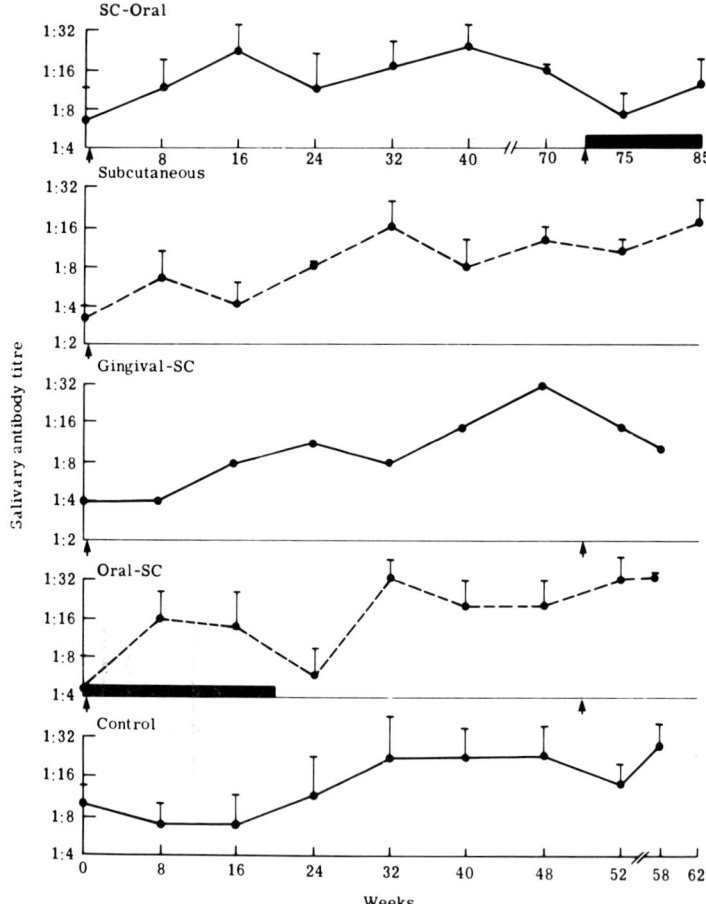

Fig. 6 Salivary agglutinating IgA antibody titres to *Strep. mutans*, with sequential immunization by subcutaneous (s.c.), oral or gingival routes. Arrows indicate subcutaneous immunization; thick bars indicate period of oral feeding.

Salivary Antibodies

Oro-intestinal immunization gave rise to a short lasting salivary IgA response, the mean titre increasing from $\log_2 2.2$ to $\log_2 4$ ($p < 0.05$, Fig. 6). The titre fell after cessation of antigen feeding, but a gradual increase in salivary antibodies was found over the remainder of the experimental period. A slight increase in antibody titre was also found in all the other immunized monkeys, from a baseline titre of $\log_2 2$–$\log_2 3$ to a titre of $\log_2 4$–$\log_2 5$ after 52 weeks (Fig. 6). None of these changes reached the 5% level of significance compared with the control monkeys, which also showed a slight increase in antibody titre from $\log_2 3.25$ to $\log_2 4.75$.

Subcutaneous immunization following o.i. (group 1) or gingival (group 2) immunization did not give rise to any detectable changes in salivary antibody titres (Fig. 6). Similarly, o.i. following s.c. immunization showed little change in titres.

Skin Delayed Hypersensitivity

There was no significant increase in skin thickness 24 h after intradermal injection of antigen and an actual decrease in skin thickness after 48 h was found in controls, o.i. immunized and gingivally immunized groups (Fig. 7). In contrast, the streptococcal cell immunized and antigen immunized monkeys showed a significant increase in skin thickness at 24 h ($p < 0.02$ and $p < 0.05$) and at 48 h with the cells alone ($p < 0.05$).

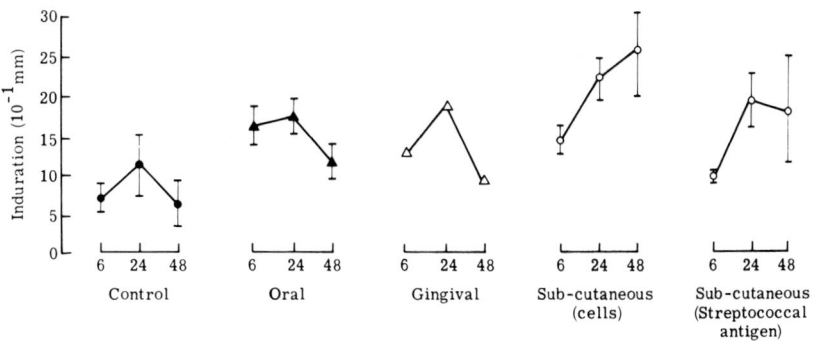

Fig. 7 Skin hypersensitivity to *Strep. mutans* in five groups of monkeys.

Passive Immunization and Caries Score

Caries was detected in the control monkeys and in those receiving either non-immune or immune serum (Fig. 8). At 39 weeks the average number of

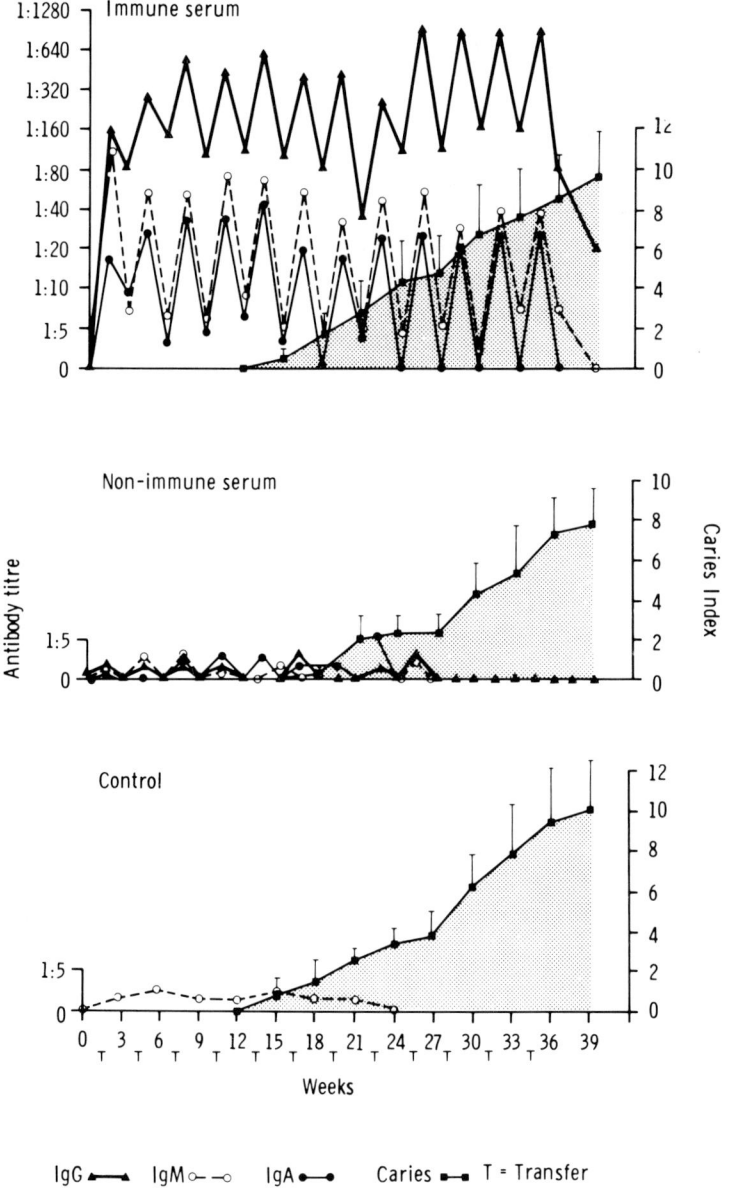

Fig. 8 Sequential fluorescent IgG, IgM and IgA antibody titres against *Strep. mutans* and the caries index in monkeys receiving intravenous injections of immune serum or non-immune serum and in sham-immunized monkeys, every 3 weeks for up to 33 weeks.

lesions per monkey in the control non-immune serum and immune serum groups were much the same. Clearly, passive transfer of immune serum failed to protect dental caries.

The least number of carious lesions was found in the group receiving separated IgG (mean of 2.0) and this increased to 5.5 with IgM and 8.5 with IgA (Fig. 9). Significant protection was induced with IgG ($\chi^2 = 15.33$, $p < 0.001$) but not with IgM, when the total number of carious lesions was

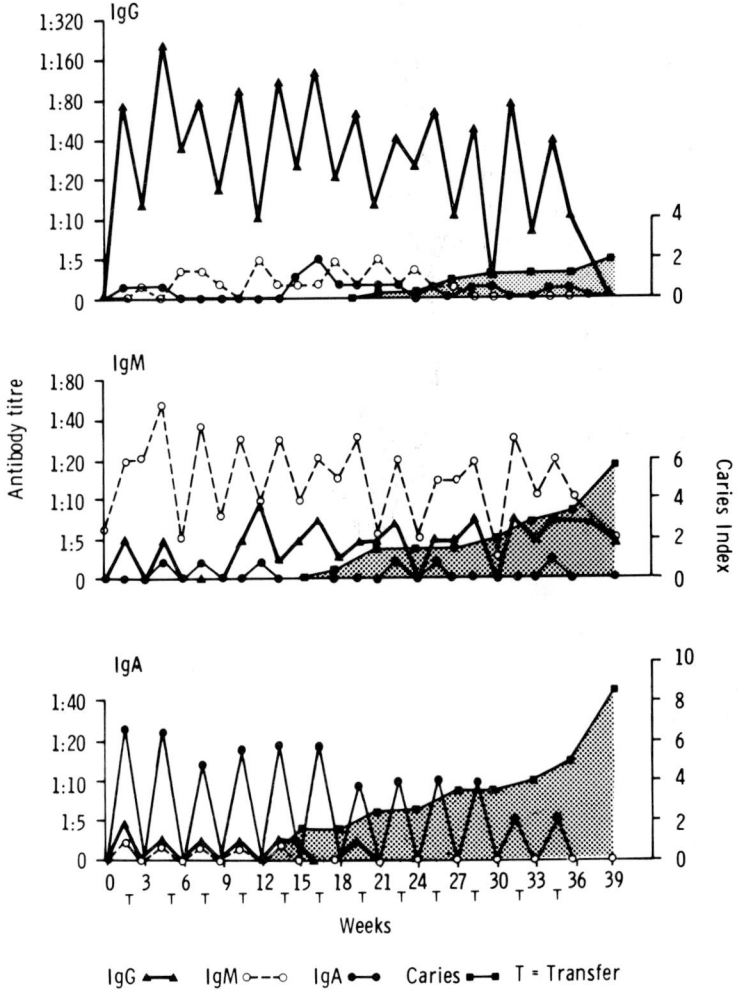

Fig. 9 Sequential fluorescent IgG, IgM and IgA antibody titres against *Strep. mutans* and the caries index in monkeys receiving intravenous injections of separated IgG, IgM or IgA sera every 3 weeks up to 33 weeks.

compared with that found in the group receiving immune serum. Comparable results were obtained with the group receiving non-immune serum or saline injections.

IgG also induced significant protection when compared with IgA (χ^2 with Yate's correction = 9.68, $p < 0.01$) but not with IgM. There was no significant difference in the CFU counts for *Strep. mutans* recovered on TYC agar.

Serum Antibodies

IgG, IgM and IgA classes of antibodies were found in the monkeys given immune plasma but there were only occasional titres of $\log_2$ 1 in those given non-immune plasma or in the controls (Fig. 8). IgG titre of mean $\log_2$ 7.5 (± 0.2) was reached after transfer of immune serum and this fell within 3 weeks by a mean of $\log_2$ 2.1 (± 0.22). IgM and IgA showed lower titres, with a mean titre after transfer of $\log_2$ 4.4 (± 0.2) for IgM and $\log_2$ 3.5 (± 0.1) for IgA and the mean fall in titre of antibodies at 3 weeks was $\log_2$ 3.2 (± 0.13) for IgM and $\log_2$ 3.0 (± 0.22) for IgA.

When separated immunoglobulin classes of antibody were injected, the resulting circulating antibody was predominantly in the same class, the titre of the other two Ig classes being usually $\log_2$ 1. One exception was the presence of some IgG after the transfer of IgM antibodies (Fig. 9). The antibody titres after transfer of the separated sera were slightly lower than those found after transfer of whole immune serum, with a difference between them of a mean $\log_2$ 2.6 (± 0.31) for IgG, $\log_2$ 1.0 (± 0.21) for IgM and $\log_2$ 1.4 (± 0.31) for IgA.

Cellular and Antibody Responses after Injection of Transfer Factor and Plasma

The two monkeys which received transfer factor showed some or all markers of cell-mediated immunity, whereas the monkey receiving non-immune transfer factor showed a negative delayed hypersensitivity but a positive leukocyte migration inhibition test. The titres of serum and salivary antibodies in the monkeys receiving immune plasma were comparable with those in the previous experiment (Fig. 10). Passive transfer of immune serum and non-immune transfer factor or non-immune serum and immune transfer factor had no effect on the caries score, which showed an identical pattern, with 10 cavities each by 39 weeks. In contrast, passive transfer of immune serum and immune transfer factor resulted in only one cavity by 39 weeks.

Salivary Antibodies

The mean salivary agglutinating antibody titres during passive transfer of serum and/or cellular immunity are summarized in Fig. 11. A small increase in titre was found in all the groups, irrespective of the caries index. However, passive transfer of serum IgA showed an unaccountable increase in salivary

12. Serum, Salivary Antibodies and Caries

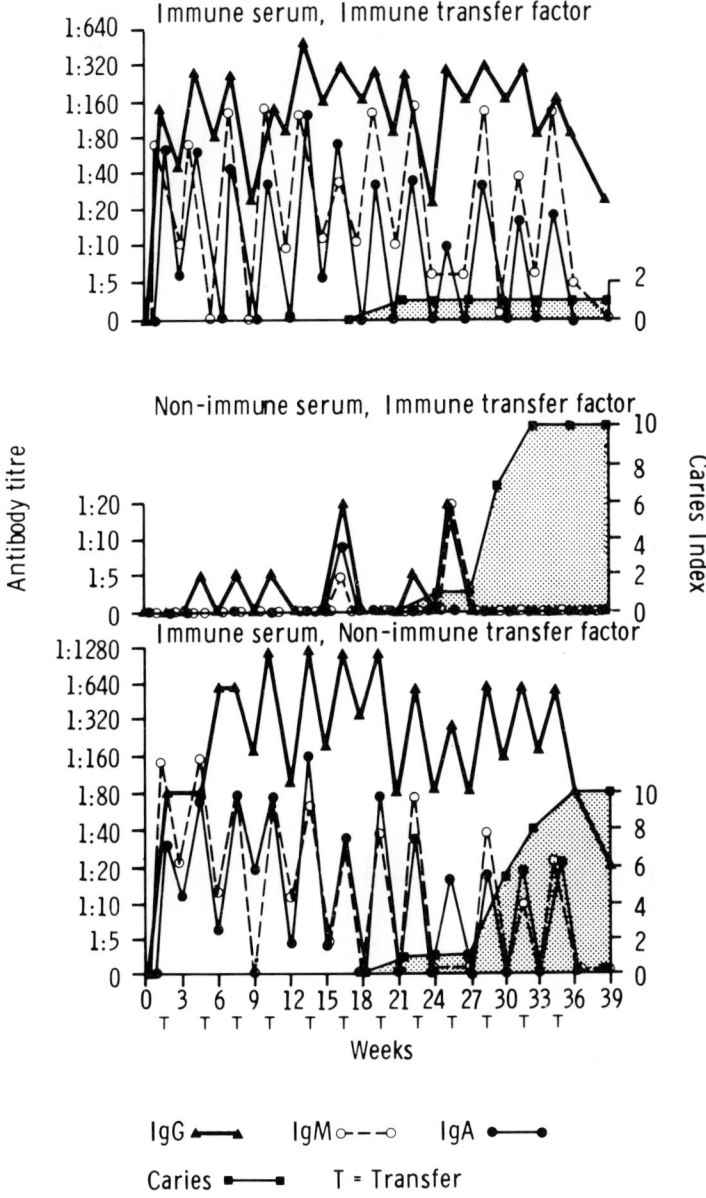

Fig. 10 Sequential fluorescent IgG, IgM, and IgA antibody titres against *Strep. mutans* and the caries index in monkeys receiving intravenous injections of separated IgG, IgM or IgA sera every 3 weeks up to 33 weeks.

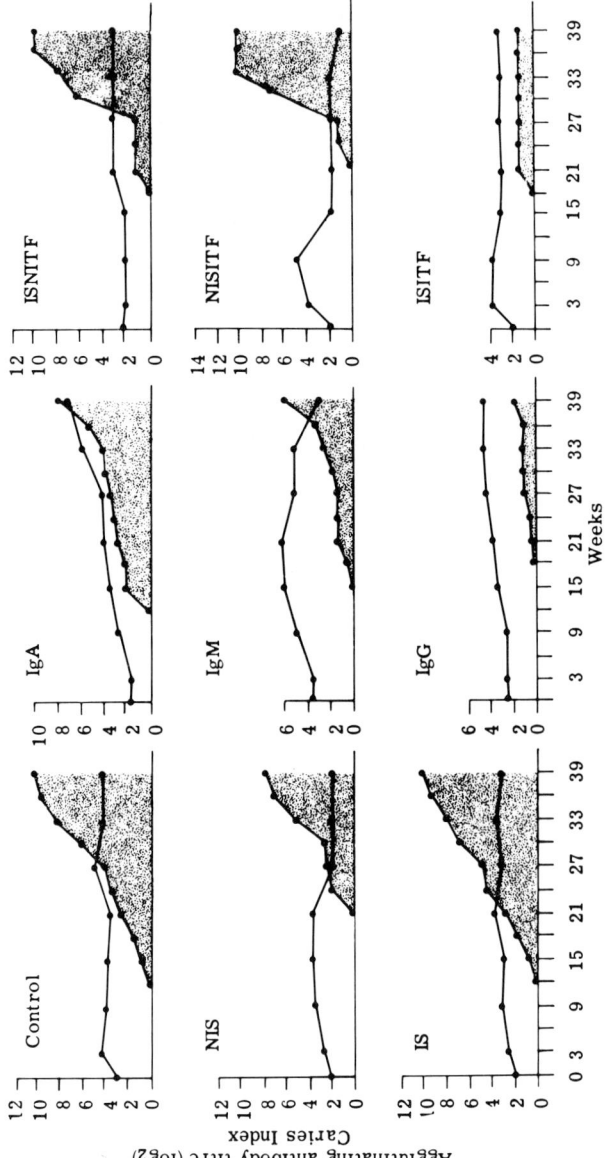

Fig. 11 Sequential salivary agglutinating antibody titres against *Strep. mutans* and the caries profiles in nine groups of monkeys receiving passive transfer of antibodies or cellular immunity.

antibody titre between weeks 33 and 39. As very little IgA passes from serum to saliva, it is assumed that the source of the IgA in whole saliva is predominantly from crevicular fluid. As in active immunization, protection against caries was not associated with an increase in salivary antibodies.

Discussion

Active Immunization

The development of dental caries was slightly reduced in monkeys immunized by the o.i. route as compared with the controls. However, this reduction was not significant and by 64 weeks the caries score in the o.i. group was 5.8 (± 1.3), compared with 8.75 (± 1.8) in the control group. Culture of *Strep. mutans* from the two groups of monkeys also failed to show significant difference in the CFU. There was a slight difference in caries between o.i. immunization, using *Strep. mutans* grown in Todd–Hewitt broth with 1% sucrose, resulting in a final caries score of 7.5, and that using *Strep. mutans* grown without added sucrose (caries score of 5). Although the reduction of caries by the o.i. route was not significant, nevertheless, there was a reduction in caries of 60–80% when s.c. immunization was used (Lehner *et al.*, 1975a, 1976b, 1977). Oral feeding of *Strep. mutans* was pursued for 18–24 weeks and it is possible that a longer or shorter schedule might have been more effective. Although the oral route is generally thought to be more acceptable than the systemic route of immunization, it is doubtful if prolonged oral administration of 5×10^{10} organisms daily would be an acceptable measure in man for a reduction of about one-third in the prevalence of caries.

Oro-intestinal immunization was not associated with an increase in serum IgG, IgA or IgM antibodies or in skin delayed hypersensitivity (DH). Salivary antibody titres were increased only from $\log_2 2$ to $\log_2 4$ during the 18–24 week period of antigen feeding, and considerable fluctuations in titres were found. Any reduction in caries would therefore be difficult to interpret in terms of systemic or salivary immune mechanisms. However, technical difficulties do not permit, as yet, direct measurement of gingival crevicular fluid antibodies, and there is a possibility of an increase in antibody formation in the gingiva. It should be noted that gastric intubation of gelatin capsules filled with 10^{11} killed *Strep. mutans* daily for 11 days induced only a transient increase in salivary IgA antibodies. A convincing secondary response could not be induced with a second series of capsules in Rhesus monkeys (Challacombe and Lehner, 1980). A comparable increase in secretory IgA antibodies of short duration was elicited in man by the ingestion of *Strep. mutans* (Mestecky *et al.*, 1978).

A surprising feature was the increase in caries in the gingivally immunized group, although only two monkeys were used. There was no associated change in antibodies or DH and the salivary antibodies showed a slight increase in titre, from about $\log_2 2$ to $\log_2 4$, comparable to that found in the o.i. group. There is no obvious interpretation for these findings, but they clearly distract from the concept of local gingival immunization.

The development of dental caries in o.i. and gingival immunization was very different from that found in s.c. immunization. Both cells and some of the protein antigens prepared from *Strep. mutans* (SA) induce significant reduction in caries of 60–80% (Lehner et al., 1975a, 1976b, 1980). This was accompanied by a prompt increase in serum IgG antibodies and the development of DH. IgA antibodies were also induced, although in the streptococcal antigen immunized monkeys this was significantly less than in those immunized with the cells. IgM antibodies were found only in the cell-immunized monkeys. Hence, protection in monkeys immunized by the s.c. route seem to show the best correlation with the IgG class of antibodies. The associated development of DH may reflect the presence of T helper cells and factors which have been elicited with the streptococcal antigen (Lamb et al., 1980). Furthermore, of the three isotypes tested in passive transfer experiments only IgG gave rise to protection against dental caries (Lehner et al., 1978a).

In view of the reports that tolerance can be readily induced in mice and rats by oral administration of a variety of antigens (Chase, 1946; Andre et al., 1975; Kagnoff, 1978; Mattingly and Waksman, 1978), the monkeys immunized by the o.i. and gingival routes were then immunized s.c. with cells of *Strep. mutans* in FIA. The serum antibody titres of all three isotypes tested promptly increased to the levels found in the monkeys immunized s.c. with the same cells and adjuvant at the start of the experiment. Clearly systemic tolerance was not induced after o.i. or gingival immunization in Rhesus monkeys. This might have been due to the long interval of 24–30 weeks between the end of o.i. and start of s.c. immunization. Tolerance induced by feeding soluble protein antigens to mice may last at least 12 weeks (Nyan and Kind, 1978), but it is not known whether particulate antigens are as effective as soluble antigens in inducing systemic tolerance, nor how long any tolerance induced may persist. Induction of tolerance has been reported in man (Lowney, 1968) but has not been characterized in a primate model. Although o.i. immunization gave rise to a weak salivary response, it is possible that concurrent systemic tolerance was not induced with the schedule used. The possibility that the oral route followed by the systemic route of immunization might affect the titre of secretory IgA antibodies in saliva was not verified.

The possibility that o.i. following s.c. immunization might alter serum or salivary IgA antibody titres was explored. This was especially pertinent as a greater degree of protection against cholera was elicited in dogs immunized with cholera toxoid by the s.c.–oral sequence than by the s.c. or oral route alone

(Pierce et al., 1977). Secretory IgA antibodies were thought to be involved in the increased and prolonged protection against cholera. *Strep. mutans* cells administered in the drinking water 70 weeks after initial s.c. immunization by streptococcal antigen had no detectable effect on any of the three classes of serum antibodies or secretory IgA antibodies in saliva. Although these results differ from those reported in dogs (Pierce et al., 1977), there was an important difference in timing of the interval between the s.c. and oral administration which was much longer in the monkey as compared with the dog experiments.

The sequence of s.c.–o.i. or the reverse sequence of immunization had no effect on the antibody titre of the three isotypes in serum or on the salivary IgA antibodies in Rhesus monkeys. However, the interval between the two routes of immunization, as well as the duration of the o.i. immunization, will need to be further explored.

Passive Immunization

Although transfer of whole immune serum resulted in IgG, IgM and IgA antibody titres to *Strep. mutans* comparable with those attained by the transfer of separated immunoglobulins, protection from caries was not achieved. In contrast significant protection was induced with IgG. This suggests that competition between the antibodies of different classes may result in lack of protection. IgA antibody could be such a candidate for competing with IgG, as IgA inhibits IgG-mediated bacteriolysis (Hall et al., 1971; Griffiss, 1975), phagocytosis (Wilton, 1978), and chemotaxis of polymorphonuclear leukocytes (Van Epps and Williams, 1976). Indeed, protection against dental caries is associated with a high IgG to IgA ratio of antibodies (Lehner et al., 1979).

We have shown that immunization with *Strep. mutans* elicits the three major classes of antibodies to this organism, but there is no certainty that the three classes of antibodies are directed to the same antigenic components. Nevertheless, transfer of IgG resulted in significantly less caries than transfer of IgA or IgM, and competition between IgG, IgA and IgM antibodies might account for the lack of protection after passive transfer of whole immune serum. The inhibitory effect of IgA is dependent on the ratio of IgA to IgG antibodies (Griffiss, 1975), so that another factor to be considered in immunization against *Strep. mutans* is the relative titre of serum antibodies of different classes. The results of passive immunization are consistent with the findings in active immunization that protection against dental caries is associated with a high IgG/IgA antibody ratio (Lehner et al., 1979).

Salivary antibodies were not related to the caries index and, at least with passive transfer of serum IgA, the salivary IgA antibodies were the highest among the nine groups; the caries index was also rather high. An alternative interpretation to serum IgA interfering with the function of serum IgG is that salivary IgA may enhance aggregation of *Strep. mutans* on the tooth surface directly or indirectly by increasing glucosyltransferase activity (Fukui *et al.*, 1974).

The part that cell-mediated immunity may play in protection against dental caries has been examined by means of transfer factor. Passive transfer of immune serum and cell-mediated immunity by means of transfer factor has induced protection against dental caries, but this was not achieved when cell-mediated immunity or immune serum alone were transferred. These results suggest that both cell-mediated immunity and antibodies are required for effective protection, as was found in monkeys actively immunized with whole cells of *Strep. mutans*.

Cell-mediated immunity is a measure of interaction of T helper cells (Lamb *et al.*, 1980) and suppressor cells (Lamb *et al.*, 1979) and the factors they release. Very low doses of the streptococcal antigen (0.01 µg) induce helper cells whereas high doses (100 µg) induce suppressor cells *in vitro*. Hence, the dose of antigen is one factor in modulating the immune response. The presence or recruitment of antigen-presenting cells (or macrophages) are essential in helper cell but not suppressor cell formation. This may be one of the reasons for the necessity for an adjuvant to elicit an effective immune response.

The helper factor released from sensitized T-cells is specific and displays similar specificities to the corresponding antibodies. It is likely that helper factor and antibodies to *Strep. mutans* share similar idiotypes. It is becoming clear that an effective immune response to *Strep. mutans* is dependent on the interaction of four sets of cells and their products (Fig. 12): macrophages

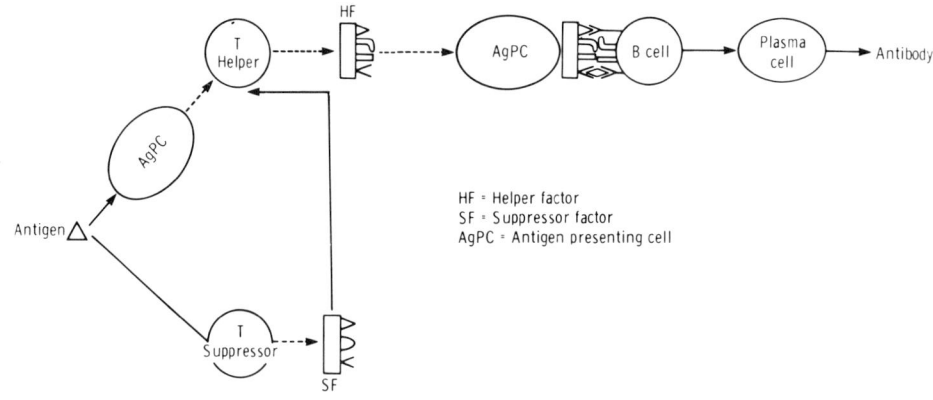

Fig. 12 A scheme of regulation of the immune response to *Strep. mutans* antigens.

releasing a genetically related factor (Erb *et al.*, 1976), T helper cells releasing helper factor, T suppressor cells releasing suppressor factor, and the B cells which transform to plasma cells and release antibodies. Every stage in this chain of reactions may be essential in eliciting the desirable end-product of a high avidity specific IgG antibody against *Strep. mutans*.

Summary

Active and passive immunization in the Rhesus monkey has been explored in order to investigate the mechanism of protection against dental caries by immunization with *Streptococcus mutans*. The oral route of immunization with *Strep. mutans* was compared with the subcutaneous route in Rhesus monkeys. Significant levels of serum IgG, IgM and IgA antibodies to *Strep. mutans* were elicited only in monkeys immunized subcutaneously. Similarly, the skin delayed hypersensitivity reaction to *Strep. mutans* was elicited only in the subcutaneously immunized monkeys. Oral immunization induced a modest increase in salivary IgA antibodies to *Strep. mutans*, although a slight increase in IgA antibodies was also found in the saliva of all other groups of immunized and control monkeys. A small, though not significant, reduction in dental caries was found in the monkeys immunized orally, whereas subcutaneous immunization with *Strep. mutans* consistently elicited a significant reduction in caries. Oral feeding of *Strep. mutans* failed to induce tolerance to a subsequent subcutaneous challenge by the same organism. Furthermore, sequential subcutaneous followed by oral immunization had little effect on the titre of salivary or serum antibodies.

Passive transfer of immune serum with IgG, IgM and IgA antibodies to *Strep. mutans* failed to induce protection against dental caries. However, when separated IgG, IgM and IgA sera were given, IgG induced significant protection but IgA or IgM antibodies to *Strep. mutans* did not. IgA and IgM may compete or interfere with the protective effect of IgG antibodies and the ratio of IgG/IgA and IgG/IgM antibodies might be an important factor in immunization against dental caries.

The role of cell-mediated immunity has been explored by the use of transfer factor. This showed that protection against dental caries can be elicited by passive transfer of whole immune serum and cellular immunity, but not by cellular immunity or immune serum alone.

The results of active and passive immunization suggest that immunoregulation is governed by four sets of cells and their products: antigen-presenting cells, T helper cells, T suppressor cells and B cells. A high avidity IgG class of antibody to *Strep. mutans* appears to play an essential part in protection against dental caries.

References

Andre, C., Heremans, J. F., Vaerman, J. P. and Cambiazo, C. L. (1975). *J. exp. Med.* **142**, 1509.
Baram, P. and Condoulis, W., (1974). *Transplant. Proc.* **6**, 209.
Caldwell, J., Challacombe, S. J. and Lehner, T. (1977). *J. med. Microbiol.* **10**, 213.
Challacombe, S. J. (1978). *Adv. exp. Med. Biol.* **107**, 355.
Challacombe, S. J. and Lehner, T. (1980). *Archs oral Biol.* **24**, 917.
Chase, M. W. (1946). *Proc. Soc. exp. Biol.* **81**, 257.
Erb, P., Feldman, M. and Hogg, N. M. (1976). *Eur. J. Immunol.* **6**, 365.
Fukui, K, Fukui, Y. and Moriyama, T. (1974). *J. Bact.* **118**, 805.
Griffiss, J. M. (1975). *J. Immunol.* **114**, 1770.
Hall, W. H., Manion, R. E. and Zinneman, H. H. (1971) *J. Immunol.* **107**, 41.
Kagnoff, M. F. (1978). *Cell Immunol.* **40**, 186.
Kirkpatrick, C. H., Rich, R. R. and Smith, T. K. (1972). *J. Clin. Invest.* **51**, 2948.
Lamb, J. R., Kontiainen, S. and Lehner, T. (1979). *Infect. Immun.* **26**, 903.
Lamb, J. R., Kontianen, S. and Lehner, T. (1980). *J. Immunol.* **124**, 1245.
Lehner, T. Caldwell, J. and Challacombe, S. J. (1977). *Archs oral Biol.* **22**, 393.
Lehner, T. Challacombe, S. J. and Caldwell, J. (1975a). *Nature, Lond.* **254**, 517.
Lehner, T., Challacombe, S. J. and Caldwell, J. (1975b). *Archs oral Biol.* **20**, 393.
Lehner, T., Challacombe, S. J. and Caldwell, J. (1976a). *J. dent. Res.* **55**, C166.
Lehner, T., Challacombe, S. J. and Caldwell, J. (1976b). *Nature, Lond.* **264**, 69.
Lehner, T., Russell, M. W. and Caldwell, J. (1980). *Lancet i*, 995.
Lehner, T., Russell, M. W., Challacombe, S. J. Scully, C. M. and Hawkes, J. (1978a) *Lancet i*, 693.
Lehner, T., Russell, M. W., Scully, C. M. Challacombe, S. J. and Caldwell J. (1979). In *Pathogenic Streptococci* (M. T. Parker, ed.), p. 215, Reedbooks, Chertsey, Surrey.
Lehner, T., Russell, M. W., Wilton, J. M. A., Chailacombe, S. J. Scully, C. M. and Hawkes, J. E. (1978b). In *Secretory Immunity and Infection* (J. R. McGhee, J. Mestecky and J. L. Babb, eds.), p. 303, Plenum Press, New York.
Lowney, E. D. (1968). *J. invest. Dermat.* **51**, 411.
Mattingly, J. A. and Waksman, B. (1978). *J. Immunol.* **120**, 861.
Mestecky, J., McGhee, J. R., Arnold, R. R., Michalek, S. M., Prince, S. J. and Babb, J. L. (1978). *J. clin. Invest.* **61**, 731.
Michalek, S. M. and McGhee, J. R. (1977). *Infect. Immun.* **17**, 644.
Michalek, S. M., McGhee, J. R., Mestecky, J., Arnold, R. R. and Bozzo, L. (1976). *Science, N.Y.* **192**, 1238.
Monte-Wicker, V., Wicker, K. and Arbesman, C. E. (1970). *Immunochemistry* **7**, 839.
Nyan, J. and Kind, Z. S. (1978). *J. Immunol.* **120**, 861.
Pierce, N. F., Sack, R. B. and Sircar, B. K. (1977). *J. infect. Dis.* **135**, 888.
Russell, M. W. and Lehner, T. (1978). *Archs oral Biol.* **23**, 7.
Stoppelaar, J. D. de, Houte, J. van and Backer Dirks, O. (1969). *Caries Res.* **3**, 190.
Taubman, M. A. and Smith, D. J. (1974). *Infect. Immun.* **9**, 1079.
Van Epps, D. E. and Williams, R. C. (1976). *J. exp. Med.* **144**, 1227.
Wilton, J. M. A. (1978). *Clin. exp. Immunol.* **34**, 423.

13. Microbial Interactions in the Mouth

J. S. VAN DER HOEVEN

Interactions in Dental Plaque

Growth at a Surface

The enamel surface of the tooth supports the formation of a thick bacterial film. In aquatic environments the adhesion of bacteria to solid surfaces and the formation of slime layers is well known. There are different mechanisms by which bacteria may adhere to solid surfaces, but extracellular polysaccharides are most often involved as polymer bridges between the bacterial and solid surfaces (Marshall *et al.*, 1971*a,b*). According to Zobell (1943), stimulation of bacterial growth at a surface results from the concentration of nutrients at that surface. He points out that there might be a further advantage to the adherent cells in the retardation of diffusion of metabolites and exoenzymes, necessary for the degradation of macromolecular substrates from the interstices between the cells and the surface.

Although the above events may explain the formation of a bacterial film in a dilute solution, these films may well develop in conditions in which there is no substrate limitation. Apparently there are advantages to cells that become adsorbed to a surface. Filip (1978) suggested that the growth rate of compost bacteria is stimulated when adsorbed to glass beads or to other solid particles. A glass rod submerged in a continuous culture of *Streptococcus mutans* is soon covered with bacteria. During formation of a film the doubling time of the attached *Strep. mutans* cells is two times higher than the doubling time of the cells in the liquid (J. S. van der Hoeven and P. J. M. Camp, unpublished observations).

When bacteria attach to the tooth surface they become exposed to saliva and will start to grow. The oral environment supports rapid growth. Following their inoculation into germ-free rats, *Strep. mutans* increases with a doubling time of 1–2 h and *Actinomyces viscosus* with a doubling time of approximately 2 h (H. J. A. Beckers and J. S. van der Hoeven, unpublished observations). The increase in thickness of plaque ceases after some time and the number of cells does not increase further. According to Pirt (1975) the development of bacterial film will be limited by the diffusion of substrates into it. Diffusion and simultaneous uptake and metabolic conversion results in concentration gradients for substrate. If the depth of a film becomes greater than the thickness of an "active" layer, then the part below may be considered to be an area either of inactivity or of lesser activity, which is controlled by a different limiting substrate. In general, there could be a series of zones in which growth is controlled by a number of different limiting nutrients.

Plaque may have a considerable thickness, but as most organisms isolated are micro-aerophilic or anaerobic it is likely that oxygen is less important than other limiting factors, such as carbohydrate, in the deeper layers of the plaque (Ellwood and Hunter, 1976). From the mixed-acid fermentation of *Strep. mutans* in mono-associated gnotobiotic rats, it would appear that the source of carbohydrate rather than the nitrogen source is limiting the growth of *Strep. mutans* (van der Hoeven, 1976). Considering the availability of ammonia and amino acids in the mouth and the efficiency with which oral streptococci utilize low concentrations of ammonia, it seems unlikely that streptococci in dental plaque are nitrogen limited (Griffith and Carlsson, 1974).

After the growth has ceased, the flow of substrate into the bacterial layer is just sufficient to maintain the bacterial population. Competition for substrate will become an important ecological determinant. Under these conditions bacteria with low maintenance energy requirements have an ecological advantage; maintenance energy is commonly used to describe the use of energy for non-growth-related functions. Differences in maintenance energy play a significant role in the competition of bacteria on root surfaces, in biological waste water treatment and on cheese (Woldendorp *et al.*, 1966), as well as in the rumen (Russel and Baldwin, 1979). In these ecosystems initially predominant fast growing species are progressively displaced by species with low maintenance energy requirements. It would be worthwhile to investigate to what extent maintenance energy determines the relative success of different populations in dental plaque.

The affinity for substrate may be another factor in the competition for substrate in the layer. Bacteria with a high affinity for the limiting substrate can grow at substrate concentrations that are too low to support the growth of bacteria with lower affinity. In mixed cultures in a chemostat, the bacterium with the highest affinity for the limiting substrate predominates at a low substrate concentration but will be displaced if the chemostat is run at a higher substrate concentration (Jannasch and Mateles. 1974). In dental plaque many bacteria can utilize the same substrates, e.g. sugars. The affinity for such components may be an important factor in the competition.

The interactions described above result from the competition for substrates in the layer. Apart from this many other types of interaction play a role in dental plaque. The general term for all these is symbiosis, although this is sometimes used as though it was synonymous with mutualism, in which both organisms are stimulated. This term includes beneficial interactions (commensalism), antagonistic interactions (competition, amensalism) or the absence of interaction (neutralism). It is important to stress that it is a continuous spectrum of interrelationships.

Commensal Relationships

Commensal relationships arise from the production of metabolites in the ecosystem. In as much as these components are excreted, they become available for other bacterial populations. There is evidence that fastidious oral bacteria such as spirochetes and *Bacteroides melaninogenicus* benefit from the complex microflora of the dental plaque, that provides a low redox potential and a series of indispensable growth factors (Socransky et al., 1964; Loesche, 1968). *Vibrio* depends for growth on hydrogen, which it can obtain directly (e.g. from *Veillonella* species) or by producing H_2 from formate. Formate can be provided by streptococci (Carlsson and Griffith, 1974) or by *Fusobacterium nucleatum* (Loesche and Gibbons, 1968).

Veillonella utilizes lactic acid as an energy source. The major lactic acid-producing bacteria in plaque are streptococci and actinomyces. The experimental association of *Step. mutans* with *V. alcalescens* in gnotobiotic rats could serve to illustrate the operation of several ecological determinants simultaneously.

The nutrient interrelationship between streptococci and veillonellae in plaque appears from the simultaneous presence of both species in plaque, as well as the fermentation pattern in plaque inhabiting both species (Mikx et al., 1972; van der Hoeven et al., 1978). *V. alcalescens* OMZ193 attains higher levels in plaque in the presence of *Strep. mutans* FIL than in combination with C67–1. This can be explained by the high lactic acid production of FIL. The simultaneous growth of veillonellae and FIL in plaque produces less plaque biomass (Fig. 1; van der Hoeven et al., 1978). This is reminiscent of the retardation of the growth of *Strep. salivarius* and *V. alcalescens* in mixed cultures (Parker and Snyder, 1961). The accumulation of veillonellae in preformed "*in vitro* plaque" of Gram-positive filamentous organisms, including *A. viscosus*, points to the significance of interbacterial attachment in colonization (Bladen et al., 1970). To test whether this mechanism operates *in vivo*, pairs of *Strep. mutans* and *V. alcalescens* strains were inoculated into germ-free rats. *V. alcalescens* establishes better in the presence of a coaggregating *Step. mutans* strain than in combination with a non-coaggregation *Strep. mutans* strain (B. C. McBride and J. S. van der Hoeven, unpublished observations). By analogy with a mechanism proposed by McCabe and Donkersloot (1977), the adherence of veillonellae may be mediated by binding of extracellular glucosyltransferase from *Strep. mutans*.

Apart from other functions, the extracellular polysaccharides in dental plaque serve as energy reserves, providing substrate to the microflora during

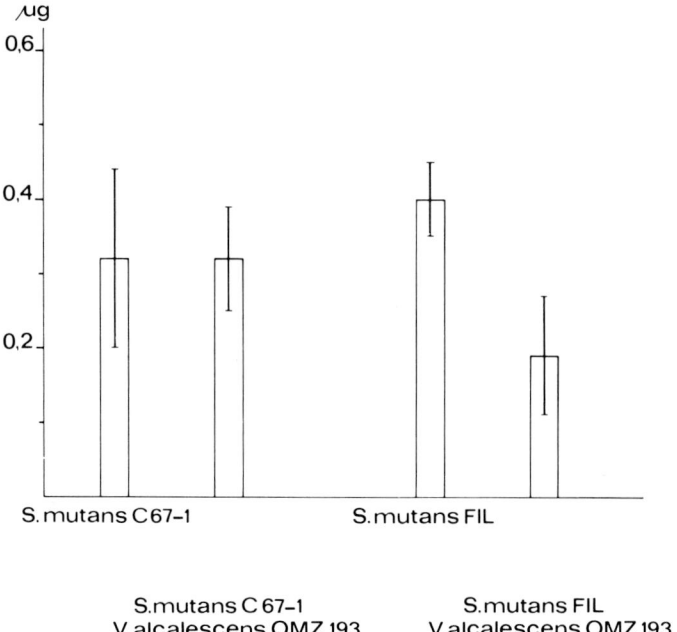

Fig. 1 DNA as an index of biomass in the fissure plaque of gnotobiotic rats associated with *Strep. mutans* C67-1 or FIL, either alone or in combination with *V. alcalescens* OMZ193. The proportions of OMZ193 are 0.05% and 16% in the combinations with C67-1 and FIL, respectively.

periods in between meals. Of the two major polysaccharides, fructans are more readily degraded by the plaque microflora than glucans that persist for longer periods of time in the plaque (Wood, 1964; Critchley, 1969; Hotz *et al.*, 1972).

The great majority of polysaccharide-producing bacteria in nature appear to be unable to utilize their own extracellular polysaccharides as carbon sources. Unrelated organisms degrade polysaccharides of other bacteria. In the mouth, organisms such as *Strep. salivarius* and *A. viscosus* are capable of both synthesis and breakdown of fructans. In addition, fructan-hydrolysing activity in dental plaque originates from oral streptococci (van Houte and Jansen, 1968), including species that do not synthesize fructans. Glucan hydrolases in plaque originate from several organisms, including streptococci (Dewar and Walker, 1975), actinomyces and bacteroides species (Staat *et al.*, 1973). Apart from *Strep. mutans*, these organisms do not synthesize glucans.

Interbacterial Aggregation

The attachment of one species to the surface of another may be of ecological importance for organisms that lack a means to become firmly attached to the surface of the tooth or the pellicle.

Certain strains and species of plaque bacteria have been shown to aggregate when mixed together (Gibbons and Nygaard, 1970). The coaggregation of *Strep. sanguis* and *A. viscosus* has recently been studied in some detail and appears to result from the interaction between protein receptors and carbohydrate moieties in the cell envelopes of both species (Ellen and Balcerzak-Raczkowski, 1977; McIntire *et al.*, 1978; Cisar *et al.*, 1979).

Few experimental data are available to demonstrate the significance of interbacterial aggregation as an ecological determinant in plaque *in vivo*. Electron micrographs of dental plaque suggest that some organisms attach to dissimilar species. The typical "corn cob" appearance (Listgarten *et al.*, 1973) indicates an association between coccoid forms, possibly *Strep. sanguis* (Takazoe *et al.*, 1978) and filamentous organisms. Data by Slots and Gibbons (1978) suggest that the attachment and colonization of *B. melaninogenicus* depends upon the presence of dental plaque containing actinomyces and other Gram-positive bacteria. As mentioned above, the experimental establishment of veillonellae in gnotobiotic rats is promoted by the presence of coaggregating *Strep. mutans* strains in the plaque.

Bacteria may adhere to plaque via polysaccharides from other bacteria. Experiments of Hamada *et al.* (1978) suggest that glucans from *Strep. mutans* mediate in the binding of some other Gram-positive and Gram-negative bacteria.

Strep mutans cells appear to have specific receptors which bind glucan (dextran) (Olson *et al.*, 1974) and dextran-induced aggregation would seem an important mechanism in the accumulation of *Strep. mutans* on teeth. The effect of dextran on the initial adherence of *Strep. mutans in vivo* is suggested by the following experiment. Rats harbouring a high proportion of dextran-producing *Strep. bovis* in their oral flora were fed either a sucrose or a glucose diet and subsequently inoculated with *Strep. mutans* strains. Subsequently inoculated dextran-aggregating strains of *Strep. mutans* attach in larger numbers to the plaque in the sucrose-fed rats than to plaque in the glucose-fed rats. There is no such difference in the attachment of *Strep. mutans* strains that do not aggregate with dextran (J. S. van der Hoeven and A. H. Rogers, unpublished results; B. C. McBride and J. S. van der Hoeven, unpublished results).

Antagonistic Relationships

Competition for substrate is likely to be an important determinant in plaque. However, as indicated above, few data are available to support this contention. A variety of inhibitory substances is produced by members of the oral microflora: bacteriocins by *Strep. mutans* and *Strep. sanguis* (Kelstrup and Gibbons, 1969; Nakamura *et al.*, 1977); hydrogen peroxide, known to be produced by *Strep. sanguis* (Holmberg and Hallander, 1973) and organic acids (Donoghue and Tyler, 1975). All these components may play a role in the regulation of the plaque microflora.

Colonization Resistance

Longitudinal sampling of dental plaque from a well-defined area of the tooth shows that the bacterial composition is qualitatively and quantitatively surprisingly constant (Bowden *et al.*, 1975). Yet, the mouth is regularly exposed to a multitude of microbiological contaminations that might be expected to upset the balance. Usually, foreign organisms disappear at a rapid rate, because they cannot become established. The aliens may lack essential characteristics to enable them to survive in the mouth. However, organisms indigenous to the mouth, that are deliberately introduced, often have difficulties in becoming established (Jordan *et al.*, 1972; Krasse *et al.*, 1967).

In analogy to other microbial ecosystems the microbial community of the dental plaque has the capacity to maintain stability; this is termed homeostasis (Alexander, 1971). Homeostasis reflects the most efficient exploitation of ecological niches. The establishment of a foreign organism suggests that a niche that it could occupy was not already filled or that a modification of the environment opens up new opportunities for the alien This is illustrated by the favourable effect of frequent intake of sucrose on the implantation of *Strep. mutans* in dental plaque (Krasse, 1965).

Colonization resistance refers to the mechanism that controls the microbial colonization of ecosystems. The colonization resistance (CR) can be expressed as the threshold dose for a contaminant to become established (van der Waay, 1979). Oral microflora's may differ considerably in (CR), depending upon their composition. For example, the (CR) of the dental plaque microflora in Osborne–Mendel rats (Animal Laboratory, University of Nijmegen) is low. Approximately 10^4 cells are required for the establishment of *Strep. mutans* OMZ176. The major components of the plaque in these rats are *Strep. bovis*, veillonellae, and some biotypes of Gram-negative rods (van der Hoeven and Rogers, 1979*b*). Supplementation of the plaque microflora with a biotype of *A. viscosus* and *Strep. sanguis* increases the (CR) (Mikx *et al.*, 1975) to a threshold dose of 10^{10} cells of OMZ176 (J. S. van der Hoeven, unpublished results). We can inoculate *Strep. mutans* at various intervals, following the supplementation of the oral flora with the (CR) components *A. viscosus* and *Strep. sanguis*. Shortly after the inoculation of the (CR) components, *Strep. mutans* strains T2 or SW31 become established in large numbers, but the longer the delay in introducing *Step. mutans* the poorer is its establishment (Fig. 2; van der Hoeven and Rogers, 1979*a*). The results suggest that the (CR)

13. Microbial Interactions in the Mouth

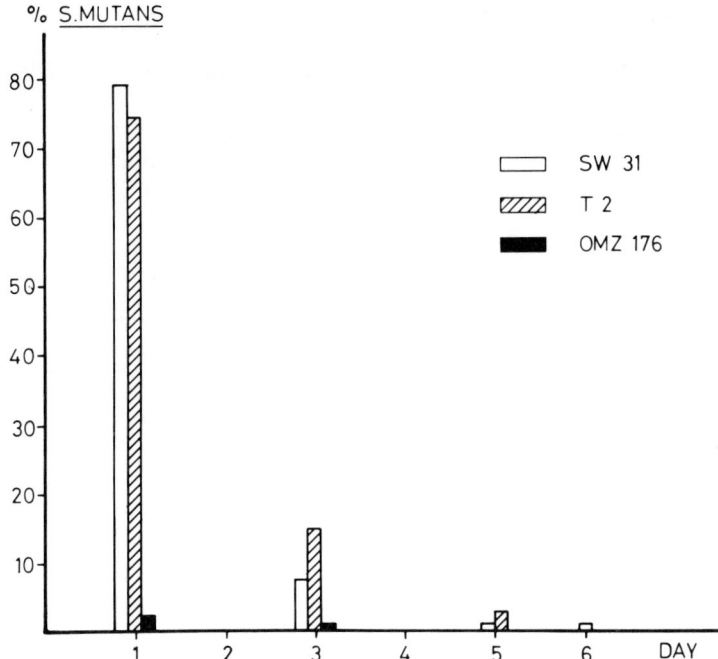

Fig. 2 Implatation of *Strep. mutans* in rats at various intervals following the inoculation of *A. viscosus* Nyl and *Strep. sanguis* Ny101. The proportion of *Strep. mutans* expressed as a median percentage of the total cultivable plaque flora is given.

components can occupy the niche of *Strep. mutans* but cannot displace *Strep. mutans*. In the transient state, when *A. viscosus* and *Strep. sanguis* only partially occupy the niche, *Strep. mutans* colonizes successfully. The difference in establishment between *Strep. mutans* T2 or SW31 and OMZ176 indicates a strain dependency of the (CR) against *Strep. mutans*. van Houte *et al.* (1976) also observe that the inocula required for infection vary considerably between different strains. Whereas a dose of 5.8×10^7 cells is not sufficient to establish *Strep. mutans* BHT, a 100-fold lower dose sufficed for E49. A study in our laboratory suggests that the successful implantation of *Strep. mutans* is related to production of bacteriocin. Strains that exhibit inhibitory activity against the resident microflora establish in greater proportions than bacteriocin-negative strains. Furthermore, bacteriocin seems to be produced in dental plaque in rats containing a high proportion of producer strain *Strep. mutans* T2 (van der Hoeven and Rogers, 1979a). The majority of freshly isolated strains, as well as laboratory strains of *Strep. mutans*, are bacteriocinogenic (Hamada and Ooshima, 1975; Rogers, 1976; Weerkamp *et al.*, 1977), which indicates the ecological importance of bacteriocin production for this organism.

Ecological Control of Pathogens

In clinical bacteriology a better understanding of the effects of antibiotic therapy has renewed an interest in ecological control of potential pathogens. Where infectious diseases such as tuberculosis, pneumococcal pneumonia and streptococcal infections were the major killers before antimicrobial therapy became available, infectious complications caused mainly by Gram-negative bacteria and *Staphylococcus aureus* are the killers of today in patients with reduced resistance. The type of microorganism responsible for the infections has changed from pathogenic non-commensal to potentially pathogenic commensal. The major source of these infections is the digestive tract. The colonization resistance of the alimentary tract plays a key role in these infections (van der Waay and Verhoef, 1979).

Studies at various body sites suggest that antagonistic components of the indigenous microflora play a role in resistance to colonization of Gram-negative bacilli of the pharynx (Sprunt and Redman, 1968), group A streptococcal colonization of the throat (Crowe *et al.*, 1973) and inhibition of *Neisseria gonorrhoea* by the endocervical flora (Saigh *et al.*, 1978).

In a number of cases phytopathogenic bacteria can be controlled by bacteriocin producer strains (Vidaver, 1976). Early attempts to suppress caries pathogens in the oral flora were based on bacteriocin production. Rutter *et al.* (1961) use *Bacillus brevis* in the mouth because this organism produces bacteriocins active against the acidogenic oral flora.

Our knowledge of the control of pathogens has not advanced greatly. Most investigations have dealt primarily with bacteriocins as controlling agents. Other traits associated with the competitive ability, such as growth rate, competition for binding sites, substrate competition, tolerance to environmental changes, etc., have not been studied.

Control of *Strep. mutans*

Irrespective of the potential significance of other bacteria in dental caries, prevention of caries would be favoured by suppression of *Strep. mutans*. The role of oral flora in the defence against caries caused by *Strep. mutans* is apparent from rat caries experiments. In one experiment, three inoculated bacterial strains counteracted the cariogenicity of *Strep. mutans* OMZ61 (Konig *et al.*, 1965). In another test the cariogenicity of *Strep. mutans* OMZ176 and E49 was significantly reduced in the presence of the indigenous microflora in SPF rats (van der Hoeven *et al.*, 1972). In these experiments the competitive mechanisms involved are not known. It is widely believed that competition is keenest between closely related strains and species. They tend to have a similar role in and demands on the environment.

Competition between strains of *Strep. mutans* is illustrated by the following experiment. Groups of germ-free rats are inoculated with *Strep. mutans* T2 (groups 1 and 2), its streptomycin-resistant mutant T2S (group 3) and its non-bacteriocinogenic mutant T2 bac$^-$ (group 4). One week later, the rats are inoculated again with T2S, T2 bac$^-$, T2 and T2 in groups 1, 2, 3 and 4, respectively. Competitive displacement of the first inoculated strain occurs only in group 4, where the parent strain has an ecological advantage over the bacteriocin-negative mutant. In groups 1, 2 and 3, the second invaders are not successful, T2S cannot displace T2 nor can T2 bac$^-$ become established in the presence of T2 or, T2 in the presence of T2S (Rogers *et al.*, 1979). Apparently, the niches that the invading strains could occupy are effectively filled. The results show that for displacement the organisms must also be dissimilar in some ecological relevant way.

A number of investigators have studied interspecific competition of *Strep. mutans* in man (Svanberg and Loesche, 1978) or in rats (Thomson *et al.*, 1979; Huis in 't Veld *et al.*, 1979; Hillman, 1978, 1979). The results of Hillman suggest that interspecific competition may be used to control *Strep. mutans*. A non-acidogenic, low cariogenic mutant of *Strep. mutans*, implanted in rats, resists colonization by the parent strain (Hillman, 1978, 1979). In these experiments, the basic capacity of *Strep. mutans* strains to compete effectively with other strains is still unknown.

In general then, colonization resistance of the microflora against *Strep. mutans* depends upon the presence of specific microorganisms. Organisms that can increase the CR of dental plaque are *Strep. mutans* biotypes (Hillman, 1978, 1979; Svanberg and Loesche, 1978) or *A. viscosus* and *Strep. sanguis* (Mikx *et al.*, 1975; van der Hoeven and Rogers, 1979*a*). The effectiveness of *A. viscosus* to compete with *Strep. mutans* suggests that the essential issue is the ecological role rather than the position in taxonomy. The role of *Strep. sanguis* in the field of competition is perhaps less pronounced (van der Hoeven and Rogers, 1979*b*).

Features that may be responsible for or contribute to the competitiveness of *A. viscosus*, or another organism, may include the following: (1) competition for binding sites to the pellicle, to the surface of other microorganisms or extracellular polysaccharides, e.g. *A. viscosus* serotype 1, which shows dextran-induced aggregation (McBride and Bourgeau, 1975), may compete with *Strep. mutans* for binding to dextran in plaque; (2) competition for substrate; (3) growth rate, e.g. preliminary results indicate that maximum growth rates of *A. viscosus* and *Strep. mutans* in plaque are similar (H. J. A. Beckers and J. S. van der Hoeven, unpublished observations); (4) ability to synthesize and store reserve substances; (5) maintenance of energy.

A. viscous does not seem to produce antibacterial substances but *Strep. sanguis* may produce inhibitory levels of hydrogen peroxide to *Strep. mutans* (Holmberg and Hallander, 1973). The displacement of cariogenic streptococci in dental plaque of rats by *A. viscosus* reduces caries development on smooth surfaces and in the fissures (van der Hoeven, 1974, 1980, unpublished data).

Ecological Control and Chemotherapy

The application of ecological control of *Strep. mutans* in man may require depression of *Strep. mutans* by chemotherapeutic agents before inoculation of bacteria that increase colonization resistance. *Strep. mutans* can be successfully depressed by a variety of chemicals such as acidulated phosphate fluoride (Loesche, 1976), stannous fluoride (Keene *et al.*, 1977), iodine (Caufield and Gibbons, 1979) or chlorhexidine (Emilson and Westergren, 1979). None of these agents is selective in depressing *Strep. mutans* only. However, application of acidulated phosphate fluoride or chlorhexidine can also increase the number of *Strep. mutans* (Loesche, 1976; Emilson and Westergren, 1979). After an ecological disturbance the outcome of the competition is difficult to predict and *Strep. mutans* may benefit from the depression of other bacteria. Ecological control of Strep. mutans may well complement chemotherapy.

Summary

The study of factors affecting microbial populations on the tooth surface may provide information of importance to the prevention of oral disease. Dental plaque is controlled by external factors such as saliva, diet and oral hygiene, in addition to the effects of bacteria on each other. A variety of bacterial interactions occur in the plaque. Interbacterial aggregation, extracellular polysaccharide-mediated attachment, commensal relationships between producer and recipient bacteria or production of bacterial inhibitors are suggested as significant determinants of the dental plaque ecosystem. Our knowledge of ecological determinants has not advanced greatly. Possible determinants of bacterial competition, such as substrate affinities or maintenance of energy requirements have not been studied so far. Much needs to be learned about the ecological niches of the individual species in dental plaque and the overlap between the niches. This knowledge might eventually be applied to ecological control of pathogens. In rats the resistance against colonization by *Streptococcus mutans* was found to be dependent upon the microbial composition of the plaque microflora. *Strep. mutans* established less well in rats that were initially colonized by *Actinomyces viscosus* which resulted in significantly reduced development of caries.

References

Alexander, M. (1971). *Microbial Ecology*, John Wiley, New York and London.
Beckers, H. J. A. and van der Hoeven, J. S. (1979). Abstract No. 32, 26th ORCA Meeting, Stirling.

Bladen, H., Hageage, G., Pollock, F. and Harr, R. (1970). *Archs oral Biol.* **15**, 127–133.
Bowden, G. H., Hardie, J. M. and Slack, G. L. (1975). *Caries Res.* **9**, 253–277.
Carlsson, J. and Griffith, J. C. (1974). *Archs oral Biol.* **19**, 1105–1109.
Caufield, P. W. and Gibbons, R. J. (1979). *J. dent. Res.* **58**, 1317–1326.
Cisar, J. O., Kolenbrander, R. E. and McIntire, F. C. (1979). *Infect. Immun.* **24**, 742–752.
Critchley, P. (1969). *Caries Res.* **3**, 249–265.
Crowe, C. C., Sanders, W. E., Jr. and Longley, S. (1973). *J. infect. Dis.* **128**, 527–532.
Dewar, M. G. and Walker, G. J. (1975) *Caries Res.* **9**, 21–35.
Donoghue, H. D. and Tyler, J. E. (1975). *Archs oral Biol.* **20**, 381–387.
Ellen, R. P. and Balcerzak-Raczkowski, I. B. (1977). *J. periodont. Res.* **12**, 11–20.
Ellwood, D. C. and Hunter, J. R. (1976). In *Continuous Culture 6. Applications and New Fields* (A. C. R. Dean, D. C. Ellwood, C. G. T. Evans and J. Melling, eds), pp. 270–282, Ellis Horwood Ltd, Chichester.
Emilson, C. G. and Westergren, G. (1979). *Scand. J. dent. Res.* **87**, 288–295.
Filip, Z. (1978). *Eur. J. appl. Microbiol. Biotechnol.* **6**, 87–94.
Gibbons, R. J. and Nygaard, M. (1970). *Archs oral Biol.* **15**, 1397–1400.
Griffith, C. J. and Carlsson, J. (1974). *J. gen. Microbiol.* **82**, 253–260.
Hamada, S. and Ooshima, T. (1975). *Archs oral Biol.* **20**, 641–648.
Hamada, S., Tai, S. and Slade, H. D. (1978). *Infect. Immun.* **21**, 213–220.
Hillman, J. D. (1978). *J. dent. Res.* **57**, special issue A, abstract no. 784.
Hillman, J. D. (1979). *J. Dent. Res.* **58**, special issue A, abstract no. 44.
Holmberg, K. and Hallander, H. O. (1973). *Archs oral Biol.* **18**, 423–434.
Hotz, P., Guggenheim, B. and Schmid, R. (1972). *Caries Res.* **6**, 103–121.
Huis in 't Veld, J. H. J., de Boer, J., Havenaar, R. and Kamp, E. M. (1979). Abstract No. 30, 26th ORCA Meeting, Stirling.
Jannasch, H. W. and Mateles, R. I. (1974). *Adv. microbial Physiol.* **11**, 165–212.
Jordan, H. V., Englander, H. R., Engler, W. O. and Kulczyk, S. (1972). *J. dent. Res.* **51**, 515–518.
Keene, H. J., Shklair, I. L. and Mickel, G. T. (1977). *J. dent. Res.* **56**, 21–27.
Kelstrup, J. and Gibbons, R. J. (1969). *Archs oral Biol.* **14**, 251–258.
König, K. G., Guggenheim, B. and Mühlemann, H. R. (1965). *Helv. odont. Acta* **9**, 130–134.
Krasse, B. (1965). *Archs oral Biol.* **10**, 223–226.
Krasse, B., Edwardsson, S., Svensson, I. and Trell, L. (1967). *Archs oral Biol.* **12**, 231–236.
Listgarten, M. A. Mayo, H. E. and Amsterdam, M. (1973). *Archs oral Biol.* **18**, 651–656.
Loesche, W. J. (1968). *Periodontics* **6**, 245–249.
Loesche, W. J. (1976). *Oral Sci. Rev.* **9**, 65–107.
Loesche, W. J. and Gibbons, R. J. (1968). *Archs oral Biol.* **13**, 191–201.
Marshall, K. C., Stout, R. and Mitchell, R. (1971a). *Can. J. Microbiol.* **17**, 1413–1416.
Marshall, K. C., Stout, R. and Mitchell, R. (1971b). *J. gen. Microbiol.* **68**, 337–348.
McBride, B. C. and Bourgeau, G. (1975). *Archs oral Biol.* **20**, 837–841.
McCabe, R. M. and Donkersloot, J. A. (1977). *Infect. Immun.* **18**, 726–734.
McIntire, F. C., Vatter, A. E., Baros, J. and Arnold, J. (1978). *Infect. Immun.* **21**, 978–988.
Mikx, F. H. M., van der Hoeven, J. S., König, K. G., Plasschaert, A. J. M. and Guggenheim, B. (1972). *Caries Res.* **6**, 211–223.
Mikx, F. H. M., van der Hoeven, J. S., Plasschaert, A. J. M. and König, K. G. (1975).

Caries Res. **9**, 1–20.
Nakamura, T., Suginaka, Y., Orata, T., Obata, N. and Yamazaki, N. (1977). *Bull. Tokyo dent. Coll.* **18**, 217–229.
Olson, G. A., Guggenheim, B. and Small, P. A. (1974). *Infect. Immun.* **9**, 273–278.
Parker, R. B. and Snyder, M. L. (1961). *Proc. Soc. exp. Biol. Med.* **108**, 749–752.
Pirt, S. (1975). *Principles of Microbe and Cell Cultivation*, Blackwell Scientific Publications, Oxford.
Rogers, A. H. (1976). *Archs oral Biol.* **21**, 99–104.
Rogers, A. H., van der Hoeven, J. S. and Mikx, F. H. M. (1979). *Infect. Immun.* **23**, 571–576.
Russell, J. B. and Baldwin, R. L. (1979). *Appl. environ. Microbiol.* **37**, 537–543.
Rutter, R. R., Ruefenacht, W. G., Chamberlain, C. R., Thomassen, P. R., Rose, M. and Scrivener, C. A. (1961). *J. dent. Res.* **40**, 1112–1115.
Saigh, J. H., Sanders, C. C. and Sanders, W. E., Jr. (1978). *Infect. Immun.* **19**, 704–710.
Slots, J. and Gibbons, R. J. (1978). *Infect. Immun.* **19**, 254–264.
Socransky, S. S., Loesche, W. J., Hubersak, C. and MacDonald, J. B. (1964). *J. Bact.* **88**, 200–209.
Sprunt, K. and Redman, W. (1968). *Ann. intern. Med.* **68**, 579–590.
Staat, R. H., Gawronski, T. H. and Schachtele, C. F. (1973). *Infect. Immun.* **8**, 1009–1016.
Svanberg, M. and Loesche, W. J. (1978). *Archs oral Biol.* **23**, 551–556.
Takazoe, I., Matsakubo, T. and Katow, T. (1978). *J. dent. Res.* **57**, 384–387.
Thomson, A. L., Bowen, W. H., Little, W. A., Kurzmiak-Jones, H. M. and Gomez, I. M. (1979). *Caries Res.* **13**, 9–17.
van der Hoeven, J. S. (1974). Thesis, Nijmegen.
van der Hoeven, J. S. (1976). *Archs oral Biol.* **21**, 431–434.
van der Hoeven, J. S. (1980). *Caries Res.* **14**, 61–66.
van der Hoeven, J. S. and Rogers, A. H. (1979a). *Infect. Immun.* **23**, 206–212.
van der Hoeven, J. S. and Rogers, A. H. (1979b). *Archs oral Biol.* **24**, 787–790.
van der Hoeven, J. S., Toorop, A. I. and Mikx, F. H. M. (1978). *Caries Res.* **12**, 142–147.
van der Hoeven, J. S., Mikx, F. H. M., Plasschaert, A. J. M. and König, K. G. (1972). *Caries Res.* **6**, 203–210.
van der Waay, D. (1979). In *New Criteria for Antimicrobial Therapy: Maintenance of Digestive Tract Colonization Resistance* (D. van der Waay and J. Verhoef, eds), pp. 43–60, Excerpta Medica, Amsterdam and Oxford.
van der Waay, D. and Verhoef, J. (eds) (1979). *New Criteria for Antimicrobial Therapy; Maintenance of Digestive Tract Colonization Resistance*, Excerpta Medica, Amsterdam and Oxford.
van Houte, J. and Jansen, H. M. (1968). *Archs oral biol.* **13**, 827–830.
van Houte, J., Burgess, R. C. and Onose, H. (1976). *Archs oral Biol.* **21**, 561–564.
Vidaver, A. K. (1976). *A. Rev. Phytopath.* **14**, 451–465.
Weerkamp, A., Vogels, G. D. and Skotnicki, M. (1977). *Caries Res.* **11**, 245–256.
Woldendorp, J. W., Giessen, Th. J. J. and Mulder, S. J. (1966). *Proc. 9th int. Congr. Microbiol. Moscow* 143.
Wood, J. M. (1964). *J. dent. Res.* **43**, 955.
Zobell, C. E. (1943). *J. Bact.* **46**, 39–56.

14. Role of Adherence in the Development of Dental Plaque

GUNNAR RÖLLA

Introduction

It is established beyond reasonable doubt that dental plaque is an essential factor in the aetiology of periodontis and caries (Löe et al., 1972; Axelsson and Lundhe, 1978) and an abundance of data has been collected concerning the microbiology of plaque. However, the exact difference between cariogenic plaque and plaque which does not cause caries is not known (Mandel, 1979), and much uncertainty has been revealed during recent discussions concerning the specific or non-specific nature of the infection causing periodontal lesions (Socransky, 1979).

An understanding of plaque development has to be based on the knowledge of surface chemistry, biochemistry, microbiology and immunology. In spite of this, very few multidisciplinary research programmes have been initiated in this field. The available information mainly represents scattered research in numerous model systems of unknown relevance to the pathological phenomena observed in the clinic.

This paper discusses the chemical properties of the target surface (i.e. the dental enamel), the bacterial cell walls and the essential factors in the oral environment, such as inorganic competing ions and proteins. Some recent data which may shed light on the relative importance of growth and adherence in plaque formation are also included.

The Enamel Surface

The inorganic phase exposed on the surface of teeth consists of hydroxyapatite. The importance of the *surface* properties of enamel and the type of interactions with macromolecules and bacteria in the oral environment has only been fully realized recently, although clearly stated 20 years ago by Neuman and Neuman (1958). Traditional dental research has concentrated mainly on the three-dimensional crystallographic aspects of dental enamel and the effect of fluoride on these. However, recent observations clearly indicate that important aspects of the cariostatic effect of fluoride may be explained in terms of the changed surface properties of enamel (Glantz, 1969; Tinanoff et al., 1976; Rölla, 1973).

A tooth in the mouth can be compared to a crystal lattice submerged in an electrolyte. It is a well-known physical principle that electrolyte ions will be absorbed to oppositely charged sites on a crystal surface. The solubility of the "salts" thus formed gives an indication of the strength of the attractive forces involved, low solubility obviously indicating high affinity. The pattern of the charges on the surface of the lattice is balanced by electrolyte ions in the hydration shell, thus securing the electroneutrality of the crystal.

The dental enamel exhibits more phosphate than calcium positions on the outer surface (it is calcium deficient) and is therefore negatively charged (Kibby and Hall, 1972; Ash *et al.*, 1971). Furthermore, it has been stated that, whereas the phosphate of the hydroxyapatite surface is charged, the corresponding calcium positions are unpolarized. Calcium in the hydration layer, however, is hydrated and charged (Neuman and Neuman, 1958). The preponderance of phosphate on the hydroxyapatite surface presumably causes a correspondingly high concentration of positively charged counterions in the Stern layer of the hydration shell (Gregory, 1980). Polyvalent cations will displace monovalent cations in these positions. There is a reason to believe that reactive calcium ions absorbed as counter-ions to the hydroxyapatite crystal is a major feature of the tooth surface in the mouth. The low solubility of calcium phosphate indicates high affinity of this cation for hydroxyapatite phosphate. Divalent cations can be absorbed to a negatively charged surface on an *equivalent* or an *equimolar* basis. The latter principle involves binding of an additional anion to maintain electroneutrality (Weiss, 1958). The principle is illustrated in Fig. 1.

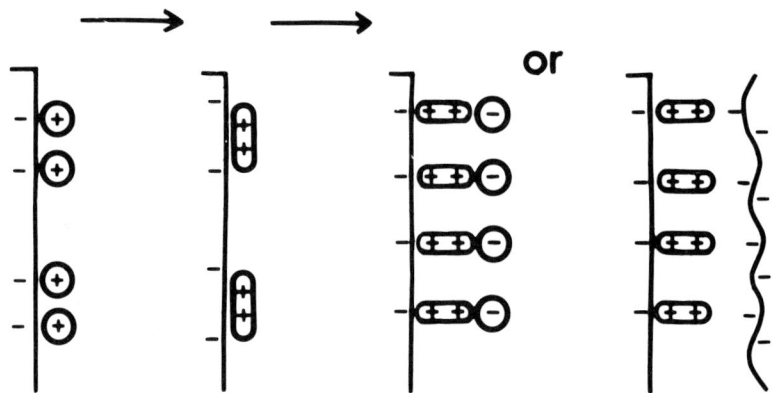

Fig. 1 An illustration to show the principles of equivalent and equimolar adsorption of calcium on hydroxyapatite, the latter changing the surface charge from negative to positive. A positive charge carried by the counter-ions appears to be the mechanism by which the acidic protein pellicle binds to the surface of teeth (Rölla and Bowen, 1978).

The equimolar adsorption of divalent cations is presumably caused by incomplete shielding of the negatively charged surface by equimolar absorbed ions. It is evidence for fluoride uptake by dental enamel through adsorption to the equimolarly adsorbed calcium, and some of the fluoride concentration taking place in plaque might be caused in this way (Rölla and Melsen, 1975a; Rölla et al., 1977a; Rölla, 1977a,b; Rölla and Bowen, 1978).

This model would predict that acidic, calcium-binding proteins and negatively charged microorganisms have high affinity for teeth, and experimental evidence for such a mechanism is available (Mandel and Concool, 1975; Belcourt, 1976; Krogstad and Rölla, 1977; Rölla and Embery, 1977).

Influence of Macromolecules Present in the Liquid Phase

Pellicle Formation

Bernardi et al. (1972) first presented the current concept of the mechanism of interaction of proteins with hydroxyapatite. This concept has been modified and extended by Rölla and Bowen (1978). The hydroxyapatite surface seems to be amphoteric; it binds acidic and basic proteins equally well (Fig. 2). Adsorbed acidic proteins can be desorbed by phosphate or other anions

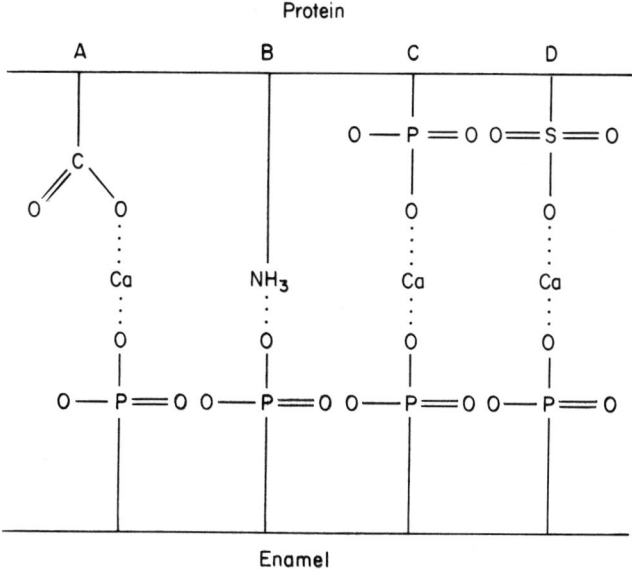

Fig. 2 The most important mechanisms by which macromolecules are bound to hydroxyapatite surfaces. The surface carries a high density of phosphate groups which determine the selectivity of the reactions with proteins.

(Bernardi et al, 1972; Rölla, 1973; Rölla et al., 1977b) and adsorbed basic proteins by calcium ions. The principle of the amphoteric nature of the hydroxyapatite surface can be accounted for by the model illustrated in Fig. 2. Acidic proteins are most likely to be adsorbed on calcium bound in the hydration layer of the crystal (Fig. 2, A, C, D) and basic proteins to phosphate groups in the crystal surface proper (Fig. 2, B). Basic proteins thus have to displace calcium ions in the hydration shell to reach their positions (Rölla and Bowen, 1978).

The oral environment contains not only enamel surface and bacteria but also a large number of salivary proteins. A number of experiments designed to study the problem of polymer adsorption to surfaces have shown that the following principles are involved in the interaction between macromolecules and solids:

(a) Soluble polymers with high molecular weight have a higher affinity for solid surfaces than polymers with low molecular weight, presumably because of the polyfunctional nature of large molecules (Fontana, 1971).

(b) Ionic polymers have a higher affinity for solids than non-ionic polymers. The reason for this may be that the ionic groups cause an extension of the molecules by the repulsion acting between the bound charged groups of the molecule (Fuerstenau, 1971).

(c) There is evidence for *chemical* interaction between polymers containing carboxyl and phosphate groups and dental enamel (Fuerstenau, 1971; Beech, 1972, Termine and Conn, 1976). Calcium counter-ions adsorbed to the surface of the enamel may react chemically with acidic groups available in the adsorbed polymer. This is presumably the principle by which polycarboxylate cements bind to dental enamel (Beech, 1972).

There is evidence for a very strong interaction of phosphate-containing macromolecules with hydroxyapatite surfaces (Termine and Conn, 1976), and phosphonates and sulphonates have been shown to function as crystal poisons in many experiments. This effect is most likely based on a strong surface adsorption to hydroxyapatite, presumably combined with a chemical reaction with the calcium ions in the hydration layer of counter-ions, permanently blocking further growth or crystallization of the hydroxyapatite crystal lattice. Data concerning selective adsorption of salivary glycoproteins to dental enamel support the concept of selective adsorption of acidic proteins.

The most likely chemical basis for selective adsorption is that tooth surfaces display numerous calcium ions by equimolar adsorption, as discussed above, which give conditions for selective adsorption of salivary polyanions.

Sulphated glycoproteins with blood group substance activity are found in the acquired pellicle on human teeth *in vivo* (Sönju *et al.*, 1974; Rölla and Embery, 1977). It seems likely that phosphoproteins may also be present. The blood group-active mucin molecules have high molecular weights and are polyanionic and thus have the physical and chemical properties for a high affinity to hydroxyapatite, even in the salivary environment of competing phosphate ions. Sulphated mucins have a general protective role on the mucosal surfaces, so that from a teleological point of view their presence on the teeth seems likely.

The Bacterium

The Cell Surface

The bacterial cell surface includes the cytoplasmic membrane, rigid wall and capsular material surrounding the cell. This fails, however, to indicate the complexity of surface components and the dynamic nature of the cell surface as it grows and divides and the relationship of the surface components to substances transiently associated with the cell surface, such as excreted proteins and polysaccharides (Shockman *et al.*, 1976).

The rigid wall in Gram-positive bacteria consists of 40–80% of peptidoglycans, and these substances appear to be responsible for the physical properties of the wall, including protection of the fragile cytoplasmic membrane against major osmotic variations. The rigid wall also contains substantial amounts of one or more anionic or neutral polysaccharides, covalently linked to the peptidoglycan. Teichoic acid or teichouronic acids and some of the Lancefield group carbohydrates of streptococci are examples of covalently linked polymers in Gram-positive bacteria. Covalently attached wall polymers provide the cell with characteristic surface properties, including serological reactivity.

Lipoteichoic acids extending from the cytoplasmic membrane through the outer wall surface are known to be found in many Gram-positive bacteria. Lipoteichoic acid consists of glycerol units linked together with phosphate diester bonds. A lipid moiety is also covalently linked to the polymer.

The Role of Lipoteichoic Acid in Adhesion, Cohesion and Pathogenicity of Sucrose-induced Dental Plaque

Teichoic acid with its numerous charged phosphate groups exhibits high affinity for hydroxyapatite (Fig. 3) (Ciardi *et al.*, 1977). Some Gram-positive bacteria are known to produce *extracellular* teichoic acid. *Streptococcus mutans* is also known to synthesize insoluble glucose polymers in the presence of sucrose. There is evidence that the dextran coat carried by sucrose-grown

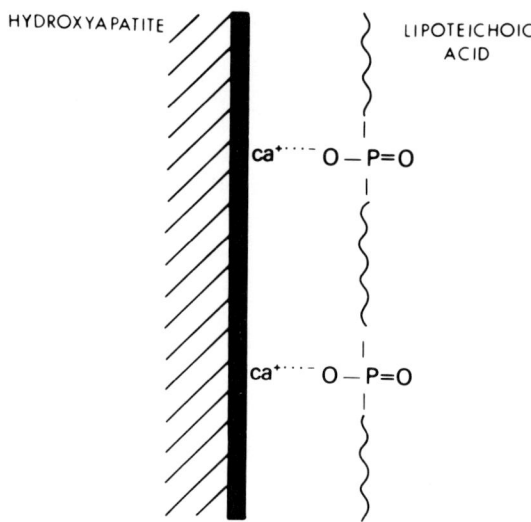

Fig. 3 The illustration shows how the phosphate polymer lipoteichoic acid can be bound to a negatively charged surface by calcium bridging. This concept suggests a mechanism by which *Strep. mutans* is bound to hydroxyapatite or glass (Ciardi *et al.*, 1977).

Strep. mutans contains large amounts of lipoteichoic acid. It seems likely that extracellular teichoic acid which is produced inside the bacteria is trapped in the polysaccharide "net" carried by sucrose-grown *Strep. mutans* (Rölla, 1976). The adhesiveness exhibited by the polysaccharide coat of *Strep. mutans* is now thought to be based on the presence of teichoic acid in this polysaccharide coat, rather than on the presence of dextran. This would give the well-known high adhesiveness of sucrose-grown *Strep. mutans* a rational chemical basis. Increased uptake of *Strep. mutans* on monkey teeth *in vivo* during high sucrose diet has been demonstrated by Kilian and Rölla (1976). Several of the *in vivo* and *in vitro* experiments indicating weak adsorption of *Strep. mutans* to teeth have been performed in systems with excessive concentrations of phosphate (0.067 M) and may thus not be necessarily relevant, because this ion inhibits uptake of bacteria by hydroxyapatite.

The first colonizers of tooth surfaces are Gram-positive bacteria. All of them carry anionic structures on their surface. These structures may be exposed to a greater or lesser extent on the outer surface. Binding to hydroxypatite or to the teeth will presumably be related to the available anionic groups *on the surface* of the bacteria. Anionic groups buried deeper in the cell wall may not necessarily give high affinity for hydroxyapatite, but may still confer negative charges on the bacterial cell on electrophoresis (Olsson *et al.*, 1976). Electrophoretic mobility will therefore

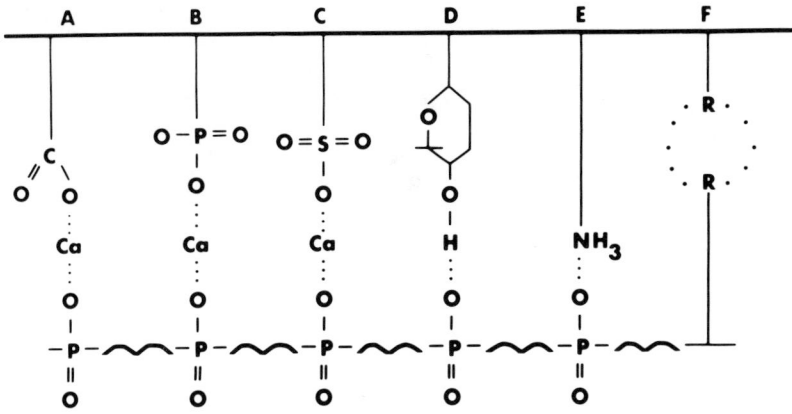

Fig. 4 Mechanisms by which lipoteichoic acids may interact with other chemical structures. F represents hydrophobic interaction through the lipid which is a part of the lipoteichoic acid molecule. Lipoteichoic acid is shown schematically at the bottom.

not be correlated with affinity for hydroxyapatite in all instances. It is possible that affinity for calcium might be a better index of affinity for tooth enamel (Rölla, 1976).

Lipoteichoic acids may bind sucrose-grown *Strep. mutans* to pellicle material and other microorganisms by a number of mechanisms including hydrophobic bonds. The pellicle protein is acidic in nature and will contain bound carboxyl, sulphate and phosphate groups which will be able to interact with lipoteichoic acids through bridging with calcium ions. Hydrophobic bonding is known to be essential in the binding of lipoteichoic acids to erythrocytes and may well be significant in establishing interbacterial adhesion and cohesion (Fig. 4). An illustration showing complex formation

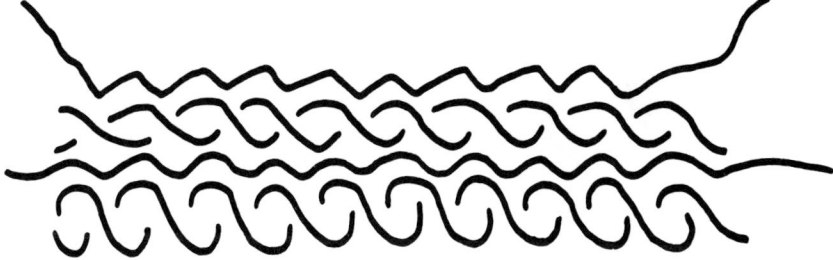

Fig. 5 Interaction between two different carbohydrates: complex is formed between a carbohydrate double helix chain and a simple chain based on steric interaction (after Rees, 1975). This may well represent a model for the lipoteichoic acid/glucan complexes in sucrose induced dental plaque.

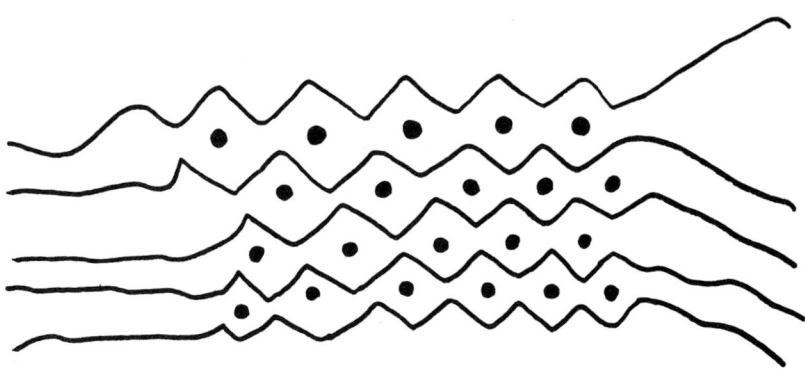

Fig. 6 Interaction between carbohydrate chains through divalent cations (after Rees, 1975). Complexes between lipoteichoic acid and other charged molecules in plaque may be formed by similar mechanisms.

between two different carbohydrate chains is seen in Figs 5, 6 and 7. Such complex formation is thought to occur in the coat of sucrose-grown *Strep. mutans* between lipoteichoic acids and glucan molecules.

Strongly anionic polymers like lipoteichoic acids may function as a diffusion barrier in the plaque matrix, inhibiting the diffusion of acid formed deep in the plaque to the outer surface, resulting in a steep pH gradient in

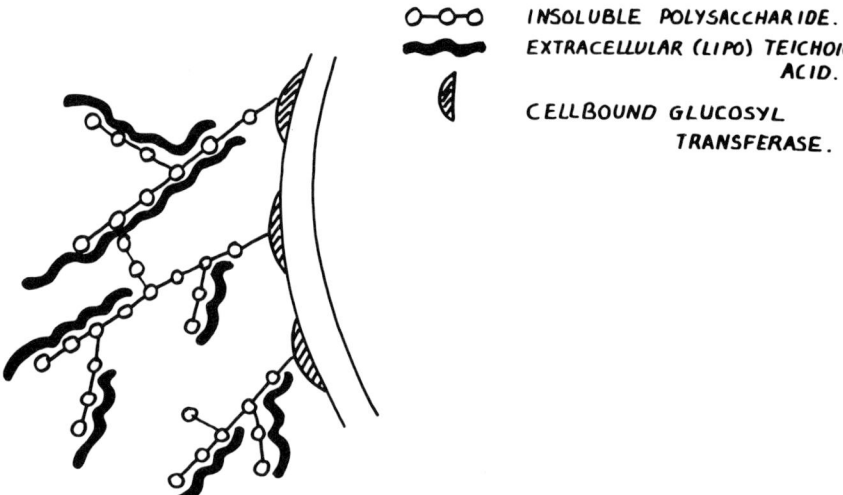

Fig. 7 A segment of a wall from a sucrose-grown *Strep. mutans* is illustrated, carrying a glucan coat with lipoteichoic acid, forming complexes with the glucans, presumably similar to those illustrated in Figs 5 and 6.

sucrose plaque. Such a polyanionic plaque matrix would also be a potential chelator of calcium ions from the enamel surface, even at neutral pH. Bacterial polymers (i.e. lipoteichoic acid and glucan) can thus render plaque cariogenic by influencing the adhesiveness, cohesion and diffusion of dental plaque.

The finding that sucrose induces the production of such polymers and at the same time represents the main factor in the aetiology of caries may not be incidental (Rölla et al., 1980).

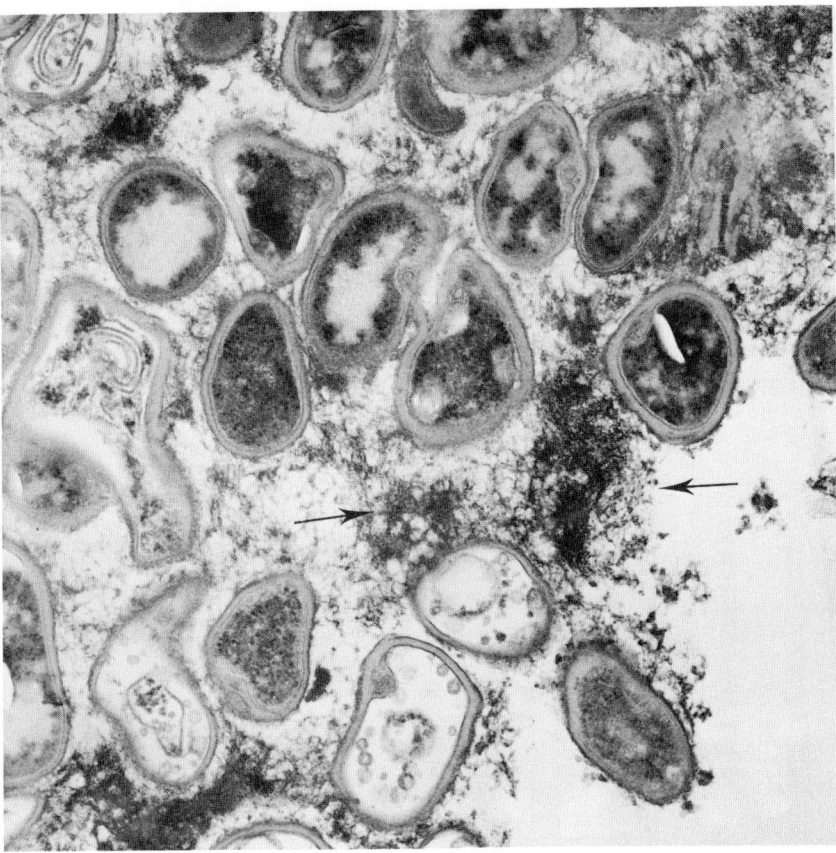

Fig. 8 A section of sucrose-induced dental plaque stained with ruthenium red, which binds selectively to anionic material. It can be seen (arrows) that the intermicrobial matrix binds large amounts of electron-dense material (ruthenium red), indicating a strong anionic character of the plaque matrix. This anionic material (presumably mainly lipoteichoic acid) can give sucrose plaque high adhesiveness, cohesion and pathogenicity (see text). (The electron micrograph was taken in cooperation with Dr O. Fejerskov.) × 27 720.

Adhesion and Growth in Plaque Development

The selectivity expressed in the adsorption of only a few species of Gram-positive bacteria on the tooth surfaces during the first phase of plaque formation indicates that adhesion based on some specific mechanism is essential at this stage. The appearance of a more complex microflora during later stages of plaque development shows that a second phase of selective adhesion takes place, but this time on a bacterium to bacterium basis. The increase in the biomass of plaque in the intermediate period might be caused by bacterial growth. Existing adsorbed bacteria may multiply and they may lay down large volumes of intermicrobial matrix, in particular if a high sucrose diet is consumed. Figure 8 shows plaque collected in a high caries group of children. The section is stained with ruthenium red. It can be seen that the intermicrobial matrix is strongly anionic because ruthenium red is known to adsorb selectively to anionic groups like phosphate and sulphate. The selectivity of the enamel surface is based on its *charge*, as discussed above. This can be clearly demonstrated by treating hydroxyapatite with cations or anions. The former increases the uptake of microorganisms and negative charged proteins, whereas the latter have the opposite effect. The principle is illustrated in the experiments described in Fig. 9.

The importance of bacterial growth in plaque development is illustrated by

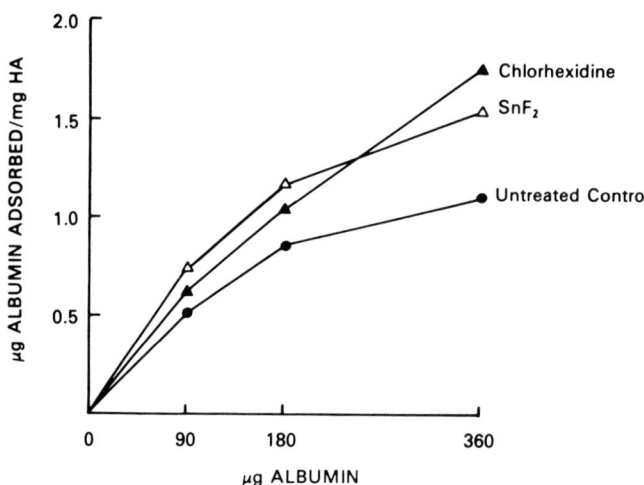

Fig. 9 The effect of charge on the uptake of acidic macromolecules by hydroxyapatite. Hydroxyapatite powder pretreated with 1 mM of either SnF_2 or chlorhexidine takes up more protein than the untreated control. (This mechanism may be partly responsible for the staining caused by these agents when used clinically due to an increased thickness of the pellicle).

14. Adherence and Dental Plaque

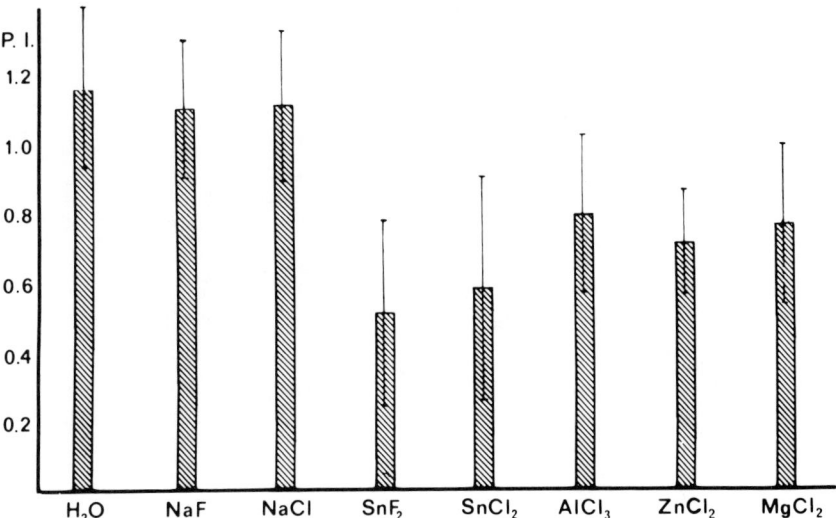

Fig. 10 Plaque inhibition by metal ions. Mean plaque index values and standard deviations are shown in the figure ($n = 6$). Plaque formation was enhanced by sucrose rinses and the mouth rinses contained 20 mM aqueous salt solutions, except the sodium salts which were used in concentrations of 40 mM (Skjörland et al., 1978).

the observation that columns of bacteria are often seen in sections of mature plaque. It has also been shown by scanning electron microscopy that plaque starts to form in cracks and pits in the enamel surface which harbour microorganisms. However, saliva is considered to be a poor medium for bacteria, and the generation time of oral bacteria is rather long (Carlsson, 1978). The ecological situation may, however, be improved in organisms which are adsorbed to a surface, compared with those floating freely.

Experiments with different cationic substances have shown that these can inhibit plaque (Fig. 10) (Rölla and Melsen 1975b; Skjörland et al., 1978; Tinanoff et al., 1976). These agents may work by changing the surface potential of salivary bacteria, as demonstrated by Olsson et al (1976), but the view that the cations may also function by influencing the metabolism of bacteria cannot be disregarded. Figure 11 shows that most of the polyvalent cations tested for plaque inhibition in Fig. 10 also reduce the metabolism of dental plaque, as measured by a pH electrode after sucrose application at time intervals after the treatment with metal ions. An exception is magnesium, which *increases* the metabolism of plaque, whilst the accumulation of plaque is decreased. This is conceivably caused by an interference with the adsorption mechanism (Fig. 10). From this experiment one could estimate that about a

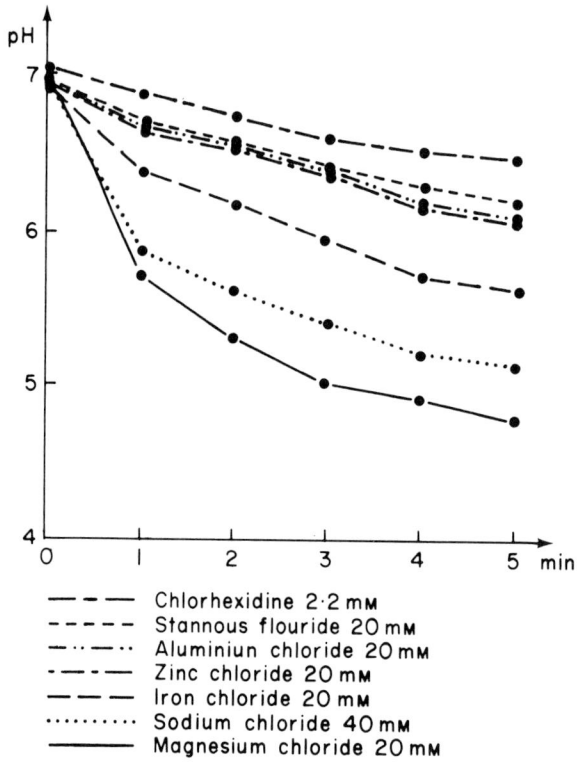

Fig. 11 The effect of metal ions on the metabolism of dental plaque causing plaque inhibition. The acidity of the plaque was tested at the given time intervals after application of 5 mM of the metal salts. (R.V. Oppermann and G. Rölla, unpublished work).

third of the increase in plaque biomass measured by the plaque index is caused by adhesion related to surface charge. No general conclusions can, however, be drawn based on this experiment alone.

If the adhesion of bacteria to teeth could be inhibited, bacterial growth would be eliminated as a factor in plaque development. Interference with bacterial adhesion to teeth, as a major method in preventive dentistry, seems to be within our reach.

Summary

This paper is concerned with chemical properties of the enamel surface and the mechanisms involved in pellicle formation. The possible role of complexes of lipoteichoic acids and glucan as the chemical basis for adhesiveness of sucrose-grown *Streptococcus mutans* is discussed. The effects of such complexes in the plaque matrix on the physical properties of dental plaque are considered. An attempt is made to assess the relative contributions by bacterial growth and adhesion in plaque development; this is based on plaque inhibition observed by using metal ions, which are known not to reduce plaque formation. It is emphasized that inhibition of bacterial adsorption to teeth as a major method in preventive dentistry seems to be within our reach.

References

Ash, R., Barrer, R. M., Butler, M. D. and Hudson, J. D. W. (1971). In *Tooth Enamel*, Vol. II (R. W. Fearnhead and M. V. Stack, eds), pp. 52–59, John Wright, Bristol.
Axelsson, P. and Lundhe, J. (1978). *J. dent. Res.* **56**, C142.
Beech, D. R. A. (1972). *Archs oral Biol.* **17**, 907–911.
Belcourt, A. (1976). *Archs oral Biol.* **21**, 717–722.
Bernardi, G., Giro, M. G. and Gaillard, C. (1972). *Biochim. biophys. Acta* **278**, 409–420.
Carlsson, J., (1978). In *Health and Sugar Substitutes* (B. Guggenheim, ed.), pp. 205–210, Karger, Basel.
Ciardi, J. E., Rölla, G., Bowen, W. H. and Reilly, J. A. (1977). *Caries Res.* **85**, 387–391.
Fontana, B. J. (1971). In *The Chemistry of Biosurfaces*, Vol. I (M. L. Hair, ed.), pp. 83–140, Marcel Dekker, New York.
Fuerstenau, D. W. (1971). In *The Chemistry of Biosurfaces*, Vol. I (M. L. Hair, ed.), pp. 143–174, Marcel Dekker, New York.
Glantz, P.-O. (1969). *Odont. Rev.* **20**, Suppl. 17.
Gregory, F. (1980). In *Dental Plaque and Surface Interactions in the Oral Cavity* (S. A. Leech, ed.), pp. 7–29, IRL Press, London.
Kibby, C. L. and Hall, K. W. (1972). In *The Chemistry of Biosurfaces*, Vol. II (M. L. Hair, ed.), pp. 663–724, Marcel Dekker, New York.
Kilian, M. and Rölla, G. (1976). *Infect. Immun.* **14**, 1022–1027.
Krogstad, S. and Rölla G. (1977). *J. Biologie buccale* **5**, 31–35.
Löe, H., van der Fehr, F. R. and Rindom Schiött, C. (1972). *Scand. J. dent. Res.* **80**, 1–9.
Mandel, I. D. (1979). *Am. Scient.* **67**, 680–688.
Mandel, I. D. and Concool, B. (1975). *J. dent. Res.* **54**, Special issue A, abstract L94.
Neuman, W. F. and Neuman, M. W. (1958). *The Chemical Dynamics of Bone Mineral*, The University of Chicago Press, Chicago.
Olsson, J., Glantz, P. O. and Krasse, B. (1976). *Archs oral Biol.* **21**, 605–609.
Rees, D. A. (1975). In *Biochemistry of Carbohydrates* (W. J. Whelan, ed.), pp. 1–42, Butterworth, London.
Rölla, G. (1973). *Coll. int. Cent. natn. Rech. scient.* **230**, 459–465.
Rölla, G. (1976). In *Microbiol Aspects of Dental Caries*, Vol. II (H. M. Stiles, W. J. Loesche and T. C. O'Brien, eds), Proceedings of a Workshop on Microbial Aspects of Dental Caries, June 1976, St. Simons Islands, pp. 309–324, IRL Press, London.
Rölla, G. (1977a). *Caries Res.* **11**, Suppl. 1, 243–261.
Rölla, G. (1977b). *J. dent. Res.* **56**, Special issue A., abstract 270.
Rölla, G. and Bowen, W. H. (1977). *Scand. J. dent. Res.* **85**, 149–151.
Rölla, G. and Bowen, W. H. (1978). *Acta odont. Scand.* **36**, 219–224.
Rölla, G. and Embery, G. (1977). *Scand. J. dent. Res.* **85**, 237–241.

Rölla, G. and Melsen, B. (1975a). *Caries Res.* **9**, 66–73.
Rölla, G. and Melsen, B. (1975b). *J. dent. Res.* **54**, special issue B, 57–62.
Rölla, G., Hsu, D. and Bowen, W. H. (1977a). *Caries. Res.* **11**, 308–312.
Rölla, G., Robrish, S. and Bowen, W. H. (1977b). *Acta path. microbiol. scand.* B **85**, 341–346.
Rölla, G., Oppermann, R. V., Ciardi, J. E., Bowen, W. H. and Knox, K. W. (1980). *Caries Res.* **14**, 235–238.
Shockman, B. D., Tsien, H. C. and Kessler, R. E. (1976). IN *Microbial Aspects of Dental Caries*, Vol. III (H. M. Stiles, W. J. Loesche and T. C. O'Brien, eds), Proceedings of a Workshop on Microbial Aspects of Dental Caries, June 1976, St. Simons Island, pp. 631–647, IRL Press, London.
Socransky, S. S. (1979). *Naeringsforskning* **23**, Suppl. 17, 680–688.
Skjörland, K., Gjermo, P. and Rölla, G. (1977). *Caries. Res.* **12**, 101.
Sönju, T., Christensen, T. B., Kornstad, L. and Rölla, G. (1974). *Caries Res.* **8**, 113–122.
Termine, J. D. and Conn, K. M. (1976). *Calcif. Tissue Res.* **22**, 149–157.
Tinanoff, N., Brady, J. M. and Gross, A. (1976). *Caries. Res.* **10**, 415–426.
Weiss, A. (1958). *Kolloidzeitschrift* **158**, 22–28.

15. Anaerobic Microorganisms in Gingival Plaque

CARL ERIK NORD

Introduction

There has been a rapidly increasing interest in anaerobic bacteriology during the last few years among both microbiologists and clinicians. This is due largely to an increasing recognition of the importance of anaerobic bacteria in the aetiology of infection in man. These developments have led to major additions to our knowledge of anaerobic methodology, taxonomy of anaerobes and the ecological and pathogenetic roles of anaerobic bacteria (Finegold, 1977).

Most anaerobic infections arise in proximity to mucosal surfaces where the anaerobes predominate as part of the normal flora. Frequent sites populated by large numbers of anaerobes are the oral cavity, colon, vagina and skin. Knowledge of this flora is clinically relevant, since it generally accounts for the frequency of certain types of anaerobic bacteria encountered in endogenous infections.

The concentrations of bacteria and the relative proportions of aerobes and anaerobes found in different anatomical sites of the human body are shown in Table I. Concentrations in the saliva are 10^8–10^9 colony forming units (CFU) per millilitre; anaerobic counts are 10 times higher than those of aerobes. On tooth surfaces, the concentrations of anaerobes and aerobes are 10^{10}–10^{11} CFU/ml, with a ratio of 100:1. Bacterial concentrations in gingival scrapings approximate to 10^{11}–10^{12} CFU/ml with anaerobes outnumbering aerobes by a factor of 100–1000:1.

The predominance of anaerobic bacteria in the gingival plaque is accounted for by the fact that the oxidation–reduction potential is low, approximately -200 mV. A significant difference is also observed between the oxidation–reduction potential of normal gingival sulci and that of deeper periodontal pockets. In the development of dental plaque a change from a simple flora to a complex flora is accompanied by a change in the oxidation–reduction potential from $+200$ mV to -200 mV (Russel and Melville, 1978). The reduced environment is highly suitable for the growth of anaerobic bacteria.

TABLE 1
Concentrations of Normal Organisms in Man

Anatomical site	Bacterial concentrations (CFU/ml or g)	Ratio of anaerobes to aerobes
Upper airways		
Nasal washings	10^3–10^4	5:1
Saliva	10^8–10^9	10:1
Tooth surface	10^{10}–10^{11}	100:1
Gingival crevice	10^{11}–10^{12}	1000:1
Gastrointestinal tract		
Stomach	10^2–10^5	1:1
Small bowel	10^2–10^4	10:1
Ileum	10^4–10^7	100:1
Colon	10^{11}–10^{12}	1000:1
Female genital tract		
Endocervix	10^8–10^9	10:1
Vagina	10^8–10^9	10:1

Laboratory Diagnosis of Anaerobic Bacteria

Collection of Specimens

Correct method of collection of specimens and rapid transport to the microbiological laboratory are essential prerequisites for satisfactory results. Appropriate specimens for anaerobic culture are those which are not contaminated by the normal flora especially from the mucosal surfaces.

Double syringes or thin swabs should be used (Berg and Nord, 1972; Newman and Sims, 1979). Because of the expense involved in anaerobic cultivation methods, every effort should be made to obtain representative specimens for laboratory studies.

Transport of Specimens

Expeditious transport of the specimen to the laboratory is essential for the recovery of anaerobic bacteria. The deleterious effects of oxygen and drying, multiplication of rapidly growing bacteria and the detrimental effects of chilling anaerobic bacteria justify rapid transport of specimens in order to ensure the recovery of fastidious bacteria. The system for transport should be so designed as to prevent drying and multiplication of microorganisms. Examples of such systems are gased-out tubes, vials or other systems which self-generate anaerobic conditions (Spiegel *et al.*, 1979). Specimens should be kept at room temperature during transport and cultures should be plated on appropriate media immediately upon arrival at the microbiological laboratory. Some extremely oxygen-sensitive anaerobic bacteria are found in the oral cavity, while potential pathogens are often more tolerant to air exposure (Tally et al., 1975).

Cultivation Techniques

Several anaerobic culturing techniques are available and there is some controversy concerning the relative merits in terms of yield, expense and ease of utilization. The three systems most frequently used for culturing anaerobic bacteria are: the anaerobic jar, pre-reduced anaerobic sterilized media and roll tubes, and the anaerobic chamber.

Anaerobic jars

The commercial anaerobic jars, Gas Pak® and Gas-Kit® are used in many microbiological laboratories. The system use a gas-generating envelope to which water is added, generating carbon-dioxide and hydrogen. A valve in the lid can also be used which, by evacuation and exchange, given an anaerobic atmosphere. In the top of the jar is a container holding palladium-coated aluminium pellets which catalyse the reaction of hydrogen and oxygen to water. It takes 10–12 h to get an oxidation–reduction potential of -300 mV.

Roll tube technique

The culture tubes are inoculated on the open bench under a stream of oxygen-free nitrogen or carbon dioxide. The tube is then closed with a butyl rubber stopper and placed in an incubator. The system permits daily inspection and fast-growing anaerobic bacteria can be easily recognized. The method is widely employed to identify anaerobes, but for primary isolation the system has gained only limited acceptance.

Anaerobic chambers

Most anaerobic chambers consist of a vinyl bag, an interchange with two doors for access, a vacuum pump to remove oxygen and different gas tanks. The anaerobic atmosphere contains 5% hydrogen, 5% carbon dioxide and 90% nitrogen which is circulated over palladium-coated aluminium pellets to remove traces of oxygen.

The advantage of the anaerobic chamber is that detailed bacteriology can be performed with standard techniques. The temperature in the chamber can serve as an incubator.

The anaerobic chamber provides the greatest flexibility for research and is therefore most suitable for studying the normal human flora, including that of the oral cavity (Heimdahl and Nord, 1979).

Media for Primary Isolation of Anaerobic Bacteria

Three different types of anaerobic media are recommended for the isolation of anaerobic bacteria: all purpose agar medium, selective agar medium and liquid medium. Selective media that can be used in studies of the anaerobic oral flora are shown in Table II.

TABLE II
Selective Media Used for Cultivation of Oral Anaerobic Bacteria

Medium	Bacterial species	Reference
Actinomyces metronidazole medium	*Actinomyces*	Kornman and Loesche, 1978
Lactobacillus selective medium	*Lactobacillus*	Sutter et al., 1975
Bifidobacterium medium	*Bifidobacterium*	Sutter et al., 1975
Phenylethyl alcohol blood agar	*Peptococci, Peptostreptococci*	Sutter et al., 1975
Rifampin blood agar	*Eubacterium*	Sutter et al., 1971
Neomycin–vancomycin blood agar	*Veillonella, Fusobacterium*	Sutter et al., 1975
Kanamycin–vancomycin blood agar	*Bacteroides*	Sutter et al., 1975
Fusobacterium nucleatum agar	*Fusobacterium nucleatum*	Walker et al., 1979

Identification of Anaerobic Bacteria

The identification of anaerobic bacteria is most often based on the criteria given in the *Anaerobic Laboratory Manual* from Virginia Polytechnic Institute by Holdeman et al. (1977). Taxonomic criteria are based on morphological appearance, fermentation pattern and analysis of fatty acids and products of glucose metabolism by gas–liquid chromatography.

Agar plates should be inspected after 48 h of incubation and again at 5–7 days in order to obtain optimal recovery. This technique allows both early detection of rapidly growing anaerobic bacteria and allows growth of some cocci, Gram-positive rods and bacteroides strains. All agar plates should be carefully scrutinized with a hand lens and each colony type picked for Gram-straining and subcultured for determination of oxygen tolerance.

Once anaerobic bacteria have been isolated in pure culture, identification can be made with schemes given in the *Anaerobic Laboratory Manual* (Holdeman et al., 1977). The identification techniques include morphological studies, gas–liquid chromatography, biochemical tests, serology, phage-typing, immunofluorescence and antibiotic susceptibility testing.

Morphology
Laboratory diagnosis of anaerobic bacteria begins with the examination of a Gram-stained smear which gives important preliminary information regarding types of bacteria present and will suggest further tests which should be carried out. Most anaerobic bacteria have a pleomorphic appearance in Gram strain.

Gas–liquid chromatography
Gas–liquid chromatography analysis is useful for identification of anaerobic bacteria to the genus level. It involves qualitative and quantitative detection of fermentation products, mainly short fatty acids. The technique can also be used for direct preliminary identification of anaerobic bacteria isolated from infections (Nord, 1977) and to follow changes in the normal anaerobic oral flora (Heimdahl and Nord, 1979).

Biochemical tests
To determine the species of an isolate it is also necessary to make other tests such as fermentation of carbohydrates. The tests are usually carried out with standard tube techniques. Several commercially available micromethods have recently been introduced. These methods can be employed with anaerobic jars or in anaerobic chambers. Comparative studies with standard methods have shown reliability with rapid growing anaerobes, but less reliability with slow growers and more oxygen-sensitive anaerobes (Nord *et al.*, 1975).

Serology
Serological techniques have been developed which make it possible to subdivide anaerobic bacteria further for epidemiological purposes into different serotypes. Useful typing schemes for oral anaerobic bacteria have been described for *Bacteroides melaninogenicus* (Lambe, 1974) and *Actinomyces israelii* (Holmberg, 1975).

Phage-typing
This technique is also useful for ecological studies of the carriage of anaerobic bacteria in various parts in the oral cavity and for studies of the mechanism and epidemiology of anaerobic infections. Phage-typing schemes have been described for *Bact. fragilis* (Booth *et al.*, 1979) and for *Propionibacterium acnes* (Webster and Cummins, 1978).

Immunofluorescence
Identification of anaerobic bacteria by immunofluorescence technique is suitable for the normal oral flora. Immunofluorescence has been used to identify anaerobic Gram-positive rods such as *A. viscosus* and *A. naeslundii*

(Lai and Listgarten, 1979) and anaerobic Gram-negative rods such as *Bact. asaccharolyticus* (Mansheim *et al.*, 1978), *Bact. fragilis* (Weintraub *et al.*, 1979) and anaerobic spirochetes (Jacob *et al.*, 1979).

Antibiotic susceptibility testing
Many anaerobic bacteria have predictable patterns of susceptibility to antibiotics. All anaerobic bacteria are resistant to aminoglycosides. Streptococci, actinomyces, arachnia and propionibacteria are resistant to metronidazole.

The number of penicillin-resistant *Bact. melaninogenicus* strains have increased during the last years. Many anaerobic bacteria also show resistance to tetracyclines (Newman *et al.*, 1979; Dornbusch *et al.*, 1979). The usual patterns of susceptibility of various oral anaerobic bacteria to the antibiotics which are most useful for anaerobic oral infections are shown in Table III.

In many cases it is important that testing of susceptibility with specific antibiotics against individual isolates is carried out. Recommendations have been made to test the susceptibility of anaerobic bacteria by the dilution method (Sutter *et al.*, 1979).

Ecology of the Anaerobic Gingival Flora

By using these techniques it is possible to isolate and identify more than 100 anaerobic bacterial species in the oral cavity and the number of recognized species will probably increase in the future. During the past few years, techniques have been developed for sampling and cultivating anaerobic bacteria from different oral sites. The finding that supragingival plaque differed from subgingival plaque is an important factor in the microbiological investigations of plaque (Socransky *et al.*, 1977). In the zone of plaque that is attached to the surface of the tooth, mainly anaerobic Gram-positive bacteria are found, whilst in the unattached zone mainly anaerobic Gram-negative rods are isolated (Newman and Socransky, 1977). Many factors within the gingival sulcus and periodontal pocket influence and select for different anaerobic bacteria.

Bacterial Retention

The anaerobic bacteria that colonize retentive sites are different from those found in the supragingival plaque. The cleansing activities in the gingival pocket are less pronounced than at other sites in the oral cavity. The gingival sulcus forms a relatively stagnant environment, where bacteria that cannot adhere to the surface of the tooth may colonize. Motile bacteria such as *Campylobacter, Capnocytophaga, Selenomonas, Spirochetes* and *Vibriospecies* also colonize these regions.

TABLE III
Susceptibility of Oral Anaerobic Bacteria to Antibiotics

Antibiotic	Streptococci	Peptococci, peptostreptococci	Actinomyces, arachnia	Propionibacteria	Bacteroides melaninogenicus	Capnocytophaga	Fusobacteria
Benzylpenicillin	+++	+++	+++	+++	+++ to +*	+++	+++
Clindamycin	+++	+++	++	+++	+++	+++	+++
Tetracycline	++	++	++	++	++	+++	+++
Metronidazole	+	+++	+	+	+++	++ to +	+++

+++, Good activity; ++, moderate activity; +, poor activity.
*Resistant strains reported.

Subgingival Anaerobic Flora

Anaerobic bacteria make up a significant part of the subgingival oral flora and therefore anaerobes are involved in different periodontal infections. The indigenous anaerobic microflora in this region include the following groups: *Peptococcus, Peptostreptococcus, Streptococcus, Acidaminococcus, Megasphaera, Veillonella, Actinomyces, Arachinia, Bifidobacterium, Eubacterium, Lactobacillus, Propionibacterium, Bacteroides, Campylobacter, Capnocytophaga, Fusobacterium, Leptotrichia, Spirochetes* and *Vibrio* (Table IV). Other, not yet classified anaerobic bacteria are also present. Most of these bacteria are isolated together with facultative anaerobic bacteria.

TABLE IV
Anaerobic Bacteria in the Subgingival Region

Cocci		Rods	
Gram-positive	Gram-negative	Gram-positive	Gram-negative
Peptococcus	*Acidaminococcus*	*Actinomyces*	*Bacteroides*
Peptostreptococcus	*Megasphaera*	*Arachnia*	*Capnocytophaga*
Streptococcus	*Veillonella*	*Bifidobacterium*	*Campylobacter*
		Eubacterium	*Fusobacterium*
		Lactobacillus	*Leptotrichia*
		Propionibacterum	*Spirochetes*
			Vibrio

Electron microscopic studies have shown that the subgingival microflora exists in several zones (Listgarten, 1976). In the gingival sulcus and periodontal pocket there is a zone of plaque that is attached to the surface. The bacteria in this zone adhere to the surface of the tooth and they are usually Gram-positive cocci and rods. Among the anaerobes, *Strep. intermedius, Actinomyces viscosus, A. naeslundii* and *Propionibacterium* species have been isolated. Anaerobic Gram-negative cocci and rods can also be recovered from this site which is continuous with the supragingival plaque and can extend to the apex of the gingival sulcus or periodontal pocket. Bacteria of the attached part are not in direct contact with the apical epithelium.

Subgingival bacteria attached to the tooth surface or to calculus form a zone harbouring a number of anaerobic Gram-negative and motile bacteria. This zone is in direct contact with the junctional and sulcus epithelium at the apical and lateral walls of the gingival sulcus or periodontal pocket. Bacteria in the gingival sulcus or periodontal lesion do not invade the tissue except in acute necrotizing ulcerative gingivitis in which anaerobic spirochetes can be found deep in the gingiva.

15. Anaerobic Microorganisms in Gingival Plaque

Subgingival Anaerobic Flora in Relation to Periodontal Infection

The distribution of the two subgingival zones differ in various forms of periodontal diseases. An increase in the zone of the unattached bacteria is observed when rapid destruction of the tissues occur. The absence of periodontal disease appears to be associated with a zone of unattached bacteria.

During periods of exacerbation, bacteria in the unattached zone proliferate, the alveolar bone is resorbed and the epithelial attachment moves apically. Anaerobic Gram-negative and motile rods dominate. During periods of remission, anaerobic Gram-positive bacteria from the attached plaque grow downward on the tooth surface and establish a stable relationship. These periods of exacerbation and remission continue until the tooth is no longer supported by bone.

Bacterial Factors Involved in Periodontal Infections

Some anaerobic bacterial strains such as *Capnocytophaga ochraceus* are capable of transporting non-motile anaerobic bacteria such as *Bact. asaccharolyticus* and *Fusobacterium nucleatum*. Thus, some bacteria can be transported by other bacteria, gain access to the subgingival area and participate in periodontal infection.

Gingival plaque containing large numbers of actinomyces and streptococci enhance the attachment and colonization of bacteroides strains. Fusobacteria and capnocytophaga also attach to certain species of *Actinomyces* and *Streptococcus* (Slots and Gibbons, 1978). The cell envelope of anaerobic Gram-positive bacteria may therefore play an important role in the subgingival colonization by anaerobic Gram-negative rods.

Bact. melaninogenicus has the ability to inhibit other anaerobic bacteria and thereby probably inhibit other anaerobes to establish themselves in the periodontal environment. *Bact. melaninogenicus* can also act synergistically to inhibit phagocytosis and kill other bacteria in the flora (Murray and Rosenblatt, 1976).

Subgingival Colonization of Anaerobic Bacteria

Electron microscopic investigations have shown that the subgingival plaque is built up in a special way. Gram-positive anaerobic bacteria are attached to the tooth surface and Gram-negative anaerobic rods are found in a layer over the Gram-positive bacteria (Listgarten, 1976). The development of subgingival plaque starts with the colonization of anaerobic Gram-positive bacteria in the gingiva. These bacteria attach strongly to the tooth surface and can resist the rinsing effect of saliva and gingival fluid. The anaerobic Gram-negative rods then attach to the Gram-positive cells and begin to colonize the periodontal pocket (Slots and Gibbons, 1978). Most of the Gram-positive bacteria which first colonize the gingival pocket are facultative anaerobic. Then an anaerobic atmosphere is created by these bacteria, allowing the anaerobic Gram-negative rods to colonize the gingival pocket.

Subgingival Anaerobic Microflora in Healthy Gingiva

The healthy gingival sulcus harbour relatively few anaerobic microorganisms. *Streptococci, Peptostreptococci, Peptococci, Actinomyces* and other anaerobic Gram-positive non-sporulating rods comprise about 85% of the cultivable microflora (Table V). Anaerobic Gram-negative rods such as bacteroides, fusobacteria, spirochetes, and vibrios are only a minor part of the cultivable flora (Slots, 1977*b*). However, many anaerobic Gram-positive rods from the healthy gingival flora can induce periodontitis in animal experiments.

Subgingival Anaerobic Microflora in Gingivitis

The development of gingivitis is followed by an increased amount of gingival plaque and an anaerobic microflora different from that found in the healthy sulcus. Gram-positive bacteria are dominating also the flora in gingivitis but Gram-negative anaerobic bacteria are isolated in an increased number (Loesche and Syed, 1978). Among the Gram-positive anaerobic bacteria, *Actinomyces, Streptococci, Peptostreptococci,* and *Peptococci* are found, and among Gram-negative anaerobic bacteria fusobacteria, bacteroides, capnocytophaga, selenomonas and campylobacter are found (Table V). Anaerobic spirochetes and vibrios are also recovered from the gingival sulcus (Slots *et al.*, 1978). The continued presence of anaerobic bacterial plaque may be associated with alveolar bone loss. However, some patients may have recurrent gingivitis without development of periodontitis. It is not clear whether these patients have a different flora from those who develop gingivitis followed by periodontitis.

Subgingival Anaerobic Microflora in Juvenile Periodontitis

Different anaerobic Gram-negative rods such as *Capnocytophaga, Fusobacterium* and *Bacteroides* species, but not *Bact. asaccharolyticus, Actinobacillus actinomycetem-comitans,* vibrios, and spirochetes (Table V) are dominating the microflora or about 65% of the cultivable flora (Slots, 1976). All bacteria in the periodontal pockets are unattached or loosely attached to the tooth surface (Listgarten, 1976). The bacterial strains isolated from these lesions differ from those found in the adult forms of periodontitis (Newman and Socransky, 1977). Many of the strains appear to be unique to juvenile periodontitis. In germ-free animals these strains cause alveolar bone loss, with an osteoclastic response within a few weeks, but no plaque formation or root

TABLE V
Prevalence of Some Anaerobic Bacteria in Different Periodontal Conditions

Periodontal condition	Peptococci, peptostreptococci, streptococci	Actinomyces	Bacteroides melaninogenicus	Bacteroides assacharolyticus	Capnocytophaga ocraceus	Fusobacteria
Healthy gingiva	++	++	±	−	−	±
Gingivitis	++	+	+	+	±	+
Juvenile periodontitis	±	±	++	−	++	+
Advanced periodontitis	+	+	+	++	+	+

++, predominantly isolated; +, frequently isolated; ±, occasionally isolated; −, infrequently isolated.

caries (Irving *et al.*, 1978). The localization of these microorganisms at the site of infection and their pathogenicity in animal experiments suggest that these bacteria may be involved in juvenile periodontitis.

Subgingival Anaerobic Microflora in Advanced Periodontitis

The apical parts of the deep pockets in advanced periodontitis also harbour anaerobic Gram-negative rods (75%), but these anaerobes are different from those found in juvenile periodontitis (Table V). *Bact. asaccharolyticus* comprises about 25–50% of the cultivable flora. Fusobacteria, other *Bacteroides* species, capnocytophaga, vibrios and spirochetes can also be recovered (Slots, 1977*a*).

In chronic periodontitis a large component of subgingival plaque is found to be attached (Listgarten, 1976). Anaerobic Gram-positive non-sporulating rods such as *Actinomyces viscosus* and *A. naeslundii* are recovered in large numbers and represent about 30–40% of the bacteria present (Darwish *et al.*, 1978). The unattached part of the subgingival plaque in chronic periodontitis contains anaerobic Gram-negative rods.

In acute periodontitis, the unattached component predominates in the apical region. The microflora associated with rapid periodontitis consists of anaerobic Gram-negative rods, including *Bact. asaccharolyticus, Bact. ureolyticum. Capnocytophaga ochraceus*, and *Fusobacterium nucleatum*.

When bacteria isolated from the unattached subgingival zone are implanted into germ-free animals, they cause periodontitis. Infection with these anaerobic Gram-negative bacteria results in a destruction of alveolar bone and a stimulation of osteoclastic activity.

In experiments with monkeys it has also been shown that the alveolar bone loss is accompanied by a marked change in the subgingival anaerobic microflora (Slots and Hausmann, 1979). The number of *Bact. melaninogenicus* strains is increasing significantly during the experimental period. The high frequency of *Bact. asaccharolyticus* in advanced periodontitis suggests that this species plays an important role in this endogenous infection. These infections are different from those caused by anaerobic Gram-positive rods since the latter form large amounts of bacterial plaque; root caries and the alveolar bone loss is associated with suppression of osteoblasts (Irving *et al.*, 1974).

Summary

The use of modern culture techniques has established the presence of anaerobic bacteria in all anatomical sites of man which are colonized by microorganisms. Concentrations of bacteria in the saliva are 10^8–10^9 (CFU) per millilitre and anaerobic bacteria outnumber aerobic bacteria by 10:1.

On the tooth surface the concentrations of bacteria are 10^9–10^{10} CFU/ml, with a dominance of anaerobes over aerobes. Bacterial concentrations in gingival scrapings are 10^{11}–10^{12} CFU/ml, with anaerobic bacteria outnumbering aerobic bacteria by 1000:1.

The oral cavity harbours more than 300 different bacterial species. These bacteria are distributed in specific anatomical locations in the mouth. In saliva and on the tongue surface, the predominant anaerobic bacteria are cocci, while in the gingival crevice large concentrations of Gram-negative rods can be recovered. The predominance of anaerobic bacteria in the gingival crecive is accounted for by the fact that the oxidation–reduction potential is very low, approximately -300 mV. A significant difference is observed between the oxidation–reduction potential of normal gingival sulci and that of deeper periodontal pockets. In the development of gingival plaque, a change from a simple flora to a complex flora is accompanied by a significant change in the oxidation–reduction potential from $+200$ mV to -200 mV after about 14 days.

The reduced environment is very suitable for the growth of anaerobic bacteria. The following genera can be recovered: *Peptococcus, Peptostreptococcus, Streptococcus, Veillonella, Acidaminococcus, Actinomyces, Arachnia, Bifidobacterium, Eubacterium, Lactobacillus, Propionibacterium, Bacteroides, Campylobacter, Capnocytophaga, Fusobacterium* and *Leptotrichia*.

References

Berg, J. O. and Nord, C. E. (1972). *Acta odont. scand.* **30**, 503–510.
Booth, S. J., van Tassel, R. L., Johnson, J. L. and Wilkins, T. D. (1979). *Rev. infect. Dis.* **1**, 325–334.
Darwish, S., Hyppa, T. and Socransky, S. S. (1978). *J. periodont. Res.* **13**, 1–16.
Dornbusch, K., Nord, C. E. and Olsson-Liljeqvist, B. (1979). *Scand. J. infect. Dis.* **19**, 17–25.
Finegold, S. M. (1977). *Anaerobic Bacteria in Human Disease*, Academic Press, London.
Heimdahl, A. and Nord, C. E. (1979). *Scand. J. infect. Dis.* **11**, 233–242.
Holdeman, L. V., Cato, E. P. and Moore, W. E. C. (1977). *Anaerobe Laboratory Manual*, 4th edn, Virginia Polytechnic Institute and State University, Blacksburg.
Holmberg, K. (1975). Thesis, Karolinska Institute, Stockholm.
Irving, J. T., Socransky, S. S. and Heeley, J. D. (1974). *J. periodont. Res.* **9**, 73–79.
Irving, J. T., Socransky, S. S., and Tanner, A. C. (1978). *J. periodont. Res.* **13**, 326–332.
Jacob, E., Allen, A. L. and Nauman, R. K. (1979). *J. clin. Microbiol.* **10**, 934–936.
Kornman, K. S. and Loesche, W. J. (1978). *J. clin. Microbiol.* **7**, 514–518.
Lai, C. H. and Listgarten, M. A. (1979). *Infect. Immun.* **25**, 1016–1028.
Lambe, D. W. (1974). *Appl. Microbiol.* **28**, 561–567.
Listgarten, M. A. (1976). *J. Periodont.* **47**, 1–18.
Loesche, W. J. and Syed, S. A. (1978). *Infect. Immun.* **21**, 830–839.

Mansheim, B. J., Solstad, C. A. and Kasper, D. L. (1978). *J. infect. Dis.* **138**, 736–741.
Murray, P. R. and Rosenblatt, J. G. (1976). *J. infect. Dis.* **134**, 281–285.
Newman, M. G. and Sims, T. N. (1979). *J. Periodont.* **50**, 350–354.
Newman, M. G. and Socransky, S. S. (1977). *J. periodont. Res.* **12**, 120–128.
Newman, M. G., Hulen, C., Colgate, J., Anselmo, C. (1979). *J. dent. Res.* **58**, 1722–1732.
Nord, C. E. (1977). *Acta path. microbiol. scand.* **259**, 55–59.
Nord, C. E., Dahlbäck, A. and Wadström, T. (1975). *Med. Microbiol. Immunol.* **161**, 239–242.
Russel, C. and Melville, T. H. (1978). *J. appl. Bact.* **44**, 163–181.
Slots, J. (1976). *Scand. J. dent. Res.* **84**, 1–10.
Slots, J. (1977*a*). *Scand. J. dent. Res.* **85**, 114–121.
Slots, J. (1977*b*). *Scand. J. dent. Res.* **85**, 247–254.
Slots, J. and Gibbons, R. J. (1978). *Infect. Immun.* **19**, 254–264.
Slots, J., and Hausmann, E. (1979). *Infect. Immun.* **23**, 260–269.
Slots, J., Moenbo, D., Langebaeck, J. and Frandsen, A. (1978). *Scand. J. dent. Res.* **86**, 174–181.
Socransky, S. S., Manganiello, A. D., Propas, D., Oram, V. and van Houte, J. (1977). *J. periodont. Res.* **12**, 90–106.
Spiegel, C. A., Minok, G. E. and Krywolap, G. N. (1979). *J. clin. Microbiol.* **9**, 637–639.
Sutter, V. L., Sugihara, P. T. and Finegold, S. M. (1971). *Appl. Microbiol.* **22**, 777–780.
Sutter, V. L., Vargo, V. L. and Finegold, S. M. (1975). *Wadsworth Anaerobic Bacteriology Manual*, UCLA, Los Angeles.
Sutter, V. L., Barry, A. L., Wilkins, T. D. and Zabransky, R. J. (1979). *Antimicrobial Agents. Chemother.* **16**, 495–502.
Tally, F. P., Stewart, P. R., Sutter, V. L. and Rosenblatt, J. E. (1975). *J. clin. Microbiol.* **1**, 161–164.
Walker, C. B., Ratkliff, D., Muller, D., Mandell, R. and Socransky, S. S. (1979). *J. clin. Microbiol.* **10**, 934–936.
Webster, G. F. and Cummins, C. S. (1978). *J. clin. Microbiol.* **7**, 84–90.
Weintraub, A., Lindberg, A. A. and Nord, C. E. (1979). *Med. Microbiol. Immunol.* **167**, 233–230.

16. Principles and Progress in the Prevention of Periodontal Disease

HARALD LÖE

Introduction

As we enter the 1980s, and as we look back to the last two decades, it is clearly seen that the total periodontal research effort has been characterized by a high degree of dynamism and much progress. Fundamental research into the aetiology and pathogenesis of periodontal diseases has disclosed broad principles and finer details relative to the mechanisms of their initiation and progression. Although there are still voids in the knowledge of microbiology, immunology and tissue responses during periodontal health and disease, our understanding of the causes and the disease characteristics has reached a point where it is possible to formulate concepts for the clinical management of these diseases. New approaches in the prevention of periodontal disease have been introduced and tested, and there are indications that in certain population groups the practice of prevention is beginning to show the expected results.

Concept of Prevention

It is now firmly established that supragingival plaque causes gingivitis (Löe *et al.* 1965) and that the active pathogenic agent in dental plaque is bacterial in nature. Also, experimental animal data (Lindhe *et al.*, 1973) and circumstantial evidence from a variety of investigations in man, suggest strongly that gingivitis is the precursor of more advanced periodontal destruction. It is now agreed that formation of plaque on teeth represents a massive accumulation of bacteria already present in the oral cavity, and that plaque formation occurs in healthy individuals relatively independent of intake of food, types of foodstuff, degrees of salivation, mastication or malocclusion. However, although plaque formation in man seems to be ubiquitous, there are strong indications that colonization of bacteria on the teeth and gingivae are not haphazard. Rather, bacterial colonization is characterized by a certain degree of selectivity, and the establishment of particular bacterial species are associated with different dental disease states.

Thus, *Streptococcus mutans* is associated with the development of caries in dental enamel (for a review, see Bowen, 1976), while different subspecies of *Actinomyces* seem to be related to caries in root cementum and to the development of chronic gingivitis (for a review, see Loesche, 1976). It has been known for many years that the development of acute necrotizing ulcerative gingivitis coincides with the presence of a fusiform-spirochaetal flora.

These plaques are essentially located at and above the gingival margin and can be eliminated, reduced or influenced by fairly simple mechanical and chemical measures. There is scientific evidence to show that if supragingival plaque is controlled, gingival health will prevail (for a review, see Löe, 1970). On the other hand, although the mechanisms are not yet understood, given time, a supragingivally located plaque will start to proliferate subgingivally (Waerhaug, 1952). As soon as subgingival plaque is established and a subgingival infection has developed, the bacterial aggregates cannot be reached by simple procedures applied by the patients themselves, and will require professional intervention. This transition from a supragingival to a subgingival infection, therefore, represents a crucial change in the disease process and from this point onwards the opportunity to deal with the disease prophylactically has virtually been lost.

Subgingival plaques are significantly different from the supragingival varieties and are characterized by relatively more Gram-negative, anaerobic organisms and more motile bacteria (Slots, 1977; Socransky, 1977). Various species of *Bacteroides* (Slots, 1976, 1977; Newman and Socransky, 1977) and *Actinobacillus* (Tanner et al., 1979) have been associated with different types of advanced periodontitis.

The last two decades have also seen the emergence of immunological research applied to the problems of periodontal disease (Lehner et al., 1974a,b, 1976; Genco, 1979). This research has provided indications that both cellular and humoral immune reactions play an important role in the tissue alterations of the periodontium during the disease process. To what extent these immunopathological mechanisms might be exploited in an attempt to increase the defence against periodontal disease is still an open question. At this time, it does not seem expedient to pursue the possibility of vaccination against gingivitis and slow developing periodontitis. However, recent developments in research on leukocyte function in juvenile periodontitis (Lavine et al., 1976; Cianciola et al., 1977) and a better account of the specificity of the bacterial antigens themselves and the antibody targets (Baehni et al., 1979) during this type of periodontal disease, may well be an important prelude to immunization against juvenile periodontitis.

The recent and more detailed understanding of dental infections and their relationship to the initiation and progress of the specific dental and periodontal diseases is indeed scientifically stimulating, and most encouraging from a clinical point of view. There is a growing awareness that dental plaque represents a multitude of bacteria in various combinations, with a variety of pathogenic potentials and systemic responses, and that some types of plaque may even be non-pathogenic. However, the concept of specific pathogenicity, which has been termed a "specific plaque hypothesis" (Loesche, 1976) is still not ready for clinical application in the prevention (and treatment) of these diseases. It is likely that, in the not too distant future, additional information on the bacterial assault, on the immunological responses, as well as other host reactions in periodontal disease, can be used in designing more selective approaches to disease control. However, the current level of knowledge and technology does not allow for such a differentiated approach to the clinical problem. Therefore, clinically, dental plaque must be dealt with as an entity; the approach to disease prevention and control must still be to attack the supragingival plaque as a whole, and the desired goal is to maintain a plaque-free dentition.

Methods of Prevention

There is substantial data to show that absence of plaque is consistent with dental and gingival health (Löe et al., 1965; Löe and Schiött, 1970; Löe et al., 1972; Axelson and Lindhe, 1977, 1978) and that any reduction in plaque is associated with a reduction in gingivitis. In the late 1950s Waerhaug and his associates (Lovdal et al., 1960) showed in a population study that individuals sustaining "good" oral hygiene over a 5 year period reduced gingivitis by 90%. Those exhibiting "fairly good" oral hygiene showed 50–60% reduction in gingivitis, and even those who continued to show "not good", but apparently improved, oral hygiene also exhibited substantial reductions in gingivitis. Since these results were published, a number of experimental clinical and epidemiological investigations have confirmed this general concept. As a matter of fact, the correlation between the amount of plaque at the gingival margin and the state of the gingiva is so strong that among several clinical measurements, the scoring of the plaque index would be highly effective in reflecting the state of gingival health (Paulson et al., 1979).

Elimination or reduction of supragingival plaque can be accomplished by mechanical and/or chemical means administered by professionals and/or by the patients themselves. The mechanical methods include cleansing with various pastes and dentifrices, dental engine-driven brushes and rubber cups, powered tooth-brushes, regular tooth-brushes, interdental brushes, toothpicks, dental floss, and various water irrigation devices.

The dental literature is replete with experimental studies, descriptions of devices and methods for mechanical removal of plaque as well as comprehensive review articles in this field. In a fundamental sense, the past decade has seen no novel developments in this area. Therefore, it would suffice to summarize the findings that each one and various combinations of these mechanical procedures have been tested in controlled studies and have proved their efficacy in reducing or eliminating dental plaque and disease, and some have shown substantial inhibition of caries as well (Axelson and Lindhe, 1977).

On the other hand, recent years have seen a reassessment of the usefulness of antimicrobial mouth-rinses in the control of dental infections. Both the acceptance of the concept that caries and periodontal diseases were infectious diseases, and the choice of a potent antimicrobial agent (chlorhexidine) during the early stages of this research, helped to promote this approach to disease control (Löe and Schiött, 1970). During the subsequent years, a great variety of short- and long-term studies on the use of this agent in the control of plaque, gingivitis, caries and mucosal lesions, in healthy or handicapped adults and children, were completed. The microbiological and ecological problems connected with frequent and prolonged use of chlorhexidine have been elucidated. Toxicological, teratogenic, metabolic and systemic effects of this drug have been accounted for, and several other fundamental aspects related to the antiseptic principle in controlling dental diseases have been tested (see Löe, 1971). In summary, this vast volume of material suggests that chlorhexidine is one of the safest and most effective antiseptics known, and that the side effects are inconsequential.

The material is now marketed both as a mouth-rinse, as a gel and as a dentifrice, and is used in most countries of the world. However, at a recent discussion of the state of this art, I struck the following cautionary note, that I would like to reiterate (Löe, 1979): "Although most of us who have been engaged in this research probably should be pleased with such a relatively short lagtime between acquisition of new data and clinical application, I am somewhat concerned about the indiscriminate use of this and other agents. This question of uncontrolled daily use of antimicrobials could easily rival nuclear energy or herbicides as an issue, and a premature introduction of these agents for over the counter purchase may defeat the long-term purpose. I strongly believe that at this point in time, the use of chlorhexidine should be based on firm diagnostic criteria, should be appropriately monitored, and the frequency of application prescribed on the basis of disease characteristics."

Clinical Assessments

Given the fact that the technologies for prevention of periodontal disease are available, have been shown to be efficacious and that most of the methods are safe, why is it that even in well-developed societies where adequate economies are available, periodontal disease is still responsible for the greatest loss of teeth in the adult population?

TABLE I
Average Number of Teeth Present in Norwegian Students and Academic Staff that Participated in all Four Surveys, 1969–1975

	\multicolumn{11}{c}{Years of age}										
	17–18	19–20	21–22	23–24	25–26	27–28	29–30	31–32	33–34	35–36	37–38
1969–70	27.38	26.92	27.50	27.68	26.46	26.00	27.23	26.78			
n	21	13	26	37	26	22	13	9			
1971		27.38	27.00	27.54	27.68	27.46	26.77	27.38	26.78		
n		21	13	26	37	26	22	13	9		
1973			27.24	26.85	27.50	27.62	27.35	26.64	27.38	26.78	
n			21	13	26	37	26	22	13	9	
1975				27.24	26.92	27.58	27.68	27.38	26.64	27.31	27.11
n				21	13	26	37	26	22	13	9
Cross-sectional means											
	27.38	27.20	27.30	27.44	27.48	27.45	27.33	27.07	26.89	27.09	27.11
n	21	34	60	97	102	111	98	70	44	22	9

Before I attempt to answer this question, let me report on a longitudinal study on the natural development of periodontal disease and tooth mortality in a selected Norwegian population.

The investigation started in Oslo, Norway in 1969. The population consisted of 565 randomly selected non-dental, male high school and university students and teachers between the ages of 17 and 35 years. The principal reasons for selecting this population and for performing the study in Oslo were that this city has had a public dental programme that offers systematic preventive, restorative, endodontic, orthodontic, and surgical therapy on an annual recall basis for all children and adolescents (ages 3–16 years) and a documented attendance record of 90% for the last 40 years. The other 10% made use of personal dental services provided by private practitioners in the area. The city of Oslo also offers a reimbursement plan for expenses incurred for dental services to persons between 18 and 21 years of age, and the university, through its health services, provides a dental programme for its students. It is, therefore, fair to state that the chosen population represents a group of individuals that has had maximum exposure to conventional dental care throughout life. It should be noted that this group of individuals has not participated in any experimental preventive programme, but represented a group of ordinary middle-class, well-educated citizens. Whatever the level of interest in, knowledge of and awareness of dental care this group had, it must have been attained through general mass media and/or dental education programmes provided to all children and students during their school years and in their continued exposure to dental professional personnel in private practice.

The group was examined in 1969, 1971, 1973 and 1975, and the time span between the first and fourth examination was 6 years and 3 months. However, due to the design of this study (Fig. 1), it is clear that the data offer the possibility of describing the longitudinal changes in periodontal health over the first 40 years of life (Löe et al., 1978a).

At the baseline examination in 1969, the group as a whole showed good to excellent oral hygiene and mild gingivitis; supragingival calculus was inconspicuous and untreated caries was rare. The 17-year-old subjects had an average of 27.4 out of a possible 28 teeth (third molars excluded) and the oldest group examined had 27.1 teeth, indicating that there had been virtually no tooth loss between 17 and 35 years. Subsequent examinations confirmed these findings and also showed that no major tooth loss took place between the ages of 30 and 40 years (Table I). The average 40-year-old individual had lost an average of less than one tooth (Löe et al., 1978b).

It is generally assumed that after the age of 35 or 40 years, most extractions will occur as a result of periodontal disease. This study, which focused primarily on the pattern (Fig. 2) and rate (Fig. 3) of progression of periodontal

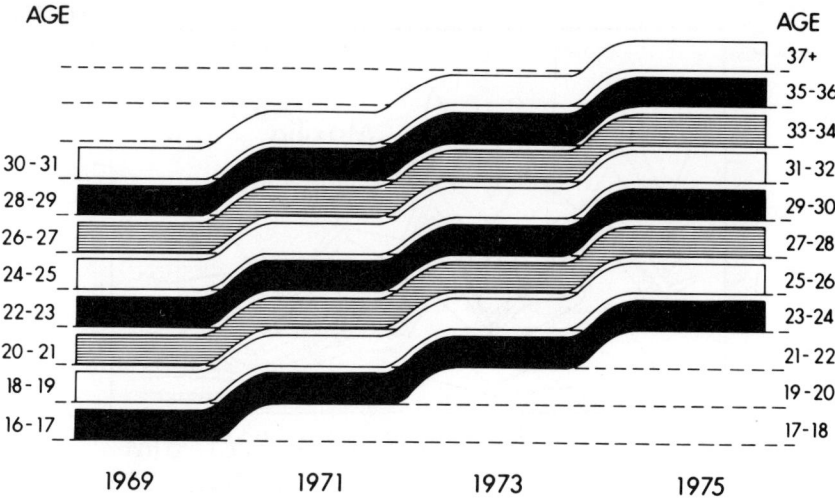

Fig. 1 The semi-longitudinal study design, the age cohorts at baseline and subsequent re-examination of the Norwegian sample. (From Löe et al., 1978a).

disease, showed that at 40 years of age less than 1.5 mm, or approximately 10% of the periodontal support had been lost (Fig. 4), and that the progress of this disease in this population is remarkably slow (approximately 0.05 mm/year) (Löe et al., 1978c).

Although none of the participants exhibited a dentition completely free of plaque, it is noteworthy that as this population reached 40 years of age, approximately 70% of all tooth surfaces exhibited no visible amount of plaque (Table II, Fig. 5) (Anerud et al., 1979). Gingival health was also remarkably high, as less than 10% of the total number of gingival units exhibited a degree of gingivitis which showed bleeding on probing (Table III). These lesions were found mainly in the interdental areas of the posterior teeth (Fig. 6) (Anerud et al., 1979).

There is no doubt that the relative cleanliness characterizing this population had resulted from active oral hygiene practices, mainly tooth-brushing. It is also interesting to note that the individual level of cleanliness was basically established before the age of 17 years and that this high level of hygiene was maintained towards the age of 40 years.

These data clearly show that within a middle-class population, a system of care which provides for access to and continuity of modern conventional dental services, including mechanical oral home care, is highly effective in reducing tooth mortality and in maintaining periodontal health. This contradicts the widespread notion that current dental care might be

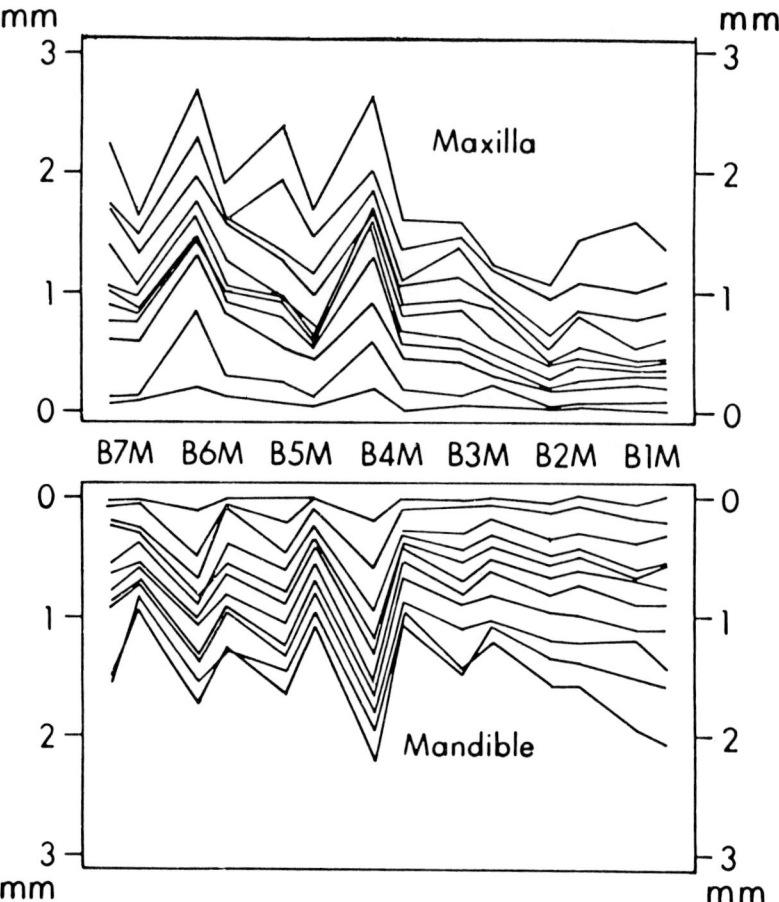

Fig. 2 Mean rate of attachment loss in buccal (B) and mesial (M) root surfaces of anterior (1,2,3) and posterior (4,5,6,7) teeth of Norwegian non-dental students and teachers between 17 and 37+ years. (Adapted from Löe et al., 1978c.)

"efficacious but not effective" and reveals a beneficial potential not usually appreciated.

Why is it then, that periodontal disease continues to be the culprit of tooth loss among adults in the Western world? The answer is that, whereas it is true that on a relative basis periodontal disease has been responsible for most of the tooth extractions in the past, the available statistics on the rate and causes of tooth mortality are probably outdated, and do not reflect the recent improvements in tooth retention. Most data on tooth loss either relate to population groups which have had little or no exposure to periodontal

16. Prevention of Periodontal Disease 263

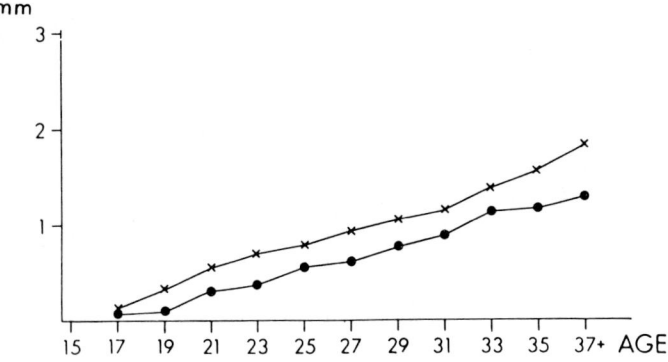

Fig. 3 Mean loss of attachment in mesial (●——●) and buccal (×——×) root surfaces in Norwegian non-dental students and teachers according to age.

prevention, or are based on population groups whose age characteristics simply rule out any reasonable benefit of modern approaches to prevention of dental diseases. The emphasis on prevention and its practice as we know it today started in earnest during the late 1950s and early 1960s. Since, in the absence of preventive measures, destructive periodontal disease (loss of attachment) will start during early adulthood, and given the fact that these subgingival lesions are generally unresponsive to existing preventive methods, it can be seen that those who had contracted the disease prior to the era of prevention, and have not been cured, would continue to show a steady progression of periodontal attachment loss and tooth mortality during their

TABLE II

Cumulative Mean and Frequency (%) of Plaque Index Scores According to Age of Norwegian Non-dental Students and Teachers who Attended all Surveys, 1969–1975

Age	Mean	S.D.	PlI = 0	PlI = 1	PlI = 2	PlI = 3
17–18	1.25	0.69	14.26	46.70	38.96	0.09
19–20	1.23	0.74	18.16	40.54	41.03	0.27
21–22	1.19	0.75	20.37	40.67	38.90	0.06
23–24	1.13	0.77	23.96	39.06	36.92	0.06
25–26	1.12	0.78	24.76	38.55	36.66	0.04
27–28	1.13	0.79	24.96	36.64	38.33	0.07
29–30	1.11	0.79	26.17	36.23	37.60	0
31–32	1.14	0.79	25.44	35.25	39.23	0.08
33–34	1.13	0.81	27.39	32.54	40.03	0.04
35–36	1.10	0.83	29.45	30.79	39.77	0
37+	0.95	0.81	35.54	33.47	30.99	0

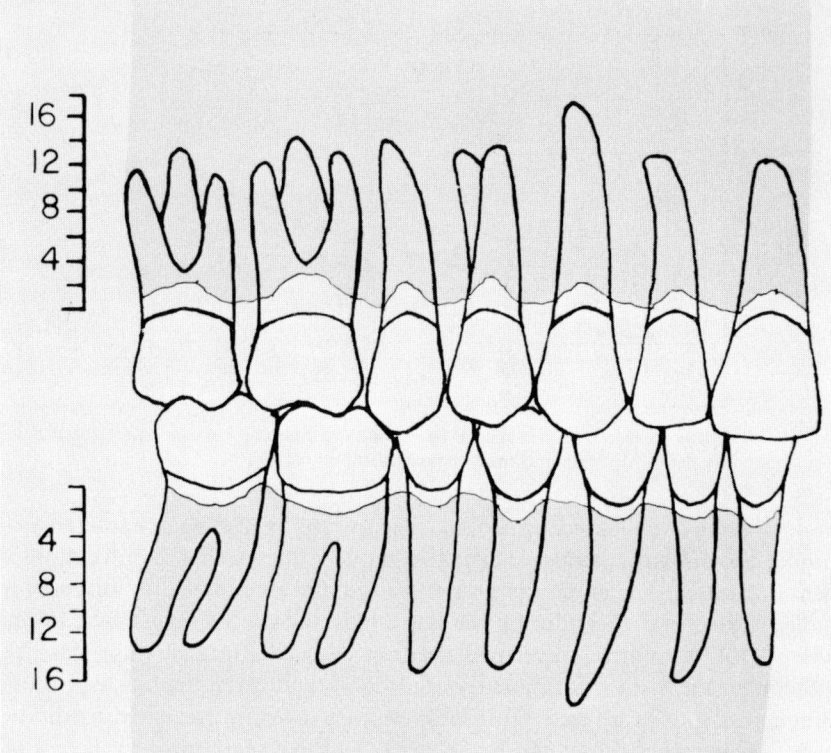

Fig. 4 Mean periodontal support of a well-educated, middle class Norwegian population at approximately 40 years of age. (From Löe et al., 1978c.)

TABLE III

Cumulative Mean and Frequency (%) of Gingival Index Scores According to Age of Norwegian Non-dental Students and Teachers who Attended all Surveys, 1969–1975

Age	Mean GI	S.D.	GI = 0	GI = 1	GI = 2	GI = 3
17–18	0.66	0.57	39.30	55.74	4.96	0
19–20	0.65	0.62	42.54	49.51	7.95	0
21–22	0.66	0.60	41.45	51.59	6.96	0
23–24	0.76	0.62	33.56	56.52	9.92	0
25–26	0.72	0.63	37.96	52.27	9.76	0.02
27–28	0.79	0.68	35.91	49.75	14.20	0.13
29–30	0.77	0.67	36.99	49.23	13.79	0
31–32	0.80	0.68	35.09	50.18	14.72	0
33–34	0.83	0.72	35.71	45.31	18.98	0
35–36	0.71	0.69	42.62	44.21	13.00	0
37+	0.70	0.61	38.22	53.72	8.06	0

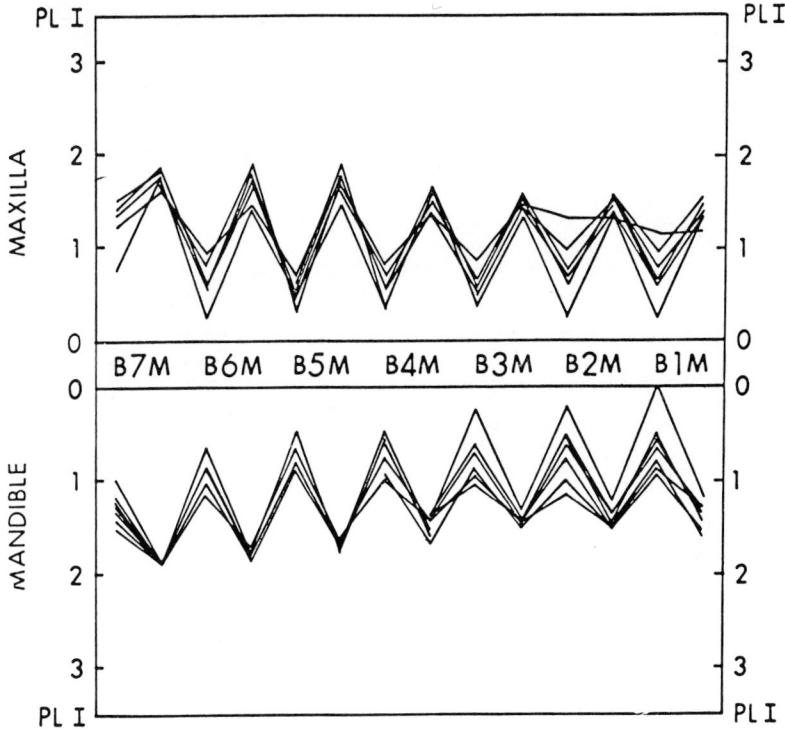

Fig. 5 Distribution of mean plaque index scores for buccal (B) and mesial (M) surfaces of all maxillary and mandibular teeth (7–1) of Norwegian non-dental students and teachers aged 17–37+ years. (Adapted from Anerud et al., 1979.)

adult life. On the other hand, those who reached adult age around 1960 or later will find themselves in a quite different circumstance, reaping the full benefit of systematic periodontal prevention. This was in part our working hypothesis and an important premise for the selection of age groups for the study, and I believe the results have vindicated this approach.

Although this study does not provide a direct explanation for the dramatic degree of tooth retention and periodontal health in this population, it may be surmised that the cumulative impact of a variety of social, behavioural and professional factors (Bailit, 1978; Burt, 1978) is responsible. It is of great importance that further studies to be made of the relative contribution of these factors. However, in the context of this discussion it seems reasonable to conclude that the current methods for the prevention of periodontal diseases, although relatively primitive, are efficacious and increasingly effective in extending the longevity of the human dentition in health.

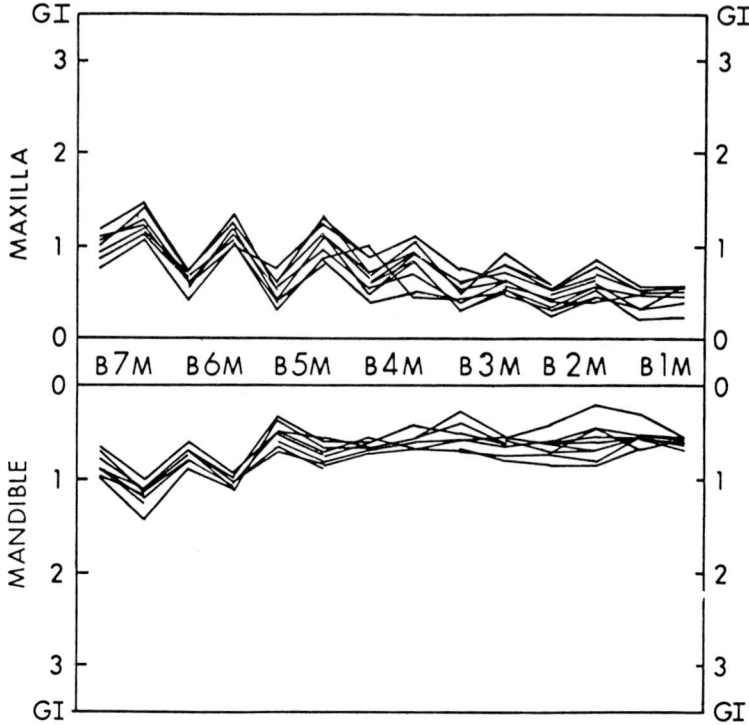

Fig. 6 Distribution of mean gingival index scores for buccal (B) and mesial (M) surfaces of all maxillary and mandibular teeth of Norwegian non-dental students and teachers aged 17–37+ years. (Adapted from Anerud et al., 1979.)

Summary

Supragingival bacterial plaque causes gingivitis in man. Animal data and circumstantial evidence strongly suggest that gingivitis is the precursor of more advanced periodontal destruction. Investigations during the last decade have revealed that dental plaque represents a multitude of bacteria in various combinations, with a variety of pathogenic and immunological potentials. These developments in microbiology and immunology have opened the way for new approaches to periodontal diagnosis, which in turn might make it possible to develop specific immunotherapeutic and chemotherapeutic methods for the control for periodontal infection, both on an individual and a population basis.

However, the concept of specific pathogenicity is not ready for clinical application and current clinical approaches to prevention of periodontal disease must be confined to plaque control. There are simple mechanical and chemical methods available which have proved their efficacy in reducing or eliminating dental plaque in individual patients or population groups. Furthermore, there are data which show that control of plaque and conventional dental care may substantially increase the longevity of the human dentition.

References

Anerud, A., Löe, H., Boysen, H. and Smith, M. (1979). *J. periodont. Res.* **14**, 526–540.
Axelson, P. and Lindhe, J. (1977). *J. dent. Res.* **56**, C142–C148.
Axelson, P. and Lindhe, J. (1978). *J. clin. Periodont.* **5**, 133–151.
Baehni, P., Tsai, C. C., Norman, M., Stoller, N., McArthur, W. P., and Taichman, N. S. (1979). *J. periodont. Res.* **14**, 279–288.
Bailit, H. L. (1978). *J. publ. Hlth Dent.* **38**, 289–301.
Bowen, W. H. (1976). *Oral Sci. Rev.* **9**, 3–21.
Burt, B. A. (1978). *J. publ. Hlth Dent.* **38**, 272–288.
Cianciola, L. J., Genco, R. J., Patters, M. R., McKenna, J, and Van Oss, C. J. (1977). *Nature, Lond.* **265**, 445.
Genco, R. J. (1979). *Näringsforskn.* **23**, Suppl. 17, 22–31.
Lavine, W., Stolman, J., Maderazo, E., Ward, P., and Cogen, R. (1976). *J. dent. Res.* **55**, B212.
Lehner, T., Challacombe, S. J., Wilton, J. M. A., and Ivanyi, L. (1976). *Archs oral Biol.* **21**, 749–753.
Lehner, T., Wilton, J. M. A., Ivanyi, L., and Manson, J. D. (1974a). *J. periodont. Res.* **9**, 261–272.
Lehner, T., Wilton, J. M. A., Challacombe, S. J. and Ivanyi, L. (1974b). *Clin. exp. Immunol.* **16**, 481–492.
Lindhe, J., Hamp, S. E. and Löe, H. (1973). *J. periodont. Res.* **8**, 1–10.
Löe, H. (1970). In *Dental Plaque* (W. D. McHugh, ed.) pp. 259–270, E. & S. Livingstone, Edinburgh.
Löe, H. (ed.) (1971). *J. periodont.* Res., Suppl. 12.
Löe, H. (1979). *Näringsforskn.* **23**, Suppl. 17, 32–36.
Löe, H. and Schiött, C. R. (1970). In *Dental Plaque* (W. D. McHugh, ed.), pp. 247–255, E. & S. Livingstone, Edinburgh.
Löe, H., Theilade, E. and Jensen, S. B. (1965). *J. Periodont.* **36**, 177–187.
Löe, H., von der Fehr, F. R., and Schiött, C. R. (1972). *Scand. J. dent. Res.* **80**, 1–9.
Löe, H., Anerud, A., Boysen, H., and Smith, M. (1978a). *J. periodont. Res.* **13**, 550–562.
Löe, H., Anerud, A., Boysen, H., and Smith, M. (1978b). *J. periodont. Res.* **13**, 563–572.
Löe, H., Anerud, A., Boysen, H., and Smith, M. (1978c). *J. Periodont.* **49**, 607–620.
Loesche, W. J. (1976). *Oral Sci. Rev.* **9**, 114–212.
Lovdal, A., Arno, A., Schei, O., and Waerhaug, J. (1960). *Acta odnot. Scand.* **19**, 537–555.
Newman, M. G. and Socransky, S. S. (1977). *J. periodont. Res.* **12**, 120–123.
Paulson, S., Holm-Pedersen, P., and Kelstrup, J. (1979). *Scand. J. dent. Res.* **87**, 178–183.

Slots, J. (1976). *Scand. J. dent. Res.* **83**, 1–10.
Slots, J. (1977). *Scand. J. dent. Res.* **85**, 114–121.
Socransky, S. S. (1977). *J. Periodont.* **48**, 497–504.
Tanner, A., Haffer, C., Brathall, D., Visconti, R. and Socransky, S. S. (1979). *J. clin. Periodont.* **6**, 278–307.
Waerhaug, J. (1952). *Odont. Tskr.* **60**, Suppl.

17. Mechanism of Action of Fluoride in the Control of Plaque in Dental Caries

G. NEIL JENKINS

In vitro Evidence that Fluoride Might Influence Pellicle or Plaque Formation

Experiments *in vitro* have shown that fluoride, either in solution or within apatite, affects the adsorption of proteins by apatite, and this has led to the suggestion that one way in which fluoride might conceivably reduce caries is by a reduction of plaque formation (Rölla, 1977).

Ericson and Ericsson (1967) first showed that when hydroxyapatite was treated with sodium monofluorophosphate (MFP) so that it contained 0.3%, or about 10% saturated with F and comparable with the concentration on the outer surface of the enamel, it took up less protein when shaken with unstimulated human saliva than the original hydroxyapatite (HA). The use of MFP to introduce F into HA is not entirely satisfactory, however, as other reactions may occur, such as the adsorption of phosphate or the incorporation of MFP itself (Ingram, 1972, 1973).

Similar experiments (Rölla and Melsen, 1975) in which HA was stirred with albumin solution, with or without various concentrations of F or MFP in solution, also showed that they partly reduced adsorption of the protein. The HA would, of course, become fluoridated, but no attempt was made to determine whether bound or free F was responsible for this effect. At each concentration MFP was the more active. The adsorption by HA of *Streptococcus mutans* labelled by growing in [^{14}C]glucose was reduced by 50% in the presence of 0.5 M (approximately 0.1%) F. Fluoride and MFP desorbed protein from HA at concentrations of 1 mM (19 p.p.m.) and 10 mM (190 p.p.m.) F, respectively.

The binding of proteins to the amphoteric substance HA is considered to arise from electrostatic forces acting on either the acidic or basic groups (Bernardi *et al.*, 1972). MFP (acting either as the anion MFP$^-$ or possibly as a source of fluoride ions usually present as an impurity) and F$^-$ bind with and block positive charges on the HA and therefore prevent anionic proteins from being adsorbed or, by competition, promote desorption of proteins already attached. The proteins of newly formed pellicle scraped off the enamel within

2 h of formation contained a preponderance of acidic amino acids (Sönju and Rölla, 1973), i.e. they are anionic, as this concept requires.

All these experiments were criticized by Moreno *et al.* (1977) mainly on the ground that, as the surface area of the HA used was not known, it was impossible to calculate whether the surface was saturated with protein and therefore whether any of the adsorption was by protein layers adsorbed earlier in the experiment, rather than by HA itself. By constructing adsorption isotherms of aspartic acid and albumen on apatite of known surface area, partly (41%) and completely saturated with F (i.e. very much higher than occurs in enamel), Moreno *et al.* (1977) overcame this difficulty. Their results were diametrically opposed to previous findings; F in apatite increased the adsorption and it was possible to calculate that this arose both by increasing the number of adsorption sites and their affinity for the two molecules tested. Later work (Moreno *et al.*, 1978), with tyrosine-rich and proline-rich peptides from human parotid saliva confirmed this conclusion and showed that a concentration of F in the apatite of 0.49% (not much greater than that of enamel) increased the affinity but not the number of binding sites. Fluoride increased the adsorption of the two peptides to different extents, suggesting that F might alter the composition as well as the amount of protein adsorbed from saliva *in vivo*.

It is difficult to judge the practical importance of such contradictory findings. The results of Moreno *et al.* (1978) would seem to be the more technically valid, by avoiding adsorption of protein by protein but, except in one experiment, they used apatites more highly fluoridated than enamel would be, even after topical application of F, and tested individual proteins rather than whole saliva. In view of the variations between the effect of F on the adsorption of different substances there is no proof that their results apply to any of the proteins involved in pellicle formation. Pellicle formation is not a monomolecular layer so that adsorption to protein already attached, as almost certainly occurred in the earlier experiments, may be more applicable to the situation *in vivo*, although it is difficult to understand how fluoridated apatite affects protein adsorption separated by many layers from the apatite.

Although adsorption by apatite seems relevant to pellicle formation, several authors have interpreted those results showing that F disfavoured adsorption as indicating that it may also reduce plaque formation. The factors involved in development of plaque are still uncertain but are more complex than adsorption and are not known to be influenced by F. This failure to distinguish between pellicle and plaque has led to much confusion (for further discussion see Jenkins, 1978).

Pellicle is now considered to be protective against caries (for the references see Moreno *et al.*, 1978) and it would be contrary to the overall anticaries effect of F if it reduced pellicle.

17. Fluoride and Plaque Control

Glantz (1969) found that enamel treated with SnF_2 had a lower surface energy, was less wettable and that protein adhered to it less readily than before treatment. Many authors quoting this work overlooked the fact that the stannous salt was used and frequently state erroneously that fluoride itself lowers the surface energy of enamel and reduces its wettability.

Clinical Data

Effects of F on Pellicle

Measurement of the amount and composition of pellicle formed under normal conditions are extremely difficult and I am unaware of any attempts to determine whether they are affected by F, either in water or in the much higher concentrations involved in topical application and dentifrices.

Effect of Fluoridated Water on the Amount of Plaque

Although some subjective observations suggest that tooth surfaces are "cleaner" in residents with optimal fluoride in their water (Ericson and Ericsson, 1967; Møller, 1965), this does not appear to have been quantified in terms of plaque weight. The impression might arise from the slightly whiter enamel surface produced in fluoride areas.

Fluoride in the concentrations present in plaque from fluoridated water has been reported by one group of workers (Broukel and Zajicek, 1974) to affect the formation of extracellular polysaccharides and presumably plaque weight. This finding has not been reported by others and is difficult to explain, as the tranferases involved in their synthesis are not inhibited by F.

Effect of High Concentrations of F, SnF_2 and Amine Fluoride on Plaque Formation

Bowen and Hewitt (1974) reported that 70 p.p.m. F as NaF affected the dry weight of four out of five strains of *Strep. mutans* during growth *in vitro* and raised the proportion of fructose to glucose in the extracellular polysaccharides that they synthesized. It is doubtful whether plaque ever contains such high concentrations of F, but as the fructosans are more readily dissolved and metabolised than the glucosans, if this difference did occur *in vivo* it might have a small influence on plaque weight.

Birkeland (1972) weighed the plaque from 147 schoolchildren who were receiving weekly mouth rinses of either 10 ml of 0.2% NaF or 0.2% NaCl. The plaque was collected double-blind 4–5 days after the last of eight rinses and was significantly smaller in the NaF group, especially in the boys who, as other workers have found, had much more plaque than the girls. Birkeland suggested that the experiments of Ericson and Ericsson (1967) or of Glantz

(1969) might explain this effect of F, but, for the reasons mentioned above, this seems unlikely. An alternative speculation is that the F slowly released from adsorption on the enamel inhibits bacterial growth in plaque. The F concentrations on the enamel surface before, and at various intervals after, topical application by NaF or NaF in H_3PO_4 (APF) show an immediate rise, but much of it is lost within a few months (the rate of loss depends on the number of applications), after which the remaining F seems permanently bound (Mellberg et al., 1966, 1977). Much of the F removed from the surface must enter plaque, at least temporarily, and presumably may exert an inhibitory effect on the bacteria. Woolley and Rickles (1971) showed that the pH drop in the plaque of schoolgirls after taking 10–15 ml of a 25% solution of mixed sugars was smaller 3–4 days after a topical application of 2% fluoride, but there was no significant difference 1 week after, by which time most of the soluble F had presumably been removed.

Loesche et al. (1973) found that the amounts of plaque scored visually was significantly reduced 6 days after between five and 10 daily applications of APF, compared with plaques treated with a placebo gel, but by 6 weeks the difference was no longer significant. The percentages of *Strep. mutans*, but not *Strep. sanguis*, in the interproximal plaques were reduced and remained so even 12 weeks after the treatment. They explained this selective effect in *Strep. mutans* as follows: The topical application would inhibit all the bacteria on the tooth surfaces but would not have much effect on soft tissues. Consequently, *Strep. sanguis* from soft tissues could rapidly reinfect the enamel surfaces whereas there is no similar reservoir of *Strep. mutans*, which is confined to the tooth surface.

Stannous Fluoride

König (1959) reported that after topical application of SnF_2 (= 250 p.p.m. F) to rats' teeth plaque formation was greatly reduced, a finding which became explicable after the work of Glantz (1969), mentioned above.

Hoffman et al. (1977) immersed pieces of enamel in 10% SnF_2 for 15 min and, after washing, incubated them with *Strep. mutans* (6715) or *Strep. sanguis* (10556) in Todd–Hewitt broth. The pH change in the medium and the bacterial colonization were all markedly less in SnF_2-treated enamel, compared with controls. Gross and Tinoff (1977) showed similar effects *in vivo* on two subjects who for periods of 48 hr wore an appliance on which cylinders of human enamel were mounted and used twice daily a mouth-rinse of SnF_2 (100 p.p.m. F) or a water control, after which the adhering bacteria were removed by sonication and counted. The numbers of bacteria were reduced by between 95 and 99% by the SnF_2 and the electron microscopic appearance confirmed a gross effect.

A similar study in which SnF_2, $SnCl_2$ and NaF (all 100 p.p.m. F^-) were compared showed that the SnF_2 was much more effective than NaF (Tinanoff et al., 1976) but that $SnCl_2$ treatment also inhibited bacterial colonization, as confirmed by Rölla in a slightly different procedure (see Chapter 14 in this volume).

White and Taylor (1978) compared the plaque scores in 20 subjects brushing and rinsing with a preparation containing SnF_2 for 6 days followed, for 5 days, by rinses only with 17 subjects who used placebos. The results showed a non-significant trend for lower scores in the SnF_2 group during the brushing and rinsing period and the scores remained at approximately the same level during the "rinsing only" period when those in the control group showed a steady rise, the difference being highly significant ($p < 0.001$).

There is therefore considerable evidence that SnF_2 does affect plaque formation, probably because it reacts with enamel to produce a complex salt such as stannous fluorophosphate, $Sn_3F_3PO_4$ (Wei, 1974; Wei and Forbes, 1974), or $Sn_2PO_4OH + CaF_2$ and fluorapatite (Hercules and Craig, 1978) which lower its surface energy, making it hydrophobic as Glantz (1969) suggests. There do not seem to be any tests on the duration in vivo either of the effect on plaque or of the complex chemical changes on the surface, although a reduction in caries continues for at least 5 years after the end of SnF_2 treatment (Houwink et al., 1974). It is likely that, in addition to the inhibition of plaque formation, a reduction of enamel solubility contributes to the well-established effect of SnF_2 on caries.

Amine Fluoride

Extensive work by the Zürich school demonstrated the antibacterial properties, power of reducing enamel solubility, low toxicity and stability of amine fluorides (for reference see König and Mühlemann, 1961). This in vitro work was followed by animal experiments and clinical trials on caries in schoolchildren (Marthaler, 1961, 1968, 1974) all of which gave positive results. This review will discuss more recent work on the effectiveness and mode of action of amine fluorides.

The effect of 6–8 p.p.m. F were compared as cetylamine hydrofluoride, NaF, SnF_2 and MFP on acid production by salivary sediment, formed into a plaque on a glass slide (Dolan et al., 1973). The amine F was much more active than the other substances but the comparison was complicated because 0.1% of calcium phosphate was added to the sediment (its function was unclear) and this would be expected to bind the F ion and react in a complicated way with MFP (Ingram, 1972, 1973) and thus reduce their concentrations.

Samples of plaque accumulated for 36 h were collected from volunteers at intervals up to 10 h after rinses with amine fluorides or NaF and their pH changes followed in vitro when incubated with 10% glucose compared with similar plaque samples collected after a saline rinse (Schneider and

Mühlemann, 1974). A marked reduction in pH drop was found up to 6 h after the rinse with the amine F whereas virtually no difference was detectable at 3 h with the NaF rinse.

The pH drop in saliva collected at intervals after mouth-rinsing with various amine fluorides, NaF or controls also showed that the amine fluorides exerted a much more powerful antiglycolytic effect than NaF (Dolan et al., 1974).

Mouth-rinses containing amine F were tested for 4 days on the formation of plaque and its microbial population in 48 college students divided into "low" and "high" plaque formers. Less plaque was formed, especially in the high formers, compared with placebo, although the difference was of marginal significance ($0.05 < p < 0.1$). There was a dramatic reduction in the number of organisms per unit volume of plaque but the proportions of the various types were not affected (Shern et al., 1974).

An 8 week clinical trial on the effect of a mouth-rinse containing a mixture of two amine fluorides (F=250 p.p.m.) in 20 male subjects, compared with a placebo rinse in 20 controls, showed no significant difference for the gingival index, but a reduction in gingival fluid (significant at 4 weeks) and lower values for plaque score and weight (Stoller et al., 1977). No explanation was offered for the lack of effect on the gingival index as an improvement might have been predicted following the reduction in plaque.

The F uptake in vitro by enamel from cetylamine HF and its penetration were much greater than from APF, NaF or Na_2SnF_6 while uptake from MFP and SnF_2 was negligible (Kirkegaard, 1977).

Weiss et al. (1977) took weighed slabs of human enamel which had been immersed with shaking in solutions of either saline, amine F, amine Cl, or MFP equivalent in F content to the amine F and attached them to orthodontic bands cemented on to the upper first molars of three volunteers. The results showed that all three treatments reduced plaque deposition in 3 days, compared with the saline controls in the ascending order: MFP (not significant), amine Cl, amine F (both significant). At 7 days all three treatments produced decreases which were not significant. The F retention by the enamel slabs from MFP and the amine F, compared with the saline, was highly significant, but the uptake from the two treatments did not differ, unlike some previous experiments in which retention from amine F exceeded that of inorganic F. In this experiment the amine moiety of the compound reduced plaque formation; the F apparently having no effect.

Effect of Amines

A series of 12 amines inhibited the attachment of colonies resembling plaque to polished enamel surfaces of extracted teeth, when incubated anaerobically

TABLE I
Effect of Various Substances on Streptococcal Deposits and F Concentrations during Incubation with Rats' Teeth (after Balmelli et al., 1974)

	Extent of deposit	F (p.p.m.) on molar surfaces
Control	126	247
NaF	114	317
Amine F	30	719
Amine Cl	43	278

with *Strep. mutans* (Warner et al., 1976). The antiplaque and antibacterial activities of the fluorides of these amines were very similar.

Balmelli et al. (1974) compared the effects of solutions of amine F, amine Cl and NaF on inhibiting bacterial growth and adhesion to enamel by dipping rats' teeth for 1, 5 and 15 min into them or a water control, then incubating for 48 h in a medium inoculated with *Strep. mutans*. The results (Table I) showed great inhibition for the amine F, somewhat less for the amine Cl and very little for the NaF and higher F concentrations on the tooth surfaces in the amine F group. Evidently the amine moiety was largely responsible, as was confirmed by the small differences in the effect of amine F and amine Cl. *In vivo*, the amine F would not only reduce adhesion of plaque but the increased F in the enamel would probably reduce its solubility.

The binding of the amines, which Balmelli et al. (1974) suggest is through carboxylic groups in the pellicle or enamel protein, would form a hydrophobic layer to which further protein and bacteria could not adhere. The binding is very tight, that might explain the high uptake of F by the enamel from amine F and the amines might possibly exert an antibacterial effect as well as preventing bacterial adhesion (Shern et al., 1974). This combination of properties of amine fluorides probably accounts for their effectiveness.

Source and Nature of Plaque F

The F concentration of plaque measured by the specific ion electrode is about 2–5 p.p.m. wet weight, i.e. approximately 100 times that of the salivary environment (0.02–0.05 p.p.m.) (Grøn et al., 1969; Agus et al., 1976; Jenkins and Edgar, 1977), but considerably lower than earlier estimates (Hardwick and Leach, 1972). Plaque F probably arises from the F in saliva or gingival fluid and is slightly higher in residents of F areas (Agus et al., 1976; Jenkins and Edgar, 1977), the additional F being probably derived from short-lived direct contact of plaque with the water, as the rise in plasma and saliva concentrations in F areas seems too small to account for the difference. There is no evidence that F incorporated into enamel during development is a source of plaque F, as enamel appears to acquire F from plaque (Weatherall et al., 1972, 1973; Charlton et al., 1974), but after topical applications some F attached temporarily to enamel may gradually diffuse into plaque.

The nature and effects of plaque F have been reviewed elsewhere (Jenkins and Edgar, 1977) and will only be briefly summarized here. It is obvious that plaque could not retain these high concentrations unless it is bound to some constituent(s).The proteins and polysaccharides of the matrix do not bind F (Birkeland and Rölla, 1972). Plaque contains high concentrations of calcium and phosphate suggesting that apatite might be present and if so, it could bind the F (Birkeland, 1972). Solubility data from my own laboratory (Edgar, 1973) are incompatible with this conclusion, however, as Ca can be extracted without F and vice versa. Many species of bacteria in pure culture, including some oral organisms, concentrate F to much higher levels than are present in their environment (Jenkins et al., 1969) and we concluded that plaque F was bound within bacteria (Table II). The F in bacteria occurs in at least three forms: free ions, what we have called "loosely bound" (released by cold perchloric acid) and "tightly bound", requiring destruction of the organic matter by hot, concentrated sulphuric or perchloric acids for its release (Jenkins and Edgar, 1977). This terminology has become confused because this loosely bound form is referred to by Kashket and Rodriguez (1975) as "tightly bound". They did not use hot acid and therefore did not realize that a further fraction is in cells grown in F media in addition to that released by cold perchloric acid.

TABLE II
Different Forms of F in Bacteria and Plaque (after Jenkins and Edgar, 1977)
(p.p.m. wet weight)

F concentration in medium	Loosely bound F	Tightly bound F
0	0.6	5.6
1	1.3	7.1
10	8.8	20.4
Typical plaque	4.1	8.5

Plaque F is also present in these three forms (Table II), strongly confirming our conclusion that it is mostly bound within bacteria (Jenkins and Edgar, 1977).

The Role of Plaque F in Caries

Anti-enzyme Effects

The fluoride taken up by bacteria usually exerts an inhibitory effect on acid production and on the synthesis of intracellular polysaccharides. This dual effect probably arises from the inhibition of enolase which reduces or prevents the formation of phosphoenolypyruvic acid, required for the enzymic uptake of sugar by many organisms (Schachtele and Mayo, 1973). Comparison of the pH drop during incubation *in vitro* with sugar of plaques from residents with and without F in their water or, in one case, of plaque collected before and some months after F was added to their water indicated that the F was inhibitory (Edgar *et al.*, 1970). The effect was small but statistically significant (Table III). A complication in the interpretation arises from two other observations: an inverse relation between the weight of plaque in an individual and (1) its F concentration and (2) its pH drop during incubation with sugar. Conceivably, those plaques with the higher F concentration had the lowest pH drop, not because the F was highest, but because their weight was lower. It is not clear why the plaque samples with lower weight produce a smaller pH drop *in vitro*: this occurs *in vivo* (Clarke and Fanning, 1971) where the effect can be explained by assuming that the smaller thickness allows more readily the outward diffusion of acid and the inward diffusion of bicarbonate to neutralize the acid.

TABLE III
pH Drop in Plaques from High and Low F Areas before and after Incubation with Sucrose (after Edgar et al., *1970)*

F of water	Mean pH		No. of experiments	p
	Before incubation	After incubation		
0	6.28	4.89	34	0.001
1.8	6.32	5.04		
0	6.30	4.88	13	Between 0.1 and 0.05
1.0	6.38	4.93		

Solubility Effects

Concentrations of F as low as 0.1 p.p.m. in an acid solvent reduce the amount of apatite or enamel dissolving (Manly and Harrington, 1959). The concentration of free F^- in plaque fluid is probably sufficient to exert this effect and thus to curtail the action of bacterial acids in dissolving enamel. The ionic fluoride may also exert some effect in favouring the partial remineralization of an early lesion which occurs when the plaque pH is rising and after it reduces its resting value.

Estimates of F on the surface of enamel on different parts of anterior teeth throughout a wide age range show that, contrary to previous findings, the concentrations fall significantly with age on most parts (Weatherall et al., 1972, 1973). The concentration rises on the plaque-covered areas near the gingival margin and presumable some of the plaque fluoride gradually, over decades, binds with the apatite—a process that would be favoured by the low pH of the plaque after sugar ingestion (Charlton et al., 1974). Little et al. (1971) reported that a proportion of the F in stained enamel from old teeth was organically bound. Unpublished work in the author's laboratory has confirmed the existence in surface enamel of bound fluoride, similar in properties to the tightly bound F of plaque, although in much lower concentration than stated by Little et al. (1971). It is tempting to speculate that some of this fraction of plaque F bound to bacteria becomes engulfed in the surface enamel of old teeth and is the source of the organically bound F.

There is therefore good and varied evidence suggesting that the F in plaque plays a part in protecting against caries but there is no obvious means of comparing its importance relative to that of fluoride bound to enamel.

Summary

Some *in vitro* experiments suggest that fluoride, either as free ions or incorporated into apatite, may reduce the adsorption of proteins by hydroxyapatite. Other experiments in which precautions were taken to ensure that only monomolecular layers were adsorbed suggest the opposite: that fluorapatite adsorbs more than hydroxapatite. The former result seems more likely to be relevant to the situation *in vivo* and may imply the formation of less pellicle. This work is sometimes quoted as evidence that F reduces plaque formation, but this process is more complicated than an adsorption of protein. The effect of fluoridated water on the deposition of pellicle and plaque does not appear to have been tested. However, clinical experiments indicate that the very high concentrations of F in "acidulated phosphate fluoride" gels or in rinses of 0.2% NaF may reduce the amount of plaque at least in some circumstances but again data on pellicle are lacking. Stannous fluoride and amine fluorides reduce plaque formation but the stannous ion or amine moiety are largely responsible.

The F concentration in plaque is much higher than that of the environment and its presence may contribute to the reduction of caries in several ways; there is evidence that it inhibits bacterial glycolysis, reduces the demineralizing effect of acid in plaque, favours remineralization and acts as a reservoir of F that may enter enamel.

References

Agus, H. M., Schamschula, R. G., Barmes, D. E. and Bunzel, M. (1976). *Community Dent. oral Epidemiol.* **4**, 210–214.
Balmelli, O. P., Regolati, B. and Mühlemann, H. R. (1974). *Helv. odont. Acta* **18**, 45–53.
Bernadi, G., Giro, M. G. and Gaillard, C. (1972). *Biochem. biophys. Acta* **278**, 409–420.
Birkeland, J. M. (1972). *Scand. J. dent. Res.* **80**, 82–84.
Birkeland, J. M. and Rölla, G. (1972). *Archs oral Biol.* **17**, 455–463.
Bowen, W. H. and Hewitt, M. J. (1974). *J. dent. Res.* **53**, 627–629.
Broukal, Z. and Zajicek, O. (1974). *Caries Res.* **8**, 97–104.
Charlton, G., Blainey, B. and Schamschula, R. G. (1974). *Archs oral Biol.* **19**, 139–143.
Clarke, N. G. and Fanning, E. G. (1971). *Aust. dent. J.* **16**, 13–16.
Dolan, M. M., Murphy, C. V., Kavanagh, B. and Yankell, S. L. (1973). *J. dent. Res.* **52**, 1323–1326.
Dolan, M. M., Harding, E. T. and Yankell, S. L. (1974). *Helv. odont. Acta* **18**, 54–56.
Ericson, Th. and Ericsson, Y. (1967). *Helv. odont. Acta.* **11**, 10–14.
Edgar, W. M. (1973). *Helv. odont. Acta* **17**, 50.
Edgar, W. M., Jenkins, G. N. and Tatevossian, A. (1970). *Br. dent. J.* **128**, 129–133.
Glantz, P.-O. (1969). *Odont. Rev.* **17**, Suppl., 1–132.
Grøn, P., Yao, K. and Spinelli, M. (1969). *J. dent. Res.* **48**, 799–805.
Gross, A. and Tinanoff, N. (1977). *J. dent. Res.* **56**, 1179–1183.
Hardwick, J. L. and Leach, S. A. (1962). *Proc. 9th ORCA Conf.* 151–158.
Hercules, D. M. and Craig, N. L. (1978). *J. dent. Res.* **57**, 297–305.
Hoffman, S., Tow, H. D. and Cole, J. S. (1977). *J. dent. Res.* **56**, 709–715.
Houwink, B., Backer Dirks, O. and Kwant, G. W. (1974). *Caries Res.* **8**, 27–38.
Ingram, G. S. (1972). *Caries Res.* **6**, 1–15.
Ingram, G. S. (1973). *Caries Res.* **7**, 315–323.
Jenkins, G. N. (1978). *Physiology and Biochemistry of the Mouth*, 4th edn, Blackwell Scientific Publications, Oxford.
Jenkins, G. N. and Edgar, W. M. (1977). *Caries Res.* **11**, Suppl. 1, 226–242.
Jenkins, G. N., Edgar, W. M. and Ferguson, D. B. (1969). *Archs oral Biol.* **14**, 105–119.
Kashket, S. and Rodriguez, V. M. (1975). *Archs oral Biol.* **21**, 459–464.
Kirkegaard, E. (1977). *Caries Res.* **11**, 16–23.
König, K. G. (1959). *Helv. odont. Acta* **3**, 39–43.
König, K. G. and Mühlemann, H. R. (1961). In *Caries Symposium, Zürich* (H. R. Mühlemann and K. G. König, eds), pp. 126–132, Hans Huber, Berne.
Little, M. F., Cooper, A. C. and Rowley, J. (1971). *Tooth Enamel*, Vol. II (R. W. Fearnhead and M. V. Stack, eds), pp. 100–118, John Wright, Bristol.
Loesche, W. J., Murray, R. J. and Mellberg, J. R. (1973). *Caries Res.* **7**, 283–296.
Manly, R. S. and Harrington, D. P. (1959). *J. dent. Res.* **38**, 910–919.
Marthaler, T. M. (1961). In *Caries Symposium, Zürich.* (H. R. Mühlemann and K. G. König, eds), pp. 14–26, Hans Huber, Berne.
Marthaler, T. M. (1968). *Br. dent. J.* **124**, 510–515.
Marthaler, T. M. (1974). *Helv. odont. Acta* **18**, 34–44.

Mellberg, J. R., Laakso, P. V. and Nicholson, C. R. (1966). *Archs oral Biol.* **11**, 1213–1220.
Mellberg, J. R., Nicholson, C. R., Franchi, G. J., Englander, H. R. and Mosley, G. W. (1977). *J. dent. Res.* **56**, 716–721.
Moreno, E. C., Kresak, M. and Zahradnik, R. T. (1977). *Caries Res.* **11**, Suppl. 1, 142–171.
Moreno, E. C., Kresak, M. and Hay, D. I. (1978). *Archs oral Biol.* **23**, 525–533.
Møller, K. J. (1965). *Dental Fluorose og Caries,* International Science Publishers, Cøpenhagen.
Rölla, G. (1977). *Caries Res.* **11**, Suppl. 1, 243–252.
Rölla, G. and Melsen, B. (1975). *Caries Res.* **9**, 66–73.
Schachtele, C. F. and Mayo, J. A. (1973). *J. dent. Res.* **52**, 1029–1215.
Schneider, Ph., and Mühlemann, H. R. (1974). *Helv. odont. Acta* **18**, 63–70.
Shern, R. J., Rundell, B. B. and Defever, C. J. (1974). *Helv. odont. Acta* **18**, 57–62.
Sönju, T. and Rölla, G. (1973). *Caries Res.* **7**, 30–38.
Stoller, N. H., Cohen, D. W. and Gandheld, S. V. (1977). *J. Periodont.* **48**, 650–653.
Tinanoff, N., Brady, J. M. and Gross, A. (1976). *Caries Res.* **10**, 415–426.
Warner, V. D., Warner, A. M., Mirth, D. B., Sane, J. S., Turesky, S. S. and Soloway, B. (1976). *J. dent. Res.* **55**, 130–134.
Weatherall, J. A., Hallsworth, A. S. and Robinson, C. (1973). *Archs oral Biol.* **18**, 1175–1189.
Weatherall, J. A., Robinson, C. and Hallsworth, A. S. (1972). *Caries Res.* **6**, 312–324.
Wei, S. H. Y. (1974). *J. dent. Res.* **53**, 57–61.
Wei, S. H. Y. and Forbes, W. C. (1974). *J. dent. Res.* **53**, 51–56.
Weiss, W., Gedalia, I. and Zilbeman, Y. (1977). *J. dent. Res.* **56**, 1345–1348.
White, S. T. and Taylor, P. P. (1978). *J. dent. Res.* **58**, 1850–1852.
Woolley, L. H. and Rickles, N. H. (1971). *Archs oral Biol.* **16**, 1187–1194.

INDEX

Acid phosphatases in crevicular fluid, 77
Acidaminococcus, 248
Actinobacillus, associated with periodontitis, 256
Actinomyces species, 83, 129–34, 244, 248–51
  israelii, 175, 245
  naeslundii, 83, 248, 252
  related to caries, 256
  viscosus, 83, 126, 248, 252
    B-cell mitogenicity of antigens, 179
    coaggregation with *Strep. sanguis*, 219, 223
    growth rate on tooth surface, 215
    immunization with, in rats, 173–92
    synthesis and breakdown of fructans, 218
Agglutinins, salivary, 160
Alveolar bone
  loss
    associated with suppression of osteoblasts, 252
    in immunized rats, 183
  resorbed, in periodontal disease, 249
Amine fluoride, 273–5
Amines, effect on plaque, 274
Aminopeptidase A in gingival sulcus, 31
Anaerobic microorganisms in gingival plaque, 241–54
  culture of specimens, 242–3
  groups present, 248
  identification, 244–6
Antibiotics, susceptibility of oral anaerobic bacteria to, 246–7
Antibodies, serum, 64
  and salivary, role in protection against caries, 193–214
α_1-Antichymotrypsin, 43
Antigens from oral bacteria, stimulation of gingival lymphocytes by, 125–34
Antimicrobials, uncontrolled use of, 258
Antiseptics, 258

α_1-Antitrypsin, 43–4
Arachnia, 246
Autoimmunity, cellular, in periodontal disease, 135–57

Bacillus brevis, 222
Bacteria
  anaerobic microorganisms in gingival plaque, 241–54
  film on enamel surface of tooth, 225
  Gram-positive, first colonizers of tooth surfaces, 232
  in oral cavity of hypogammaglobulinaemic patients, 159–73
  locomotion of, 116
  maintenance energy requirements, 216
  oral, antigens from, 125–34
  reactions with oral fluid components, 161
Bacterial adhesion of teeth, prevention, 238
Bacterial cell surface, structure, 231
Bacterial colonization of teeth and gingivae, 111, 115, 255
Bacteriology, clinical, ecological control of pathogens, 222
Bacteroides, 244, 248
  melaninogenicus, 83, 217, 219, 245–6
    in gingivitis and periodontitis, 250–52, 256
    inhibition of other anaerobic bacteria, 249
  asaccharolyticus, 119, 246, 249, 252
  fragilis, 245–6
  ureolyticum, 252
B cells, 213
Bifidobacterium, 244, 248
B lymphocytes, self-reactive, 155
5-Bromodeoxyuridine, 152

Calculus, dental
  in young adult males, 13
  and history of bleeding, 26

Calculus, dental—*continued*
  intraoral distribution, 10, 12
  subgingival, 115
Campylobacter, 246, 248
Candida albicans, 76
Capnocytophaga, 246, 248
  ochraceus, 249, 252
Carboxyl groups, interaction with dental enamel, 230
Carboxylendopeptidases, 32
Caries
  control of *Strep. mutans*, 222
  fluoride control of plaque in, 269–80
  gingival region, in, correlation with gingivitis and loss of tooth attachment, 12
  gingivitis in schoolchildren and, 19–23
  high-risk subjects, 13
  immune mechanisms of protection, 193–294
  immunization with
    A. viscosus in rats, 175–92
    Strep. mutans in monkeys, 193–214
  immunoglobulins and, 51
  susceptibility due to deficiency, 161
  in same subjects as periodontal disease, 9–29
  intraoral distribution, 10
  pellicle, protective effect, 270
  phagocytosis, protection from, 79
  plaque development and properties, 227–40
  prevalence in
    industrialized and developing countries, 1–2
    young adult males, 13–19
      frequency of toothache and, 26
  research requirements, 6
  world health problem, 1–7
Cathepsin D, gingival, 32–4
  in crevicular fluid, 79
Cathepsin G, properties, 38–9
Cathepsins, B, H, L and S, 32
Cetylamine hydrofluoride, 273
Chlorhexidine
  in depression of *Strep. mutans*, 224
  use of, 258
Collagen
  action of elastase on, 33
  breakdown by collagenase in inflamed gingiva, 40
Collagenase, 78
  gingival, 35, 40–43
  granulocyte, 32, 40
  role in periodontology, 31
  vertebrate, 32, 40
Colonization resistance, microbial, 220
Commensal relationships, 217
Complement (C3)
  bound to crevicular PMN is gingival fluid, 94
  components, 35
  importance in chemotaxis, 95
  in saliva, 61
    concentration, 63
Corynebacterium levaniformis, 86, 89, 92
Crevicular fluid
  cathepsin D in, 32
  collagenase in, 41
  composition, 64
  host protective systems in, 159
  immunoglobulins in, 77, 160, 193
  lysosomal enzymes in, 79
  of immunized monkeys, 70, 77
  PMNL in, 193
  transport and function of, 69–81
  proteolytic activity, 35
  source of immunoglobulins, 51, 60, 159
  study of effect on blood PMNL, 70
  volume of, 61–3
Cytotoxicity of lymphocytes, 137–40
  T-cell mediated, specificity, 149–51

Dental operator/population ratio, 2
Dentist, frequency of visits to
  and oral health, 23, 25, 27
  by young adult males, 13
Dextran coat of sucrose-grown *Strep. mutans*, 231
Dextran-induced aggregation in accumulation of *Strep. mutans* on teeth, 219
Dextran, inflammatory effect on leukocytes in mouse, 83, 86, 90, 91, 94
DFS (decayed, filled surfaces) score in schoolchildren, 20
DMF (decayed, missing, filled) index, 1–5
  higher in West, 9
  in young adult males, 13, 19, 24

Index

increased with regular brushing, 10
negative correlation with gingival index, 10
world goal for year 2000, 4
DMFT (decayed, missing, filled teeth) index, 24
DNA synthesis by gingival lymphocytes enhanced to *Veillonella*, 130

Ecological control of pathogens, 222
Edentulousness in industrialized countries, 3
Education, length of and oral health, 23
Elastase of polymorphonuclear leukocytes, 33–5
  action on collagen, 35, 43
  gingival, 35–8
  role in periodontology, 31
Enamel
  dental, properties, 229–40
  solubility, effect of fluorides on, 273
  surface, bound fluoride in, 278
Endopeptidases in gingival sulcus, 31–2
Enolase, inhibition by fluoride taken up by bacteria, 277
Enzymes in gingival crevice, 31–49
Epithelial cell population in dental plaque, 153
Epithelial cell surface, role of, 149–51
Epithelial structures, rate of renewal and concentration of enzymes in gingival crevice, 31
Epithelium, junctional, 31, 119
Eubacterium, 244, 248

Fibrin strands in inflammatory exudate, 111
Fibrinolytic system in human crevicular exudate, 39
Fluoridated water, effect on amount of plaque, 271
Fluoride
  action in control of plaque in dental caries, 269–80
  cariostatic effect, 227
  effect on
    extracellular polysaccharides, 271
    pellicle, 271
  in bacteria, 276
  in drinking water, and oral health, 23–5

Fluorides
  in control of *Strep. mutans*, 224
  use of, 2–3
Fructans, synthesis and breakdown by oral bacteria, 218
Fusobacterium nucleatum, 244, 248, 249, 252

Gingiva, healthy, subgingival anaerobic microflora in, 250
Gingival bleeding
  after probing
    correlation with
      caries, 16, 18
      number of filled teeth, 19
    in schoolchildren, 20, 21
    and past caries, 22
    in young adult males, 13, 15
  history of, and oral disease, 25–6
Gingival crevice, *see also* Crevicular fluid
  migration of PMNL through epithelium, 69, 76
  passage of immunoglobulins through, 59, 63
  proteinases, 31–49
  source of complement, 61
Gingival cultures, 36
  lymphocyte, 126, 128
Gingival fluid
  α_1-antitrypsin and α_2-macroglobulin in, 44
  immunoglobulins and complement in, 94
Gingival index, 264, 266
  and volume of crevicular fluid, 62
  correlation with *A. viscosus* and *A. israelii*, 175
Gingival lymphocytes, 125–34
Gingival plaque, microorganisms in, 241–54
Gingival pockets, 99–123
Gingival sulcus
  colonization by bacteria, 246–8
  effect of experimental neutropenia in dogs, 100
  healthy, anaerobic microflora, 250
  oxidation-reduction potential, 241
Gingivitis
  acute necrotizing ulcerative, 248
    associated with fusiform-spirochaetal flora, 256

Gingivitis—*continued*
and caries in schoolchildren, 19–23
and dental plaque, 83
and gingival bleeding in schoolchildren, 21
and loss of tooth attachment, 17
correlation with caries in gingival region, 12
causes of, 95
chronic, associated with *Actinomyces*, 256
dissolution of collagen fibrils in, 79
experimental
  in dogs, 99
  neutral protease production in, 36
high-risk groups, 13
immunocompetent cells in, 35
possible precursor of periodontal destruction, 255
subgingival anaerobic microflora in, 250
transition from supra- to subgingival infection, 256
Globulins, identification by immunoelectrophoresis, 43
Glucans
  action of oral bacteria on, 218
  from *Strep. mutans*, binding activity, 219
  in bacterial coat, 234
Glucosyltransferase
  activity increased by salivary IgA, 212
  extracellular from *Strep. mutans*, 217
  inhibition of, 64, 160
  preparation, 51
β-Glucuronidase in crevicular fluid, 79
Glycoproteins
  salivary, adsorption to enamel, 230
  sulphated, in pellicle, 231
Gram-positive cocci in subgingival plaque (experimental), 111–13, 116
initiating pocket formation, 117
Granulocytes, neutrophil, 116, 119

Histocompatibility antigens, 151, 153
Hydroxyapatite, 269
  adsorption of *Strep. mutans*, 269
  interaction with proteins, 229–31
  on tooth surface, 227–40
Hypogammaglobulinaemic patients, oral condition, 159–73

Immune reactions, in periodontium during disease, 256
Immunity, cell-mediated, against dental caries, 212
Immunization against juvenile periodontitis, 256
Immunoglobulin deficiencies and susceptibility to caries, 161
Immunoglobulins, 159
  bound to crevicular PMN in gingival fluid, 94
  functional activity, 64
IgG
  concentration in mixed saliva, 63
  human, sensitivity of, to PMN elastase, 35
  in crevicular fluid, 59, 77
  in plaque, 63–4
  in saliva, 168
  serum, passage into oral cavity in Rhesus monkey, 51–67
Inflammatory exudate adjacent to subgingival plaque in dogs, 111
Insulinase, 32

K (Killer) cells, 137

Lactobacilli, concentration in saliva, 166–7
Lactobacillus, 244, 248
 fermentii, 86, 89
Lactoferrin, 78, 159
Lactoferrin peroxidase, 159
Leptotrichia, 248
Leukocyte function in juvenile periodontis, 256
Leukocytes, *see also* Polymorphonuclear leukocytes
  mononuclear, 32
Levan, inflammatory effect on leukocytes in mouse peritoneal cavity, 83, 86, 89, 91–4
Lipopolysaccharide, inflammatory effect on leukocytes in mouse peritoneal cavity, 83, 86, 88, 92–3
Lipoteichoic acid, 160
  inflammatory effect on leukocytes in mouse peritoneal cavity, 83, 86, 89, 90, 93
  role in dental plaque, 231–3

Lymphocytes
  gingival, stimulation by antigens from oral bacteria, 125–34
  stimulation by elastase and cathepsin D, 35
Lymphocytotoxicity of periodontal disease for oral epithelial cells, 137
Lysosomal enzyme release in chronic periodontal disease, 155
Lysosomes, cathepsin D in, 32
Lysozyme, 159
  in crevicular fluid, 79
α_2-Macroglobulin, 43
Macrophages, 83, 212
  regulatory effect of complement system on, 95
Megasphaera, 248
Metalloendopeptidases, 32
Microbial interactions in the mouth, 215–26
Mononuclear leukocytes, 100
  human, cathepsin D in, 32
Mouse peritoneal cavity, comparison of inflammatory effect of plaque bacterial products, 83–97
Mouth rinses
  antimicrobial, 258
  containing fluoride, study, 271, 274
Mucins, 231

NK (Natural killer) cells, 149

Opsonic activity in oral fluids, 71, 73
Opsonization, avoidance of, by bacteria, 116
Oral bacteria, antigens from, 125–34
Oral defence mechanisms, 159
Oral disease
  intraoral distribution, 10–13
  plaque-induced, 9
  relation with various background variables, 23
Oral fluid
  importance of antibodies and agglutinins in, 159
  reaction of bacteria with components, 161
Oral health, 6
  and length of education, 23

Oral hygiene
  gingival and periodontal conditions improved by, 10
  importance, 257
  school supervised, 3

Pathogens, ecological control of, 222, 224
Pellicle formation
  confusion with plaque, 270
  influence of fluoride on, 269–71
  mechanisms involved, 229–31
  protective against caries, 270
Peptidases, 31
Peptidoglycans in bacterial cell wall, 231
Peptococci, 244, 248, 250, 251
Peptostreptococci, 244, 248, 250, 251
Periodontal disease
  cause of extractions after age 35–40 years, 260
  cellular autoimmunity in, 135–57
  development, natural, study, 260–66
  immunization with *A. viscosus* in rats, 175–92
  in same subjects as caries, 9–29
  in young adult males, 13–19
  increase in unattached bacteria, 249
  inflammatory, 78, 79
  loss of teeth due to, 1
  lymphocyte
    cytotoxicity, 144, 151
    response to plaque antigens, 133
  microflora associated with, 175
  more prevalent than dental caries, 6
  plaque and
    correlation, 10, 83
    development and properties, 227–40
  PMNL protection against, 78
  pocket formation, 99–123
  initiation by bacteria spreading subgingivally, 117
  prevention, 5, 255–68
  research requirements, 6
  result of numerous pathological mechanisms, 187
  role of enzymes in gingival crevice, 31
  subgingival anaerobic microflora, 249–52
  world health problem, 1–7
Periodontal health goals, 5
Periodontal index, 61, 125, 145

Periodontal inflammatory reaction, 79
Periodontal pockets, 99–123
  bacterial flora, 248
  colonization, 250
  formation of, theories, 115
  in young adult males, 13, 17
  and history of bleeding, 26
  and frequency of toothache, 26
Periodontitis
  acute and chronic, microflora in, 252
  advanced, anaerobic bacteria in, 251–2
  juvenile
    immunization against, 256
    microflora in, 250–51
    PMNL functional defects in, 78
  participation of immunocompetent cells in, 35
  raised IgG levels in saliva, 61
  rapidly progressive, PMNL functional defects in, 78
Phagocytosis, bacterial resistance to, 116
Phosphate-containing macromolecules, interaction with enamel, 230
Phosphate fluoride, acidulated, for depression of *Strep. mutans*, 224
Phosphoenolypyruvic acid, 277
Phosphoproteins, 231
Phytohaemagglutinin, stimulation of gingival lymphocytes by, 130
Plaque, dental
  adherance, role in development of, 227–40
  bacterial growth a factor, 236–8
  aetiological factor in caries and periodontal disease, 9
  agglutinin interference with formation, 160
  antigens from, response of lymphocytes to, 125
  bacteria, previously undescribed, 83
  bacterial antigen, 151
  distinction from pellicle, 270
  effect of brushing teeth regularly, 10
  enzymes in, action on immunoglobulins, 59
  epithelial cell population, 153
  fluoride control of, 269–80
  gingival, microorganisms in, 241–54
  host response to, 78
  immunoglobulins in, 63–4
  index, 263, 265, 273
  and gingival health, 257
  inflammatory effect, on leukocytes in mouse peritoneal cavity, 83, 85, 88
  inhibition by metal ions, 237
  interactions in, 215–20
  lysosomal enzyme release, 155
  pathogenicity of, 83
  PMNL accumulation on, 69
  presence in young adult males, 13
  relationship to severity of gingivitis, 10
  subgingival, in dogs, experimental, 100, 111, 113, 116
  supragingival, 117, 246, 256
    cause of gingivitis, 255
    removal, 257
  symbiosis in, 216
  visible, in schoolchildren, 20
Plasminogen activators, 39
Polymorphonuclear leukocytes (PMNL)
  blood, migration into oral cavity in monkeys, 70, 71, 76
  cathepsin D in, 32
  enzyme release from, by *A. viscosus*, 83
  in crevicular fluid
    immunoglobulins and complement bound to, 94
    transport and function, 69–81
    viability and function, 71–76
    predominant cells in gingival crevice, 95
    regulatory effect of complement system on, 95
  salivary, 69
    viability and function, 71, 76
Polysaccharide capsule, bacterial resistance to phagocytosis, 116
Polysaccharide coat of *Strep. mutans*, 232
Polysaccharides, extracellular, in adherence of bacteria, 215, 217
  bacterial cell wall, 231
  plaque, source of energy, 217
Prevention of periodontal disease, 255–68
Preventive care
  dental operator requirements, 2
  fluorides, use of, 2–3, 23–5, 269–80
  goals, 5–6
  interference with bacterial adhesion to teeth, 238
Propionibacterium acnes, 245, 248

Protease, neutral, in gingival washings, 36
Proteinase inhibitors of gingival crevice, 44–6
Proteinases of gingival crevice and their inhibitors, 31–49

Saliva
  concentrations of bacteria in, 241
  host protective systems in, 159, 168
  mixed
    and parotid, of immunized monkeys, examination for opsonic activity towards Strep. mutans, 70
  parotid, bacterial aggregation induced by, 168
  secretory IgA in, 160
  subject variability of, 161
Salivary agglutinins, 159–61
Salivary antibiotics, 160, 193–214
Salivary glands, source of antibodies, 51, 159
Salivary glycoproteins, adsorption to dental enamel, 230
School-supervised oral hygiene, 3, 5
Selenomonas, 246
Serine endopeptidases, 32
Serine proteinases of PMNS, bactericidal properties, 35
Serum immunoglobulins, passage into oral cavity, 51–67
Serum proteinase inhibitors, 43
  concentration in gingival crevices, 44
Skin-hypersensitivity test to *Strep. mutans* in monkeys, 202–3
Sodium monoflurophosphate, 269
Spirochetes, 217
  anaerobic, 246, 248
Stannous fluoride, 272–3
  depression of *Strep. mutans*, 224
  inhibition of plaque formation and reduction of enamel solubility, 273
Staphylococcus aureus, 222
Streptococcus, 248–51
  bovis, 220
  intermedium, 245
  mutans
    adhesiveness of, 232–5
    adsorption by hydroxyapatite, 269
    antibody levels, 167, 209
    associated with caries, 256
    bacteriocin, 220, 221
    commensal relationships, 217
    competition between strains, 222–3
    concentration in saliva, 166–8
    control of, 222–4
    culture, 196
    dental implantation in rats, 193
    effect of
      amines, 274–5
      fluoride, 271–2
    glucans synthesis, 218
    growth rate on tooth surface, 215
    immune response to, 212
    immunization with, 51
    in experimental caries, 175
    inhibition of adherence by antibodies, 64
    opsonic activity of, 73–6
    opsonization of, 70
    synthesis of glucose polymers, 231
    transmissible, caries-inducing, 159
  salivarius, 217
    synthesis and breakdown of fructans by, 218
  sanguis, 75
    antibody levels, 167, 169
    bacteriocins, 220
    coaggregation with *A. viscosus*, 219, 220, 223
    effect of fluoride, 272
    hydrogen peroxide production, 220
Streptolysin production by bacteria, 116
Subgingival anaerobic microflora in relation to periodontal infection, 249–52
Sucrose intake
  and oral disease, 23
  favourable to implantation of *Strep. mutans* in plaque, 220
Symbiosis in dental plaque, 216
Synergistic association between
  dental caries and periodontal disease, 9
  prevalence of decay and
    gingival bleeding, 17–18
    gingivitis, 15

Teichoic acid, 231
Teichouronic acid, 231

T helper cells, 212
Thio endopeptidases, 31
Thymidine, 35
T-lymphocytes, 133, 140, 144
 blastogenesis, 153
 rat, purification of, 180
 self-reactive, 155
Tooth attachment, loss of, in population, 12
 correlation with caries in gingival region, 12
Toothache, frequency, in young adult males, 26
Tooth-brushing frequency and oral health, 23, 27

Transfer factor, 198
 in cell-mediated immunity, 212
Treatment, dental, *see* Preventive care
Tropocollagen, 34
Trypsin, role in cytotoxicity, 144–9
T suppressor cells, 212

Veillonella, 244, 248
 alcalescens, 84, 86–8, 126–34
 use of lactic acid as energy source, 217
Veillonellae, commensal relationships, 217
Vibrio, 217, 246, 248

WHO Oral Disease Data Bank, 1